AAC Strategies for Individuals
with Moderate to Severe Disabilities

AAC Strategies for Individuals with Moderate to Severe Disabilities

by

Susan S. Johnston, Ph.D.
University of Utah
Salt Lake City

Joe Reichle, Ph.D.
University of Minnesota
Minneapolis

Kathleen M. Feeley, Ph.D.
C.W. Post Campus
Long Island University
Brookville, New York

and

Emily A. Jones, Ph.D.
Queens College
City University of New York
Flushing

with invited contributors

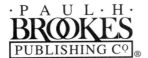

·P·A·U·L·H·
BROOKES
PUBLISHING CO.®

Baltimore • London • Sydney

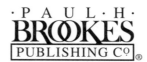

Paul H. Brookes Publishing Co.
Post Office Box 10624
Baltimore, Maryland 21285-0624
USA

www.brookespublishing.com

Typeset by Integrated Publishing Solutions, Grand Rapids, Michigan.
Manufactured in the United States of America by
Sheridan Books, Inc., Chelsea, Michigan.

The individuals and situations/descriptions in this book are based on composites. In most instances, names and identifying details have been changed to protect confidentiality. Real names and likenesses used by permission.

Library of Congress Cataloging-in-Publication Data

AAC strategies for individuals with moderate to severe disabilities / by Susan S.
    Johnston . . . [et al.]; with invited contributors.
        p.   cm.
    Includes bibliographical references and index.
    ISBN-13: 978-1-59857-206-3 (pbk.)
    ISBN-10: 1-59857-206-7 (pbk.)
    1. Communication devices for people with disabilities.   2. People with
    mental disabilities — Means of communication.   I. Johnston, Susan S.
    II. Title.
    RC429.A33 2011
    616.85'503—dc23   2011023481

British Library Cataloguing in Publication data are available from the British Library.

2015   2014   2013   2012   2011

10   9   8   7   6   5   4   3   2   1

Contents

I   Establishing the Framework for Intervention

II   Establishing Functional Communication

Contents of the Accompanying CD-ROM

About the Authors and Contributors

Susan S. Johnston, Ph.D., Professor, Department of Special Education, University of Utah, 1705 East Campus Center Drive, Room 221, Salt Lake City, Utah 84112

Dr. Johnston conducts research, teaches, and provides technical assistance in the areas of augmentative and alternative communication, early language and literacy intervention, and early childhood special education. During her tenure at the University of Utah, Dr. Johnston served as Associate Dean for Academic Affairs for the College of Education and currently serves as Director of International Initiatives for the College of Education. She received her master of arts degree and doctorate in speech-language pathology from the University of Minnesota in Minneapolis.

Joe Reichle, Ph.D., Professor and American Speech-Language-Hearing Association (ASHA) Fellow, Department of Educational Psychology, Special Education Area, University of Minnesota, 250 Educational Sciences Building, 56 East River Road, Minneapolis, Minnesota 55455

Dr. Reichle holds a joint appointment in the Departments of Speech-Language-Hearing Sciences and Educational Psychology at the University of Minnesota. He is an internationally recognized expert in the areas of augmentative and alternative communication and communication intervention for individuals with significant developmental disabilities, with more than 55 articles in refereed journals. He has coedited 10 books focused on his areas of expertise and has served as an associate editor of the *Journal of Speech-Language-Hearing Research.* During his tenure at the University of Minnesota, Dr. Reichle served on the executive committee of the dean of the graduate school, was associate chair of the Department of Speech-Language-Hearing, and was training director of the Center on Community Integration. He has also served as a principal investigator, coprincipal investigator, and investigator on numerous federally funded research and training grants.

Kathleen M. Feeley, Ph.D., Associate Professor, Department of Special Education and Literacy, C.W. Post Campus, Long Island University, Brookville, New York 11367

Dr. Feeley is the clinical coordinator for the Certificate in Autism and Special Education Program at C.W. Post Campus, Long Island University. As the founder and director of the Center for Community Inclusion at C.W. Post Campus, Dr. Feeley provides training and technical assistance to families, school districts, and adult service agencies as they include individuals with developmental disabilities within their communities. She is also Senior Editor for the journal *Down Syndrome Research and Practice* and is a member of the international research group Research Action for People with Down Syndrome (RAPID), sponsored by Down Syndrome International.

Emily A. Jones, Ph.D., Assistant Professor, Department of Psychology, Queens College, City University of New York, Flushing, New York 11367

Dr. Jones received her doctorate in clinical psychology from the State University of New York Stony Brook. She was Associate Professor in the Department of Psychology at C.W. Post Campus, Long Island University. Dr. Jones teaches courses in applied behavior analysis and developmental disabilities. She also provides training and technical assistance to families, school districts, and other service providers to support children with developmental disabilities in inclusive settings. Dr. Jones's research involves the development and demonstration of interventions to address early emerging core deficits in young children with developmental disabilities such as autism and Down syndrome. Her current interests are in the area of social and communication skills, including joint attention in children with autism and early requesting skills in children with Down syndrome.

CONTRIBUTORS

Meredith Bailey-Orr, M.A., CCC-SLP, Speech-Language Pathologist, Alternatives for Children Preschool, 14 Research Way, East Setauket, New York 11733. With two master's degrees—one in English writing and one in speech-language pathology—Ms. Bailey-Orr has more than 10 years of experience working as a practicing speech and language clinician. Her clinical work has encompassed the entire lifespan from neonatology to geriatrics. Currently, she works as an augmentative communication specialist at Alternatives for Children, advocating for the augmentative needs of children ages birth through 5.

Nancy C. Brady, Ph.D., Associate Research Professor, Life Span Institute, University of Kansas, 1052 Dole Building, 1000 Sunnyside Drive, Lawrence, Kansas 66045. Dr. Brady is Assistant Professor in the Department of Speech-Language-Hearing: Sciences and Disorders at the University of Kansas. She conducts research about communication development and disorders in individuals with developmental disabilities, including Down syndrome, autism, and fragile X syndrome, and individuals with dual sensory impairments. Her research focuses on promoting the use of augmentative and alternative communication and the transition to symbolic communication.

Albert M. Cook, Ph.D., Professor, Department of Speech Pathology and Audiology, University of Alberta, 3-79 Corbett Hall, Edmonton, Alberta, Canada. Dr. Cook teaches augmentative and alternative communication (AAC) and conducts research relating to the use of robots and cognitive development in the Faculty of Rehabilitation Medicine at the University of Alberta. He also serves as Associate Dean, Research, for the Faculty of Extension. He is the father of Brian, an individual who uses AAC.

Joanna Cosbey, Ph.D., Assistant Professor, Department of Educational Specialties, Special Education Program, University of New Mexico, MC05 3040, Hokona Hall Room 282, 1 University of New Mexico, Albuquerque, New Mexico 87131. Dr. Cosbey has worked with individuals with severe disabilities as an occupational therapist in a variety of school and community settings. She currently conducts research and teaches courses related to the communication of individuals with severe disabilities, the school-based assessment and diagnosis of children with disabilities, and inclusive teaching strategies for children with severe disabilities.

Patricia Dowden, Ph.D., CCC-SLP, Clinical Assistant Professor, Speech and Hearing Sciences, University of Washington, 1417 NE 42nd Street, Seattle, Washington 98105. Dr. Dowden has worked with children and adults with severe disabilities for more than 20 years. She is currently teaching two graduate-level courses in augmentative and alternative communication at the University of Washington and conducting research in early signals of communication in infants and toddlers with severe motor impairments.

Joan Schumann, M.S., Doctoral Student, Department of Special Education, University of Utah, 1705 East Campus Center Drive, Salt Lake City, Utah 84112. Ms. Schumann is currently completing her Ph.D. in special education at the University of Utah. She has taught students with and without disabilities in a variety of school settings, including preschool, elementary school, and high school.

Christopher E. Smith, Ph.D., BCBA-D, Clinical Psychologist, Positive Behavior Support Consulting & Psychological Resources, P.C., 68 Oakdale Road, Centerport, New York, 11721. Dr. Smith is a New York State Licensed Psychologist. He has worked with children and adults with a variety of disabilities for more than 20 years. His clinical and research interests include assessing and treating challenging behavior and functional communication training.

Krista M. Wilkinson, Ph.D., Professor, Department of Communication Sciences and Disorders, Pennsylvania State University, 308 Ford Building, University Park, Pennsylvania 16802. Dr. Wilkinson holds an adjunct associate scientist position at the University of Massachusetts Medical School Eunice Kennedy Shriver Center. She studies communication and language in children with and without disabilities. Dr. Wilkinson's primary area of interest includes the role of visual attention and processing in aided augmentative and alternative communication interventions with individuals with intellectual and developmental disabilities.

Preface

This book addresses the same population that was addressed in *Implementing Augmentative and Alternative Communication: Strategies for Learners with Severe Disabilities* (Reichle, York, & Sigafoos, 1991). In the late 1980s, Dr. Reichle and a group of his doctoral students, along with postdoctoral fellow Dr. Jennifer York, began drafting chapters for an augmentative and alternative communication (AAC) methods book that exclusively focused on individuals with severe and multiple developmental disabilities. At that time, there were few survey books that provided an overview of AAC. Thus, the book provided part overview of AAC and part methods. As the years passed, the authors elected to allow that book to go out of print. For a number of years after it was out of print, Dr. Reichle continued to receive requests for a second edition. As a result, he contacted the generation of his doctoral students that followed some of the original authors (with a little poaching of Ted Carr's doctoral talent) to coauthor a second methods book in AAC addressing individuals with severe disabilities. Although there are a number of topics that require more elaboration than can be provided in this text, we have attempted to select areas that frequently result in requests for technical assistance that many of the educators with whom we interact have found useful. We hope that you will find them helpful as well.

THE PURPOSE OF THIS BOOK

This book is intended as a methods book for special educators and speech-language pathologists who either serve or plan to serve learners with severe developmental disabilities. Its purpose is to bridge the gap between research and practice by presenting a compendium of empirically validated procedures to establish a beginning functional communicative repertoire. In addition to describing implementation procedures, we have reviewed some of the basic principles on which the procedures are based. We hope that doing this will assist readers in their implementation of evidence-based practices with individuals who experience severe disabilities.

THE CHAPTER FORMAT

Most of the chapters contain sections titled "What Does the Research Say." These sections provide a summary/synthesis of a body of research and/or a summary of intervention studies. They emphasize the evidence-based nature of the procedures discussed and are designed to help bridge the gap between research and practice. Case studies are also presented in each chapter in order to illustrate the application and results of the strategies, provide examples of how to monitor progress, and offer guidelines regarding ways to troubleshoot interventions that are not providing anticipated results.

THE CONTENT OF THE CHAPTERS

There is a range of individuals with severe disabilities who may benefit from AAC applications. These include not only individuals with severe intellectual delay but also those with accompanying autism spectrum disorders, vision impairments, and motor impairments.

From the planning stages of this book, our goal has been to emphasize the benefits of AAC. In the early chapters of the book, we establish a practical framework for intervention. Critical features of the framework include understanding issues related to 1) social functions/communication intentions, 2) communicative means, 3) features of AAC systems, 4) the design of AAC systems, 5) options to consider if direct selection isn't effective or efficient, and 6) AAC instructional strategies. Later chapters of the book provide the reader with empirically based strategies for establishing functional communication. These chapters include strategies for teaching individuals with severe disabilities 1) to use graphic symbols to communicate, 2) to gain access to desired objects and activities, 3) to escape and avoid activities, and 4) to gain and maintain access to others. The final chapters of the book provide empirically based strategies for addressing the use of AAC to enhance the intelligibility of spoken language (speech supplementation) and the use of organizational aids (within activity and across activity schedules, contingency maps, and shopping lists). Although much of the methodology addressed in this book will appear to be somewhat "behavioral," the authors embrace a wide range of intervention strategies. We believe that a developmental (sociopragmatic) approach serves many learners incredibly well.

One area that we believe requires much more consideration than it currently receives is the level of instructional intrusiveness required for a learner to acquire functional communication skills. This is an empirical issue that can, and should, be objectively examined. Warren, Fey, and Yoder (2007) articulated parameters of treatment intensity that need to be further explored within subject experimental designs in order to establish a mechanism to evaluate the level of intensity that best suits a given learner. Until this happens, we suspect there will continue to be non–data-based "camps" specifying the density and control of environmental variables needed for learners to acquire functional communication.

Next is a brief overview of the chapters that we have chosen to include in this book. Note that we have not attempted to directly address sensory disabilities. In addition, we have not attempted to address positioning and handling issues for individuals with significant developmental disabilities. Although these are vitally important areas, we simply did not have the space or the expertise to adequately address these areas in the methodological detail required to match the explicitness of other chapters.

Part I: Establishing the Framework for Intervention

Chapter 1 provides an overview of communication functions and includes a discussion of the way in which individuals move from nonintentional to intentional communicative acts. Reichle and Brady describe what we know developmentally about early communicative intents and how they are distinguished from social functions. Strategies for identifying existing communicative intents are presented. Finally, information regarding the use of different conversational functions to initiate, maintain, and terminate interactions are provided.

Information describing modes of communication (verbal, gestural, graphic) is provided in Chapter 2. Johnston and Cosbey provide a discussion of the development of gestural and graphic modes of communication among typically developing individuals as well as individuals with developmental disabilities. In addition, the authors describe the influence of one communication mode on other modes (e.g., impact of graphic mode of communication on speech).

Chapter 3 provides an overview of features associated with AAC systems. Johnston and Feeley discuss features related to speech-generating devices as well as non-electronic communication aids and provide information regarding how individual features may enhance communication. Finally, they present information regarding how research related to AAC system features can be used to support evidence-based practice.

Chapter 4 describes intervention options for individuals with severe motor impairments. Dowden and Cook discuss uses of technology for early communicators who might benefit from alternative selection methods and present interventions to make existing selection methods (scanning or other alternative methods) more efficient. Finally, they provide strategies for improving the communicative competence of individuals who use alternative selection methods.

In Chapter 5, Feeley and Jones provide readers with information related to 1) planning interventions to increase the likelihood of generalization and conditional use, 2) describing the foundation on which instruction is based, 3) developing and implementing effective prompting and reinforcement procedures, 4) implementing instructional procedures to shape behavior and to teach chains of behaviors, and 5) developing and implementing procedures to maintain and to enhance spontaneous use of communication skills.

In Chapter 6, Jones and Feeley pose a series of questions related to intervention intensity. The answers to these questions are used to inform the context for instruction. To help tailor AAC intervention to each learner's needs, the authors describe a continuum of intervention intensities with three general anchor points of empirically based contexts for instruction.

Chapter 7 addresses issues related to monitoring learner performance. Specifically, Feeley and Jones present different measurement systems followed by a discussion of when to use each. This is followed by a discussion of how to use measurement systems for monitoring learner performance and how to measure intervention integrity and response reliability.

Part II: Establishing Functional Communication

Chapter 8 offers intervention strategies for individuals who have difficulty using graphic symbols to represent objects or events. The chapter includes content related to the importance of the ability to match real objects to graphic symbols when considering the use of a graphic communication mode. Reichle and Wilkinson provide a description of the difference between identify and nonidentity matching and the role it plays in establishing a rudimentary graphic mode communication system. This chapter provides interventionists with troubleshooting procedures for learners who are having difficulty matching symbols to objects.

Chapter 9 describes procedures that are effective in establishing functional communication to gain access to desired objects and activities. Johnston and Schumann provide a review of empirically validated procedures. Specific procedures addressed include teaching requests for objects or activities, teaching requests for continued engagement in an activity, and teaching requests for assistance.

Chapter 10 describes procedures that are effective for establishing functional communication to escape and avoid activities. Jones and Smith provide a review of empirically validated procedures. Specific procedures addressed include teaching rejecting, teaching requests for assistance, teaching requests for a break, and teaching requests for a work check.

Chapter 11 describes how an individual's ability to establish and maintain communicative interactions facilitates social relationships among family members, classmates, co-workers, and others in the community. Feeley and Jones provide a discussion of initiating, maintaining (including repairing communication breakdowns), and terminating interactions. The chapter includes procedures to support AAC users' interactions.

In addition to being used as an expressive tool, AAC is also an important tool to enhance a learner's role as a listener. The role of listener requires an ability to comprehend the communicative behavior produced by a partner. In Chapter 12, Jones and Bailey-Orr describe the importance of comprehension, discuss the use of augmented input when using the learner's AAC system, and provide readers with information regarding developing and implementing visual supports to enhance comprehension and adaptive functioning.

Chapter 13 focuses on procedures related to using AAC systems to enhance the intelligibility of individuals who rely primarily on verbal communication. Specifically, Feeley and Jones focus on identifying factors that affect intelligibility, assessing intelligibility, and using a multimodal approach to enhance comprehensibility.

REFERENCES

Reichle, J., York, J., & Sigafoos, J. (1991). *Implementing augmentative and alternative communication: Strategies for learners with severe disabilities.* Baltimore: Paul H. Brookes Publishing Co.

Warren, S.F., Fey, M.E., & Yoder, P.J. (2007). Differential treatment intensity research: A missing link to creating optimally effective communication interventions. *Mental Retardation and Developmental Disabilities Research Reviews, 13,* 70–77.

Acknowledgments

It is a pleasure to thank those who made this book possible.

We are indebted to the individuals with severe disabilities, their families, and the professionals who serve them who have allowed us to be a part of their journey. Their willingness to share their thoughts and experiences has shaped our research as well as our practice.

We thank our families, who love us for who we are and are generous with their patience, understanding, and support.

We acknowledge our graduate students, who dedicate time and effort to our projects and whose enthusiasm for contributing to our field is one of our most powerful reinforcers.

We acknowledge mentors Dr. David Yoder, Dr. Jon Miller, Dr. Tom Longhurst, and Mr. William Keogh who spent countless hours attempting to teach Dr. Reichle. And thanks to Dr. Reichle, who, in turn, has served tirelessly over the years as a mentor, role model, and colleague to the coauthors of this book.

We especially acknowledge our esteemed and beloved colleague and mentor, Dr. Edward Carr, whose seminal work shaped so much of what we do and had an impact on the lives of countless individuals with disabilities.

Finally, thanks to the professional and editorial staff at Paul H. Brookes Publishing Co., especially to Melissa Behm, Executive Vice President, who has supported Dr. Reichle through his involvement in its Communication and Language Intervention Series and its Augmentative and Alternative Communication Series over the years.

Establishing the Framework for Intervention

Teaching Pragmatic Skills to Individuals with Severe Disabilities

Joe Reichle and Nancy C. Brady

▷ CHAPTER OVERVIEW

This chapter focuses on how young children move from making no attempts to influence the actions of others to becoming active communicators. Although some methodological procedures are described in this chapter, an effort has been made to provide an understanding of how **communicative intents** emerge in typically developing children, provide caveats regarding how early conversation develops, and discuss implications that this pattern of emergence has for structuring early intervention strategies. We believe that pathways in typical development that lead to communication advances can inform the design and implementation of intervention strategies with individuals who have severe developmental disabilities (carefully recognizing that some aspects of intervention strategies cannot be fully informed by typical development).

Children learn to use the same **communicative form** to express a multitude of functions (Bloom & Lahey, 1978). For example, a child may comment on an interesting object to share attention, request an out-of-reach object, or greet a peer (each of the preceding being a **communicative function**). Communicative functions represent the reasons why someone communicates. How do these different functions develop? Are interventionists teaching learners with severe disabilities to communicate different functions? The answers to these questions are addressed within this chapter. In addition, the development of early conversational parameters, such as how to **initiate, maintain,** and **terminate** an interaction, and research that has targeted these conversational parameters will be discussed. Together, communicative intents and conversational parameters have been described as **pragmatic** aspects of language (Prutting & Kirchner, 1987).

▷ CHAPTER OBJECTIVES

After studying this chapter, readers will be able to

- Describe the environmental relationships that put a learner in a position to discover that his or her behavior can control the actions of others
- Distinguish between unintentional acts, intentional behavioral acts that are not communicatively intentional, and **intentional communicative acts**
- Describe why beginning communicators may attempt to manipulate the actions of others
- Discuss challenges that interventionists face when learners acquire intentional communicative acts that are effective, but socially marginal or idiosyncratic, and that must be replaced by more socially acceptable and conventional communicative alternatives
- Describe empirically demonstrated intervention strategies to establish different beginning communicative functions

- Discuss the importance of establishing the **conditional use** of newly acquired communicative acts
- Address the extension of **social interactions** using newly acquired conventional communicative functions, including strategies to increase intentional communicative acts, initiations, turn taking, and repairs of communication breakdowns

▷ **KEY TERMS**

- ▶ behavior regulation
- ▶ comment
- ▶ communicative breakdown
- ▶ communicative form
- ▶ communicative function
- ▶ communicative intent
- ▶ conditional use
- ▶ conversational function
  - ▷ initiate
  - ▷ maintain
  - ▷ terminate
- ▶ escape/avoid

- ▶ intentional communicative act
- ▶ joint attention
- ▶ line of regard
- ▶ obtain/maintain attention
- ▶ obtain/maintain goods and services
- ▶ Picture Exchange Communication System (PECS)
- ▶ pointing gesture
- ▶ pragmatic
- ▶ preference assessment

- ▶ prelinguistic
- ▶ protests
- ▶ protodeclarative
- ▶ protoimperative
- ▶ request assistance
- ▶ requests
- ▶ responsivity
- ▶ showing
- ▶ social function
- ▶ social interaction
- ▶ video modeling

IDENTIFYING ENVIRONMENTAL RELATIONSHIPS AND CONSEQUENCES THAT LEAD TO THE EMERGENCE OF INTENTIONAL ACTS

Young children are aware of their environment during the first several months of life. They are influenced by the actions of their social partners. For example, in a series of experiments, Hood, Willen, and Driver (1998) found that infants as young as 3 months of age shifted gaze to focus in the same direction as the eyes of a digitized adult face. Young children's actions are also influenced by subtle aspects of their interaction with items and events that are part of their daily routine. For example, by 16 weeks of age, infants have a propensity to fuss just prior to scheduled feedings. By 4 months of age, children begin to anticipate aspects of familiar routines, such as cleaning up after mealtimes. Watson (1978) reported a game in which 8-week-old infants could control a crib mobile by turning their heads to control a simple switch. Table 1.1 displays relationships between child and caregiver at very early ages (see also Gesell & Ilg, 1937).

Table 1.1. Predictable infant reactions to environmental events that emerge during the initial half year of the infant's life

Avoid and escape events

Draws head away when full after being offered more nutriment

Spits out less preferred food

When offered disliked item during mealtime

- Avoids eye contact with person delivering the food item
- Exhibits more leakage/spillage from mouth
- Averts head, moving it side to side to avoid delivery of food via spoon

Obtain/maintain access to desired objects and events

If crying, quiets when placed in mother's lap

Vocalizes loudly (or fusses) when nutriment lost during mealtime

Fusses before mealtime but often waits until it is almost feeding time to do so

Over time, consistent partner responses likely result in children's early intentional communicative overtures (Bates, Benigni, Bretherton, & Camaioni, 1979; Bell & Ainsworth, 1972; Stillman, Alymer, & Vandivort, 1983). Identifying early learner reactivity to environmental events provides the basis for adults to begin to consistently react to child behaviors. It is relatively easy for adults to provide predictable consequences because the child's behaviors tend to be matched to predictable environmental events. Usually this results in the adult providing positive or negative reinforcers. By providing reinforcement, the partner creates an opportunity to teach the child that his or her behaviors can influence the actions of others.

☛ *Helpful Hint*

Background Definitions

Positive reinforcer: A consequence involving the delivery of a stimulus that increases the probability of a behavior's occurrence in the future

Example: Suppose that John places a book in his mother's lap and his mother reads it. If John's placement of books in his mother's lap occurs with increasing probability, then we can infer that listening to a book being read by his mother functions as a positive reinforcer for John.

Negative reinforcer: A consequence involving the removal of an undesired stimulus that increases the probability of a behavior's occurrence in the future

Example: Suppose that Sally's mother offers her cheese (which Sally dislikes). Sally shakes her head "no," and her mother immediately removes it. Across similar opportunities of offers of undesired food, if the probability of Sally saying "no" increases, then it is likely that the food items are negative reinforcers.

☛ *Helpful Hint*

Adults should be responsive to any learner action they believe can be prompted or shaped into a more acceptable communicative form. In reinforcing a learner's actions, it is important to attempt to provide a consequence that is appropriate for the context (e.g., provide nourishment when a child vocalizes near mealtime). Opportunities will be easier to create in the context of frequently occurring, natural routines.

☛ *Helpful Hint*

Consider environmental relationships within familiar routines:

- What naturally occurring routines occur at a predictable time each day?
- What learner behaviors are produced during these routines?
- What events occurred immediately prior to the learner's behaviors?

Establishing Predictable Responses to Environmental Events

Evidence suggests that when an environmental consequence is important to a child, he or she can be taught to produce behavior associated with the event. For example, Rheingold, Gewirtz, and Ross (1959) demonstrated that children who were several months old learned to associate vocal behavior with the delivery of desired social events. In their study, contingent on the child's vocalization, an experimenter leaned forward, smiled, tickled the infant's tummy, and produced a soothing clicking sound. As a result, the frequency of children's vocalizations increased dramatically.

How Important Is Partner Responsivity?

Hart and Risley (1995) reported that parents who produced the greatest cumulative number of child-directed spoken utterances had children with the most extensive language skills. Parents did not just produce more utterances, however; they were also far more responsive to their children's initiated communicative acts. Children's early reaction to social events provides an impetus for caregiver **responsivity.** Reactions to environmental events are driven by a host of emerging learner skills. Adults are apt to be more responsive to children who appear to be responsive to adult communicative overtures. **Line of regard** is an emerging skill that provides clear indication of child responsivity (Baldwin, 1991; Campos & Sternberg, 1981). Line of regard is produced when an adult and infant establish eye contact. Subsequently, when the adult looks in another direction, the child follows the adult's gaze, anticipating that there will be an event of interest (even though nothing may have occurred to attract the child's attention). Being competent in following another's eye gaze, or line of regard, permits children to be easily directed to events of interest just prior to an adult's communicative utterance that corresponds to the event. This allows the adult to prompt the child to react to subtle environmental events that may not yet be part of a predictable routine. Children who engage in line of regard may be better able to take advantage of adult-produced vocabulary models that occur in natural environments (Tomasello & Farrar, 1986; Wetherby, Alexander, & Prizant, 1998). Sometimes adults also use gesture and vocalization to establish **joint attention** with a child. Responsive joint attention (RJA) occurs when a child is responding to adult direction for joint attention.

What Does the Research Say?

Joint Attention and Language Acquisition

Both mothers and children talk more during periods of joint attention, and the dyad engages in longer conversations. Mothers produce more comments during episodes of joint attention focus. Joint attention focus has been shown to directly relate to the child's subsequent language development. Finally, early vocabulary acquisition is facilitated because children who followed an adult's gaze to an object are more apt to be looking at an object when the adult produces its name (Tomasello & Todd, 1983).

How Do You Teach Line of Regard?

Relying on the learner's auditory and visual localization skills is one strategy for teaching line of regard. During initial teaching opportunities, the interventionist obtains the learner's attention. Then, immediately, the interventionist looks in the direction of an event. As soon as this happens, the interventionist (or someone else) activates the referent to create an attention-gaining display (e.g., a toy might make a sound, move, or light up). Initially, the child's visual and/or auditory localization to the adult may result in a gaze shift to the display. Across success-ful opportunities, the interventionist should increase the time interval between the shift in his or her eye gaze and the activation of the event. This creates opportunities for the child to learn to anticipate the outcome of the interventionist's eye gaze.

Typically developing children begin to attend to and act on an adult's **pointing gestures** by approximately 9 months of age (Butterworth, 2003). However, at this early age their attention will only be to referents that are in close physical proximity to the pointing gesture. Between 9 and 14 months, children become increasingly more adept at following points. By 2 years of age, they will be able to follow a pointing gesture that is 8 feet away from the target of the pointing gesture. Following a pointing gesture enables adults to call a learner's attention to items and events that can be the focus of modeled (or more intrusively prompted) communicative behavior (Franco & Butterworth, 1996; Morissette, Ricard, & Decarie, 1995).

☞ Helpful Hint

Suggestions for Teaching Line of Regard

Step 1: During initial teaching opportunities, the interventionist obtains the learner's attention (e.g., moves face in front of learner, calls learner's name to obtain localization).

Step 2: Next, the interventionist looks in the direction of the target event.

Step 3: The interventionist activates the referent to create an attention-gaining display (e.g., a toy might make a sound, move, or light up).

Across successful opportunities, the interventionist gradually increases the time interval between the shift in his or her eye gaze and activating the event. This creates opportunities for the child to learn to anticipate the outcome of the interventionist's eye gaze.

How Can a Learner Be Taught to Follow a Pointing Gesture (Receptive Joint Attention)?

By around 2 years of age, when a referent can be out of the learner's field of vision across the room, a partner's pointing gesture is often effective in directing a child's attention. In teaching this skill, we have found it useful to implement this strategy using remote-controlled toys. Prior to the child entering the room, a remote-controlled toy is placed in an inconspicuous area near the learner. The interventionist brings the learner to the room and engages him or her in a planned activity. As interest wanes, the interventionist establishes eye contact with the learner and then abruptly looks in the area of the toy as he or she points in that direction. Within a second or so, the toy is activated to ensure that the learner's attention is attracted. Across instructional opportunities, the delay between the interventionist's pointing and activating the toy is increased. In addition, across successful opportunities, the distance between the learner and the item of interest is increased. Finally, the distance between the learner and the interventionist begins to be increasingly varied.

☞ Helpful Hint

Suggestions for Teaching

Teaching a learner to follow a pointing gesture (receptive/responding joint attention)

- Before the child enters the room, a remote-controlled toy is placed in an inconspicuous area.

- The interventionist brings the learner to the room and engages him or her in the planned activity (that does not involve using the remote-controlled toy).

- As interest begins to wane, the interventionist abruptly looks in the area of the toy while pointing at it.

- Within a second or so, the interventionist activates the toy to ensure that the learner's attention is attracted.

- Across instructional opportunities, increase the delay between the pointing gesture and activating the toy.

- In addition, across successful opportunities, increase the distance between the learner and the item.

- Finally, the distance between the learner and the interventionist should be increased.

Next, we will more closely examine making the transition from unintentional to intentional communicative behavior that occurs between birth and the first 9–11 months in most typically developing children.

MAKING THE TRANSITION FROM UNINTENTIONAL TO INTENTIONAL COMMUNICATION

Prior to using symbols, most children begin consistently using their motor and vocal behavior to influence the actions of those around them. In this portion of the chapter, we discuss children's initial intentional communicative repertoire.

What Is the Distinction Between Communicative Function and Nonintentional and Intentional Communicative Acts?

Communicative function has become a frequently used term in discussing a learner's beginning communicative repertoire. A function describes the outcome that a learner's behavior produces. If the learner repeatedly produces a particular behavior, then it is clear that he or she is interested in the predictable effect that follows. Some interventionists talk about communicative intentions, however. Let's see if these two terms can be related.

Wetherby and Prizant (1989) defined *communicative intentionality* as deliberately pursuing a goal produced for the benefit of another individual. Bates et al. described it as "signaling behavior in which the sender is aware a priori of the effect that a signal will have on his listener" (1979, p. 36). Although this all seems straightforward, it is fairly difficult to directly measure communicative intentionality. Instead, intentionality must be inferred from the learner's behavior and his or her social partner's reactions. Learners may engage in intentional behavior without engaging in intentional communicative behavior. It is not unusual to see a 7- to 8-month-old child intentionally attempt to open a container. After struggling to solve the problem, however, the child may not realize that he or she can use an adult as an agent to gain access. Consequently, observing a learner produce goal-directed behavior does not necessarily indicate that he or she is yet intentionally producing intentional behavior intended for the benefit of others (i.e., intentional communication).

Function describes the outcome resulting from a child's behavior. For example, after crying, a child may receive a bottle. If hunger precipitated the crying and if the sequence described occurs repeatedly, then we would expect the probability of crying to increase around mealtime. If this occurred, then the function of the child's behavior would be to obtain a desired object/event (e.g., a bottle). Even though a child's action can be associated with a particular function, it does not necessarily mean that it is an intentional communicative act. In the example, crying can have a clear function for others even though it never occurs until the learner feels a pain in his or her stomach and cries in reaction to that pain. The act only becomes communicatively intentional when it is produced for the benefit of a listener and addresses at least several of the markers outlined in Table 1.2. Rather than relying on any single marker described in Table 1.2, most researchers use a collective set of criteria in making this determination. The greater the number of markers that can be observed in an interpersonal exchange, the stronger the case for an intentional act. Although specific criteria employed have differed (see Harding & Golinkoff, 1979; McLean, McLean, Brady, & Etter, 1991; Wetherby & Prizant, 1989), there appears to be some agreement. Some of these markers and the challenges that they create for people who experience significant developmental disabilities are explored next.

Alternating Gaze Between Goal and Listener

Compelling evidence of intentionality is evident if a learner alternates his or her gaze between the goal and the listener in com-

Table 1.2. Features associated with intentional communicative acts

| Alternating eye gaze between goal and listener |
| Signaling persistently until a goal is accomplished or failure indicated |
| Waiting for a response from a listener |
| Changing the signal quality until the goal has been met |
| Ritualizing or conventionalizing communicative forms |

From Wetherby, A., & Prutting, C. (1984). Profiles of communicative and cognitive-social abilities in autistic children. *Journal of Speech and Hearing Research, 27,* 364–377; adapted by permission.

bination with some vocalization or gesture. Can a communicative act be intentional without visual regard? There is little evidence that visual regard is a necessary prerequisite for intentional communicative acts. Shifting gaze is one way to indicate attention to both the referent and communication partner. In speech, the speaker need only coordinate his or her gaze between referent and listener to establish visual regard. For people who use alternate forms of communication (e.g., line-drawn symbols), however, the demands of the symbol array (e.g., several line-drawn symbols of preferred items) make it more challenging to shift gaze. The learner may be so occupied with selecting a message (i.e., a symbol) that gaze shifts are asynchronous because gaze must be shifted between the referent (i.e., the actual item), his or her symbol display, and his or her communicative partner. The **Picture Exchange Communication System** (**PECS;** Bondy & Frost, 1994) has been explicitly designed to address this challenge. In PECS, the learner must select a symbol and proffer it to a listener whom he or she has approached. Consequently, shifting attention from referent to board or from a communication board/wallet to a listener is taught as a specific chain of behavior.

Persistent Signaling Until the Goal Is Accomplished

Persistence is related to motivation. The persistence of communicative attempts may be easily missed because of the idiosyncrasy of strategies used by some augmentative and alternative communication (AAC) users who experience significant developmental disabilities. For example, consider a child who walks into the kitchen and waits for his or her mother to find the food item that he or she wants. In this example, walking into the kitchen is the communicative overture, and waiting represents persistence. If a history builds in which the child's parent does not identify this as communicative persistence, then the child's communicative overture may be extinguished over time. In general, most researchers agree that parents are responsive to their typically developing children's early vocal and gestural overtures. The interactional patterns of many parents who have children with significant disabilities, however, differ significantly. For example, some parents of children with developmental disabilities appear to be overly responsive, whereas others are less responsive to their child's communicative signaling (Linfoot, 1994). Overresponsiveness includes anticipating so many of the learner's wants and needs that it limits the learner's opportunities to initiate communicative acts.

Changing the Signal Until the Goal Is Met

Typically developing learners have a large repertoire of motor and vocal behavior at their disposal. For example, consider Sally, who first tugs at her father's shirt sleeve to obtain attention. When that is unsuccessful, she vocalizes loudly, which causes him to look at her. Changing a communicative form may be less problematic for typically developing individuals than it is for those with developmental disabilities who may have a much smaller range of different socially acceptable symbols/gestures. Further discussion of changing signals is provided in the upcoming section on communicative repairs.

Directing Communicative Overture to a Variety of Listeners

Having a significant motor impairment may make it more difficult for a learner to estab-lish close physical proximity to a variety of prospective listeners. Learners with significant developmental disabilities have a propensity to come in physical contact with a far more restricted range of prospective listeners. Consequently, when encountering someone outside of his or her immediate family, a learner with disabilities may lack the experience of seeking the attention of a wide range of individuals. In addition, knowing when to refrain from initiating a social overture may also be a limitation for people with developmental disabilities.

Each of the areas just described is helpful in determining whether a learner is failing to engage in intentional communicative acts or whether his or her acts are intentional but not expressed using conventional communicative means. The next section addresses how these responsive reactions to learner behavior, when done consistently, are a viable tool to establish intentional communicative behavior.

Distinguishing Between a Social Function and a Communicative Intent

Descriptions of intentional social/communicative functions in the positive behavior support literature typically involve three **social functions** that include **obtain/maintain attention, obtain/maintain goods and services,** and **escape/avoid.** Within the speech-language literature (see Wetherby and Prizant, 2003), there is discussion of intentional communicative acts, specifically **requests, protests, comments,** and so forth (see the next section for a detailed discussion). Unfortunately, there may not be a direct correspondence between these two sets of terms. For example, requests for assistance can be produced with a social intent of "obtain desired objects," as when a learner has difficulty opening a toy in a cellophane wrapper. Alternatively, the same learner could **request assistance** to more quickly finish an undesired task, as when a young child asks for help picking up toys in order to end the task.

Types of Communicative Intents

Wetherby and Prizant (2003) described taxonomy of communicative intents based, in part, on Bruner's work (1975, 1977) that has gained widespread acceptance in describing typical, delayed, and atypical development of communicative intent. They identified three general communicative intents that included **behavior regulation**, **joint attention**, and **social interaction**. Each of these functions or reasons for producing a communicative act is described next.

Behavior Regulation

During behavior regulation communicative acts, the learner is interested in influencing the actions of others involving the delivery, maintenance, or removal of goods or services. Specific communicative functions associated with behavior regulation include requesting objects, requesting actions, and protesting. **Protoimperative** is a term that has been used to refer to early emerging behavior regulation communicative acts (Bates et al., 1979; McLean et al., 1991). In a protoimperative act, the learner engages in vocal and/or gestural behavior to direct a communicative partner's attention toward a referent that the learner wishes to obtain, or with which he or she desires to maintain contact, escape, or avoid. For example, a child may see a toy on a shelf that he or she cannot directly reach. After looking at the toy, he or she may reach for it and vocalize. Then the child may immediately shift his or her eye gaze to his or her mother. As soon as the child has his or her mother's attention, he or she may again look at the referent and repeat the action. Among children who are not yet producing spoken words (i.e., **prelinguistic**), behavior regulation communicative acts account for approximately 36% of their total communicative acts (Wetherby & Prizant, 2003).

Joint Attention

During joint attention communicative acts, the learner is interested in directing a communicative partner's attention to objects/

events for the purpose of sharing attention. **Protodeclarative** is a term that has been used to describe early developing joint attention acts (Bates et al., 1979; McLean et al., 1991). To illustrate a protodeclarative act, specific communicative functions associated with joint attention include commenting on objects, commenting on actions, requesting information, providing clarification, and transferring (placing an object in another person's hand). Joint attention acts account for approximately 49% of typically developing children's total communicative acts (Wetherby & Prizant, 2003).

Social Interaction

Wetherby and Prizant (2003) referred to social interaction as a third general communicative intent. Communicative acts intended to result in social interaction involve the learner's attempts to attract or maintain another person's attention to him- or herself. Specific examples of social interaction communicative functions offered by Wetherby and Prizant include greetings, showing off, requesting a social routine (e.g., requesting Peekaboo), calling, acknowledging the comments produced by another, and expressing mood or feeling.

What Does the Research Say?
Communicative Intents

Bates et al. (1979) and Carpenter, Mastergeorge, and Coggins (1983) reported that declarative (joint attention) gestures emerged prior to imperative gestures (behavior regulation). Specifically, Carpenter et al. reported that among the 24 children they studied, joint attention communicative acts emerged at approximately 10 months of age, but behavior regulation gestures were not produced until approximately 12 months of age (with a substantial range of performance across participants). Yet, Perucchini and Camaioni (1993) observed that behavior regulation communicative functions emerged prior to joint attention functions, although some of their participants acquired both functions within a fairly comparable time frame.

A study by Crais, Douglas, and Campbell (2004) found that gestures used to communicate behavior regulation
(continued)

were seen earlier than gestures used to convey joint attention or social interaction, but there was broad overlap between categories of functions. Crais and her colleagues observed that approximately half acquired behavior regulation acts prior to joint attention or social interaction acts (although not statistically significant). Social interaction communication intents emerged significantly earlier than joint attention acts. By the time that children were using words, there was no clear hierarchy across different communicative intents.

Patterns in the proportional use of communicative intents have been used to differentiate populations of individuals with developmental disabilities. Children with autism have been reported to use a much larger proportion of behavior regulation communicative acts with a substantially lower proportion of joint attention acts (McEvoy, Rogers, & Pennington, 1993; Mundy, Sigman, & Kasari, 1994). Children with Down syndrome use social interaction and joint attention communicative acts more readily than acts communicating behavior regulation (Mundy, Kasari, Sigman, & Ruskin, 1995). McLean et al. (1991) and McLean et al. (1998) found a preponderance of behavior regulation communication acts produced by learners with severe disabilities, regardless of etiology.

Teaching Behavior Regulation Acts

Often, behavior regulation has been introduced as the initial focus of intervention (Bondy & Frost, 1994; Reichle, York, & Sigafoos, 1991). Within behavior regulation, requesting objects/activities has been a frequently chosen initial communicative function (Reichle, Beukelman, & Light, 2002). Typically, the interventionist performs an ecological inventory of activities for which the learner cannot independently gain access (Reichle et al., 1991). Objects associated with these activities are used in a reinforcement **preference assessment.** Subsequently, intervention begins (see Chapter 6 for a detailed discussion of strategies to evaluate reinforcer preference).

Few investigations have examined protests as an early intervention target. Communicative acts produced to convey escape or avoidance can occur in different contexts. When offered dreaded corn at mealtime, a child may produce a symbol or headshake "no." The subsequent removal of the aversive item serves as negative reinforcement, and the learner escapes/avoids corn. Suppose the same child is in a playgroup, however, and another child attempts to steal a toy. In this example, if the victim says "no," then the desired outcome is reestablishing toy play.

Chapter 9 provides information regarding teaching requests, including detailed instructional strategies.

There is virtually no evidence directly examining the degrees to which beginning communicators see these two situations being part of the same class of situations that calls for the production of a protest. Sigafoos et al. (2004) suggested that there are a number of plausible situations that learners encounter on a regular basis that call for protests. These are summarized next in the contexts for teaching protests.

CASE EXAMPLE

Reichle, Drager, and Davis (2002)

Learner: Individual with significant developmental disabilities

Method: Taught to use requests for assistance when presented with a task that was undesirable due to the level of difficulty. At the outset of the investigation, a group of activities that were preferred but could not be independently accessed by the learner were identified as well as a final set of tasks that, like the initial set, were undesirable due to the level of difficulty.

Results: The learner generalized the request for assistance from examples involving nonpreferred materials to nonpreferred activities that had not been the focus of intervention to other items not yet trained that represented

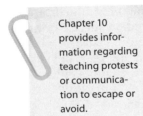

Chapter 10 provides information regarding teaching protests or communication to escape or avoid.

difficult and nonpreferred activities. Yet, no generalization of the requesting assistance act was observed during activities that consisted of preferred but difficult-to-access objects.

Discussion: Results provided tentative evidence that some learners may struggle generalizing at least some communicative intents across social function boundaries. Consequently, it may not be sufficient to think of generalization across only perceptual boundaries such as color, shape, and the size of referents. It also suggests that interventionists may need to be aware that teaching a request for assistance to a situation where the learner's goal may be to get something done as soon as possible so that he or she can escape may not generalize to situations where the request is used to obtain goods and services.

↦ Helpful Hint

Teaching Joint Attention Communicative Acts

Teaching a joint attention communicative act to many children with severe disabilities can be challenging because it can be difficult to find effective reinforcers. A typical reinforcer for a comment (one type of joint attention) would be acknowledging the comment by the communication partner. Initially, however, commenting may not be reinforcing, particularly for learners with autism. Kasari, Freeman, and Paparella (2006), however, demonstrated the effectiveness of an intervention program that combined successive practice opportunities with naturally occurring teaching opportunities in increasing joint attention for children with autism. Initially, children were prompted to point to toys and objects during structured opportunities conducted during a tabletop activity. After approximately 10 minutes, teaching occurred during floor play. Participants showed significantly more gains in joint attention than children who did not have

this intervention. A combination of repeated practice with more naturalistic teaching procedures has been demonstrated by others to teach joint attention (e.g., Jones, Carr, & Feeley, 2006; Whalen & Schreibman, 2003).

Addressing Communicative Intents with Intervention

It is clear that a range of different communicative intentions emerges during a short time span among typically developing children. Often, intervention strategies designed for individuals with developmental disabilities have focused on establishing a number of representational symbols within a single communicative function (often behavior regulation) prior to introducing a second communicative intent. An example of concurrently implementing different communicative intents follows.

CASE EXAMPLE

Reichle, Rogers, and Barrett (1984)

Participant: Fifteen-year-old girl with severe developmental disabilities

Method: Taught to produce a manual sign (WANT) to request objects and a different manual sign to indicate NO when she was offered nonpreferred items. To teach NO, the interventionist selected items that were not accepted when offered. While offering a tray containing nonpreferred items, the interventionist asked, "Want one?" Producing the sign NO resulted in the removal of the array. If NO was not produced, then the interventionist directly offered one of the nonpreferred items to the learner. When the learner showed behavioral indications of resistance (e.g., turning away from item), a physical prompt to produce the sign for NO was delivered. Prompting was systematically faded across successive teaching opportunities.

Results: A protesting communicative act was quickly acquired and appeared to be controlled by the presentation of nonpreferred items. The learner was able to use the protest response when offered a nonpreferred object and a different response (WANT) when offered a preferred object.

Discussion: The protesting skill just described was taught after first teaching the learner to request. Consequently, the learner was able to discriminate between situations that called for requesting and those that called for protesting.

Conditional use is when the learner discriminates when to use different intents while he or she is being taught multiple communicative intents. For example, Hung (1980) described an intervention strategy to teach requesting and protesting to two elementary-age children with autism. Interventionists taught participants to say "yes" when offered preferred food items and to say "no" when they were offered nonpreferred food items. The interventionist offered an item and asked, "Do you want [name of food item]?" When the child said "yes," he or she received the item. When the child said "no," interventionists removed the item. Modeling, error correction, and differential reinforcement were utilized. Both children learned to say "yes" or "no" under the appropriate conditions. Duker and Jutten (1997) also taught yes/no responses to beginning communicators.

Typically developing individuals often use the same vocabulary item when they engage in conditional communicative acts (i.e., using a communicative act when it is appropriate and refraining from using it when it is inappropriate) that involve several different communicative intents. For example, a child might say "Snoopy" while pointing to the neighbor's dog as it runs in the front yard in an effort to call his or her mother's attention to it (joint attention communicative act) while also pointing to the dog and saying "Snoopy" in an effort to get the dog to approach him or her (behavior regulation). Relatively few investigations have attempted to teach this type of multiple use with a single vocabulary item.

Learning to Use Newly Acquired Communicative Acts Conditionally

Conditional use among beginning communicators often involves choosing whether to produce a more conventional communicative act or use an idiosyncratic communicative act. Sometimes this decision involves selecting between socially acceptable and socially unacceptable behavior.

What Does the Research Say?
Establishing Conditional Use

In an effort to establish conditional use of early communicative acts, Reichle and Johnston (1999) taught two boys with significant developmental disabilities to conditionally request snack items. When items were in another person's possession or when they were distant, the boys were taught to request assistance. When the items were nearby, they were taught to refrain from requesting them and instead to reach for them.

CASE EXAMPLE

Drasgow, Halle, and Ostrosky (1998)

Participants: Three children with autism spectrum disorders and severe language delays

Baseline: Showed that the children had existing requests (reaching, grabbing, and leading)

Intervention: Each of the three children was taught to produce a replacement request (signing PLEASE) in one setting. Unfortunately, they rarely used it at home, which represented the generalization setting.

Intervention in home: The interventionists implemented differential reinforcement of alternative behavior (DRA) PLEASE and extinction of competing requests at home instead of using the intervention that had been successful at school.

> Chapter 10 provides procedures for teaching requests.

Discussion: This intervention resulted in increased use of PLEASE in generalization setting for each child. That is, the children started using their new socially acceptable communicative act as soon as the old familiar and socially unacceptable form was no longer successful in obtaining materials.

In establishing conditional use, it is important to make sure that the new communicative act being taught will be more efficient than the behavior that is already part of the learner's repertoire. When teaching a request, one cannot assume it is the only available act that the learner associates with a successful communicative episode. Consequently, a competing form may interfere with generalization of new communicative acts.

Intuitively, it makes sense that if a learner already has a conventional communicative means, then the interventionist should attempt to extend it to other situations in which a more idiosyncratic means is used. For example, an interventionist discovers that a learner shakes his head "no" to refuse offers of more juice at snack time after he has just consumed 8 ounces.

Winborn, Wacker, Richman, Asmus, and Greir (2002) examined the use of existing requests as a replacement for challenging behaviors with two toddlers who had developmental delays, seizures, and problem behaviors. Results revealed that when reinforcement for either request was concurrently available, the children used existing requests more than new requests. These children, however, also produced higher levels of problem behavior with existing requests. At first glance, it seemed as though it would be more efficient to teach a learner to extend a newly acquired behavior currently associated with challenging behaviors. Maintenance of new requests, however, may be compromised if there are relationships between existing requests and problem (or more idiosyncratic) behavior. Thus, one cannot always say that it is best to attempt to extend the use of an existing socially acceptable behavior rather than establishing a new form.

Summary of Communicative Intents

Thus far, much of the chapter has focused on the communicative intents and functions of early emerging vocal, gestural, and graphic communicative acts. The function of any particular communicative act is the purpose that single act serves in the context of the situation in which it is produced. One can also consider, however, how the learner begins to extend social interactions in conversations that involve initiating, maintaining, or terminating interactions.

PHASES OF CONVERSATION

In addition to its communicative intention, each communication act can be described in terms of its **conversational function.** How does the communicative act operate within the social interaction? How does one initiate, maintain, and terminate an interaction?

Beyond Responding: The Importance of Initiating Conversations

Typically, early communication interventions for learners with severe disabilities have addressed responding (Anderson & Spradlin, 1980; Carr, Binkoff, Kologinsky, & Eddy, 1978; Hupp, Mervis, Able, Conroy-Gunter, 1986; Salmon, Pear, & Kuhn, 1986). Typically developing children may use newly acquired symbols across conversational functions (e.g., saying, "I went to see Batman" could be used either to initiate or maintain a social interaction). Among many beginning communicators with severe disabilities, however, this does not occur unless specific teaching steps are included (Hundert & Houghton, 1992; Luciano, 1986; Warren & Rogers-Warren, 1980).

A number of interventions have been developed to improve individuals' abilities to initiate and maintain conversations. The following sections describe research on interventions that have been developed to improve initiations and maintenance of conversations and offer suggestions for implementing these and similar interventions during daily interactions.

Typically, the start of a social interaction is marked by one individual making some type of overture to a communicative partner (which could be a spoken or nonverbal greeting). Usually, face-to-face interactions include one or more of the following: close physical proximity; a history of interaction; a common focus of attention; and a goal of obtaining goods or services, gaining information, or sharing an experience.

It can be difficult to determine when an episode of social interaction is initiated within real-world interactions. For example, some individuals with slow responses due to motor impairments may require a longer amount of time to respond to their partner's communication, making it difficult to determine if the individual is responding to or initiating a new interaction. For example, the response SLIDE CLOSED following the question, "What are you doing this weekend?" would appear to be an initiation of a new topic rather than an appropriate answer to the question. But, in this case, the individual had a history of going to the pool on weekends and was not going this weekend because the slide would be closed. Therefore, it can more accurately be described as a topic-maintaining utterance.

Assessing Initiations

Sometimes, situations similar to those that occur in the natural environment can be "set up" to assess communicative initiations. For example, materials may purposefully be placed in containers that are difficult to open to provide for requesting, or an ordinary object can be replaced by a highly unusual object to provide for joint attention. If the individual acts on these contextual cues, then typically he or she is credited with an initiation. Assessments such as the Communication Temptations portion of the Communication and Symbolic Behavior Scales™ (CSBS™; Wetherby & Prizant, 2003) or the Early Social Communication Scales (ESCS; Mundy et al., 2003) encourage initiations by

manipulating contextual cues and creating a context to request or engage in joint attention. Similar procedures were used by Brady, McLean, and colleagues (Brady et al., 1995; McLean et al., 1991, 1998) to assess communication in adults with severe disabilities and evaluate development of early communication over time (Brady, Marquis, Fleming, & McLean, 2004). Desirable items in closed containers or unusual and enticing objects are presented within a series of activities in all of these assessment protocols. Adult communication partners follow a script that directs them to wait for a specified period of time before providing a prompt for communication. The purpose of the wait time is to allow time for the individual to initiate communication.

⚐ Helpful Hint

Example script for joint attention communicative intent assessment

1. The teacher places goo in the child's hand.
2. The teacher takes the goo from the child, plays with it, then passes it back to the child.
3. The teacher and the child take turns playing with the goo.
4. The teacher surreptitiously replaces the goo with similar goo that has a toy object inside.
5. After passing the goo with object to the child, the teacher waits up to 10 seconds for the child to comment about the toy in the goo.
6. If child initiates a "comment" about the toy in the goo through gesture, vocalization, or symbolic means, then the teacher responds to the comment.
7. If the child does not initiate, then the teacher takes the goo back and continues with another activity.

Example script for behavior regulation assessment

1. The teacher introduces a switch-operated vibrating bumble ball. The teacher gives the ball to the child.
2. After a few seconds, the teacher takes the ball and plays with it for a few seconds.
3. The teacher hands the ball back to the child to play with for a few more seconds.

4. The teacher takes the ball back and, while playing with it, turns the switch off.

5. The teacher hands the ball to the child with the switch in the off position.

6. The teacher waits up to 10 seconds.

7. If the child initiates a request for help by gesturing, vocalizing, or symbolic means, then the teacher turns the ball back on and allows the child to play with the ball for several more seconds.

8. If the child does not initiate a request, then the teacher takes back the ball and turns it on and gives it to the child.

Teaching/Facilitating Initiations

Halle, Marshall, and Spradlin (1979) taught beginning communicators to initiate requests at mealtimes by providing extensive contextual cues (all of the activities associated with going through a cafeteria line) and then waiting until the individuals initiated requests for their food tray. In these studies, if the individuals did not initiate requests after a specified amount of time, then a teaching prompt was provided.

> Chapter 6 provides information regarding a time delay procedure.

☞ Helpful Hint

Suggestions for teaching initiated requests

- Identify highly motivating items for each individual.

- Identify the average amount of time required for the individual to form the targeted communication response.

- Increase the opportunities for the individual to initiate requests for motivating items by making the individual aware that they are available (e.g., within visual line of regard for those who can see) but unobtainable without assistance.

- Wait for the specified amount of time before providing a teaching prompt.

- Provide reinforcement after a response approximation.

A facilitative interaction style (Miranda & Donnellan, 1986) that includes allowing the child to control and initiate topics, as well as adults following the child's lead and encouraging the child to contribute to the ongoing conversation, was found to result in a greater number of topic initiations. In contrast to a directive style in which adults controlled the interaction, assumed the lead in conversations, and structured the child's contributions to the conversation, adults were instructed to wait up to 30 seconds for a child to communicate.

Thus, it appears that allowing children sufficient time to initiate is one of the most effective strategies for teaching initiations to beginning communicators. Long wait times such as 45 seconds may feel uncomfortable for communication partners. This wait time can be shortened for most learners after the child experiences positive consequences for his or her initiations. Several intervention packages, such as the Hanen program for parents (Girolametto & Weitzman, 2006) and parent-implemented enhanced-milieu teaching (Kaiser, Hancock, & Nietfeld, 2000), have been developed to teach communication partners to wait and to be more facilitative. For example, one of the strategies taught to parents in the Hanen program is referred to as OWLing, which stands for *observe, wait,* and *listen*. Parents learn to observe their children, wait before providing the children with a consequence or a prompt, and listen or recognize all forms of communication (including gestures and nonspeech vocalizations).

A variety of situations arise in the natural environment that promote the initiation of communicative acts, including joining an ongoing routine, beginning well-established routines, calling attention to novel events, and protesting the actions of others. In these contexts, several strategies have been developed that focus on promoting initiations through visual supports, such as written scripts, picture cues, **video modeling**, and live modeling. Much of the research on visual supports has focused on children with autism because they frequently show severe impairments in social initiations (Landa, 2007). A number of investigators have taught literate children to follow a social script with written prompts when interacting with peers (Goldstein, Wickstrom, Hoyson, Jamieson, & Odom, 1988; Sarokoff, Taylor, & Poulson, 2001; Thiemann & Goldstein, 2004). Scripts enable children to learn to expect each event in the routine, and an opportunity for an initiation is created when the occurrence of one event is interrupted with an expectant delay. Initially, child communications are written into a script that remains available for self-cueing. Scripted interactions have also been effective for nonreaders, presumably by ensuring a predictable sequence of events (Sack, McLean, McLean, & Spradlin, 1992; Short-Meyerson & Abbeduto, 1997).

Video modeling has been used to teach social communication to children with autism and other developmental disabilities (Buggey, 2005; Delano, 2007; Hepting & Goldstein, 1996; Maione & Mirenda, 2006; Sherer et al., 2001). The basic procedure includes **showing** the child a video of a peer or themselves successfully producing the behavior prior to a live interaction. For example, Maione and Mirenda showed tapes of peers making comments about play activities to a child with autism prior to observing the focus child and two to three peers playing with the same items. Video feedback was later added to the intervention and included review of the video just recorded along with evaluations of whether the child was engaged in "good talking." Additional verbal prompts ("Remember to talk when you are playing") and visual prompts (the printed word *talk*) were added to improve effectiveness of the video modeling and feedback. Similar procedures may also be helpful for teaching social initiations through AAC, but research has yet to document the effectiveness.

☞ *Helpful Hint*

Suggestions for teaching with video modeling

- Identify social situations where the learner is not performing as expected.

- Videorecord competent social communicators performing the basic communication exchanges involved in the social situation (e.g., asking for their turn in playing a game).

- Show this video to the learner before intervention sessions.

- Point out the target behaviors that are displayed by the competent communicators on the video.

Maintaining Interactions

Once conversations have been initiated, competent communicators typically maintain numerous exchanges depending on the purpose of the conversation and specific interaction history between the participants. In contrast, a conversation between two old friends reminiscing about a shared past experience may last many turns and span minutes or hours. Thus, the appropriate number of turns or exchanges within a conversation is not absolute and depends on many contextual variables.

Chapter 12 provides information regarding visual supports.

Usually, young children with significant developmental disabilities have a limited range of communicative partners as a result of their dependence on caregivers and the more limited range of environments that they tend to access. They may have limited opportunities to learn strategies for maintaining conversational exchanges because they are usually interacting with familiar individuals who are willing to assume a significant role in keeping a social exchange going.

Turn Taking

Unfortunately, conversations with beginning communicators are often composed of too few turns and dominated by partners without disabilities (Buzolich & Wiemann, 1988; Light & Binger, 1998; Light, Collier, & Parnes, 1985). This is particularly true for children who use AAC because formulating an utterance often requires more time, and this latency disrupts the flow of a conversation. Communication breakdowns are also a frequent problem in conversations with beginning communicators, including beginning AAC users (Brady & Halle, 2002).

Increasing Turn Taking

Teaching nonobligatory communication responses is one way to increase the number of turns per topic. Nonobligatory responses start a conversation or follow a partner's comment or statement (Light & Binger, 1998). For example, a learner can be taught to produce responses such as "awesome" or "uh-oh" in response to interesting or surprising occurrences. Turns can also be increased by using a conversation notebook or picture book. The purpose of such a book is to provide additional conversation topics that are of interest to the beginning communicator and help cue successive turns. For example, Hunt, Alwell, and Goetz (1991) taught three beginning communicators to initiate conversations by producing a small notebook containing pictures of high-interest items. Once a conversation was initiated, participants were prompted to take additional turns by indicating a picture in the notebook and talking about the picture. Prompts were gradually faded and intervention was extended to additional partners and contexts. All three participants increased their number of conversational turns using this procedure. Teaching tools discussed in the previous section (e.g., using nonobligatory turns modeled by a peer) are also relevant here.

Maintaining Conversations After Communication Breakdowns

Communication breakdowns frequently occur with beginning communicators for many reasons. Sometimes one communication partner does not understand something communicated by a partner and, thus, asks for clarification. On other occasions, one communication partner may fail to respond to a message because he or she is not attending. Also, a partner may want to steer the conversation in another direction and either fail to respond or respond with a remark that changes the topic. **Communicative breakdowns** occur after approximately 30% of communication acts produced by beginning communicators that are directed to their caregivers (Brady & Fleming, 2007b; Calculator & Dollaghan, 1982). Brady and Fleming studied young children with developmental disabilities (including Down syndrome or autism) who used fewer than 10 words or symbols to communicate expressively. Calculator and Dollaghan (1982) observed a similar proportion of breakdowns in interactions between older AAC users and teachers in classroom settings.

Teaching Repairs of Communication Breakdowns

Repairing communication breakdowns includes repeating a communication attempt using the same words, symbols, gestures, or vocalizations or revising the communication act. Revisions could include an additional word or gesture or changes in volume or intensity. Sigafoos et al. (2004) taught two beginning communicators with severe disabilities to repair communication breakdowns by using a voice output communication aid (VOCA). At the start of intervention, learners initiated communication by reaching directly for what they wanted. The teachers created a communication breakdown by ignoring this initiation and then providing a VOCA programmed with a short phrase (i.e., "I want more"). The learners used the VOCA to request and also began initiating requests with the VOCA (rather than just using the VOCA to repair).

An alternative strategy is to encourage partners to specifically request repairs. For example, Weiner (2005) taught peers of children with developmental disabilities (two with autism and one with Down syndrome) to request clarification (e.g., "Huh?" "What?") during conversations. The intervention consisted of talking to the peers about communication breakdowns and how to respond to unintelligible communication acts by the peers with disabilities. Subsequently, the investigator prompted the peers (if needed) with questions (e.g., "Do you understand that?") during intervention and then with specific prompts to request repairs, if necessary. Results showed increases in peer repair requests, turn taking, and proportion of intelligible utterances by the children with disabilities.

Brady and Steeples (2007) also focused on teaching repair requests to communication partners. Partners were mothers of three young children with relatively high proportions of unresolved communication breakdowns. The children communicated with gestures but little to no symbolic communication. Unresolved breakdowns were those in which the mother did not appear to understand or respond appropriately to the child's communication, often after several repair attempts. Mothers were first taught to be more responsive to their child's communication by recognizing early attempts including gestures, vocalizations, and idiosyncratic communication acts. Next, they were taught to respond to unintelligible utterances with clarification requests. Two of the three children showed increases in both their proportions of initiated communication acts and successful communication acts following intervention.

In summary, conversations can be maintained by teaching beginning communicators specific communication behaviors and/or by teaching communication partners to interact in specific ways. It may be most efficient to combine both strategies. Interventions that teach children to use multiple modes of communication to repair breakdowns while also encouraging partners to increase repair requests are likely to increase the number of turns per communication episode and lead to better maintained social interactions.

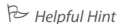 *Helpful Hint*

Suggestions for Maintaining Conversations After Communicative Breakdowns

Learner-focused strategies

- Teach multiple response topographies (e.g., graphic symbol, gesture, vocalization) so that

an alternative response can be attempted when a partner does not respond to a learner's initiation.

Partner-focused strategies

- Provide recognizable cues to communication breakdowns (e.g., say, "What?" and look confused).

- Wait for a response to a communication breakdown.

- Respond to repair attempts, including nonsymbolic gestures and vocalizations.

Terminating Interactions

Terminating interactions appropriately is just as important as initiating and maintaining interactions. Learning to terminate interactions may be challenging because there may be no clear reinforcer for terminating. In fact, the next activity may be nonpreferred. Consequently, it may be necessary to establish reinforcing events that can be delivered contingent on politely terminating pleasurable activities to proceed to an activity of more neutral or nonpreferred interest.

Users of graphic mode AAC systems face a number of challenges in terminating social interactions that are not apt to be challenges for speaking individuals. It may be difficult for an AAC user to secure the speaking floor to end an interaction because graphic mode communication is much slower. In other instances, the learner may not have an appropriate symbol available to terminate an interaction.

SUMMARY

In conclusion, we have described how individuals in the beginning stages of communication development learn to communicate for different reasons and during different phases of conversational exchanges. It is our contention that communication teaching strategies are ultimately more effective for learners when they take these pragmatic aspects of communication into account. It is not enough to teach individuals a small set of communication responses that are only used to communicate limited functions. We suggest that interventionists implement a programmatic approach that targets across pragmatic aspects of communication in order to facilitate communication development that will lead to greater participation and fulfillment.

REFERENCES

Anderson, S.R., & Spradlin, J.E. (1980). The generalized effects of productive labeling training involving common object classes. *Journal of The Association for the Severely Handicapped, 5,* 143–157.

Baldwin, D. (1991). Infants' contribution to the achievement of joint reference. *Child Development, 63,* 875–890.

Bates, E., Benigni, L., Bretherton, I., & Camaioni, L. (1979). *The emergence of symbols: Cognition and communication in infancy.* San Diego: Academic Press.

Bell, S., & Ainsworth, M. (1972). Infant crying and maternal responsiveness. *Child Development, 43,* 1171–1190.

Bloom, L., & Lahey, M. (1978). *Language development and language disorders.* New York: Wiley.

Bondy, A., & Frost, L. (1994). The Picture Exchange Communication System. *Focus on Autistic Behavior, 9,* 1–19.

Brady, N., & Fleming, K. (2007a, March). *Early communication by young children with autism: Breakdowns and repairs during mother–child interactions.* Symposium on Research in Child Development, Boston.

Brady, N., & Fleming, K. (2007b, March). *Persistence in early communication by young children with Down syndrome and other developmental disabilities.* Gatlinburg Conference on Research and Theory in Mental Retardation and Developmental Disabilities, Annapolis, MD.

Brady, N.C., & Halle, J.W. (2002). Breakdowns and repairs in conversations between beginning AAC users and their partners. In D. Beukelman & J. Reichle (Series Eds.) & J. Reichle, D.R. Beukelman, & J.C. Light (Vol. Eds.), *AAC Series: Exemplary practices for beginning communicators: Implications for AAC.* (pp. 323–351). Baltimore: Paul H. Brookes Publishing Co.

Brady, N., Marquis, J., Fleming, K., & McLean, L. (2004). Prelinguistic predictors of language growth in children with developmental disabilities. *Journal of Speech, Language, and Hearing Research, 47,* 663–667.

Brady, N., McLean, J., James, E., Mclean, L., Lee, K., & Johnston, S. (1995). Initiation and repair of intentional communication acts by adults with severe to profound cognitive disabilities. *Journal of Speech and Hearing Research, 38,* 1334–1348.

Brady, N., & Steeples, T. (2007). *Interventions to increase successful communication interactions between young children with disabilities and their mothers.* Unpublished manuscript.

Bruner, J. (1975). The ontogenesis of speech acts. *Journal of Child Language, 2,* 1–19.

Bruner, J. (1977). Early social interaction and language acquisition. In R. Schaffer (Ed.), *Studies in mother–infant interaction* (pp. 271–289). San Diego: Academic Press.

Buggey, T. (2005). Video modeling applications with students with autism spectrum disorder in a small private school setting. *Focus on Autism and Other Disabilities, 20,* 52–63.

Butterworth, G. (2003). Pointing is the royal road to language for babies. In S. Kita (Ed.), *Pointing: Where language culture and cognition meet* (pp. 9–33). Mahwah, NJ: Lawrence Erlbaum Associates.

Buzolich, M.J., & Wiemann, J.M. (1988). Turn taking in atypical conversations: The case of the speaker/augmented-communicator dyad. *Journal of Speech and Hearing Research, 31,* 3–18.

Calculator, S., & Dollaghan, C. (1982). The use of communication boards in a residential setting: An evaluation. *Journal of Speech and Hearing Disorders, 47,* 281–287.

Campos, J., & Sternberg, C. (1981). Perception, appraisal and emotion: The onset of social referencing. In M. Lamb & I. Sherrod (Eds.), *Infant social cognition: Empirical and theoretical considerations* (pp. 273–314). Mahwah, NJ: Lawrence Erlbaum Associates.

Carpenter, R., Mastergeorge, A., & Coggins, D. (1983). The acquisition of communicative intentions in infants 8–15 months of age. *Language and Speech, 26,* 101–116.

Carr, E.G., Binkoff, J.A., Kologinsky, E., & Eddy, M. (1978). Acquisition of sign language by autistic children: I: Expressive labeling. *Journal of Applied Behavior Analysis, 11,* 489–501.

Crais, E.R., Douglas, D., & Campbell, C. (2004). The intersection of the development of gestures and intentionality. *Journal of Speech, Language, and Hearing Research, 47,* 678–694.

Delano, M. (2007). Video modeling interventions for individuals with autism. *Remedial and Special Education, 28,* 33–42.

Drasgow, E., Halle, J.W., & Ostrosky, M.M. (1998). Effects of differential reinforcement on the generalization of a replacement mand in three children with severe language delays. *Journal of Applied Behavior Analysis, 31,* 357–374.

Duker, P., & Jutten, W. (1997). Establishing gestural yes–no responding with individuals with profound mental retardation. *Education and Training in Mental Retardation and Developmental Disabilities, 32,* 59–67.

Franco, F., & Butterworth, G. (1996). Pointing and social awareness: Declaring and requesting in the second year. *Journal of Child Language, 23,* 307–336.

Gesell, A., & Ilg, F. (1937). *Feeding behavior of infants.* Philadelphia: Lippincott Williams & Wilkins.

Girolametto, L., & Weitzman, E. (2006). It takes two to talk—The Hanen program for parents: Early language intervention through caregiver training. In S.F. Warren & M.E. Fey (Series Eds.) & R.J. McCauley & M.E. Fey (Vol. Eds.), *Communication and language intervention series: Treatment of language disorders in children* (pp. 77–104). Baltimore: Paul H. Brookes Publishing Co.

Goldstein, H., Wickstrom, S., Hoyson, M., Jamieson, B., & Odom, S. (1988). Effects of sociodramatic script training on social and communicative interaction. *Education and Treatment of Children, 11,* 97–117.

Halle, J.W., Marshall, A.M., & Spradlin, J.E. (1979). Time delay: A technique to increase language use and facilitate generalization in retarded children. *Journal of Applied Behavior Analysis, 12,* 431–439.

Harding, C., & Golinkoff, R. (1979). The origins of intentional vocalizations in prelinguistic infants. *Child Development, 50,* 33–40.

Hart, B., & Risley, T.R. (1995). *Meaningful differences in the everyday experience of young American children.* Baltimore: Paul H. Brookes Publishing Co.

Hepting, N.H., & Goldstein, H. (1996). Requesting by preschoolers with developmental disabilities: Video-taped self-modeling and learning of new linguistic structures. *Topics in Early Childhood Special Education, 16,* 407–427.

Hood, B., Willen, D., & Driver, J. (1998). Adults' eyes trigger shifts of visual attention in human infants. *Psychological Science, 9,* 131–134.

Hundert, J., & Houghton, A. (1992). Promoting social interaction of children with disabilities in integrated preschools: A failure to generalize. *Exceptional Children, 58,* 311–320.

Hung, D. (1980). Training and generalization of yes and no as mands in two autistic children. *Journal of Autism and Developmental Disorders, 10,* 139–152.

Hunt, P., Alwell, M., & Goetz, L. (1991). Interacting with peers through conversation turn taking with a communication book adaptation. *Augmentative and Alternative Communication, 7,* 117–126.

Hupp, S.C., Mervis, C.B., Able, H., & Conroy-Gunter, M. (1986). Effects of receptive and expressive training of category labels on generalized learning by severely mentally retarded children. *American Journal of Mental Deficiency, 90,* 558–565.

Jones, E.A., Carr, E.G., & Feeley, K.M. (2006). Multiple effects of joint attention intervention for children with autism. *Behavior Modification, 30,* 782–834.

Kaiser, A.P., Hancock, T.B., & Nietfeld, J.P. (2000). The effects of parent-implemented enhanced milieu teaching on the social communication of children who have autism. *Early Education and Development, 11,* 423–446.

Kasari, C., Freeman, S., & Paparella, T. (2006). Joint attention and symbolic play in young children with autism: A randomized controlled intervention study. *Journal of Child Psychology and Psychiatry, 47,* 611–620.

Landa, R. (2007). Early communication development and intervention for children with autism. *Mental Retardation and Developmental Disabilities Research Reviews, 13,* 16–25.

Light, J.C., & Binger, C. (1998). *Building communicative competence with individuals who use augmentative and alternative communication.* Baltimore: Paul H. Brookes Publishing Co.

Light, J., Collier, B., & Parnes, P. (1985). Communicative interaction between young non-speaking physically disabled children and their primary caregivers: Part II: Communicative function. *Augmentative and Alternative Communication, 1,* 98–133.

Linfoot, K. (1994). *Communication strategies for people with developmental disabilities: Issues from theory and practice.* Baltimore: Paul H. Brookes Publishing Co.

Luciano, M.C. (1986). Acquisition, maintenance, and generalization of productive intraverbal behavior through transfer of stimulus control procedures. *Applied Research in Mental Retardation, 7,* 1–20.

Maione, L., & Mirenda, P. (2006). Effects of video modeling and video feedback on peer-directed social language skills of a child with autism. *Journal of Positive Behavior Interventions, 8,* 106–119.

McEvoy, R., Rogers, S., & Pennington, B. (1993). Executive function and social communication deficits in young autistic children. *Journal of Child Psychology and Psychiatry, 34,* 563–578.

McLean, J.E., McLean, L.K., Brady, N.C., & Etter, R. (1991). Communication profiles of two types of gesture using nonverbal persons with severe to profound mental retardation. *Journal of Speech and Hearing Research, 34,* 294–308.

McLean, L.K., Brady, N.C., McLean, J.E., & Behrens, G.E. (1998). Communication forms and functions of children and adults with severe mental retardation in community and institutional settings. *Journal of Speech and Hearing Research, 42,* 231–240.

Mirenda, P., & Donnellan, A. (1986). Effects of adult interaction style on conversational behavior in students with severe communication problems. *Language, Speech, and Hearing Services in Schools, 17,* 126–141.

Morissette, P., Ricard, M., & Decarie, T.G. (1995). Joint visual attention and pointing in infancy: A longitudinal study of comprehension. *British Journal of Developmental Psychology, 13,* 163–175.

Mundy, P., Delgado, C., Block, J., Venezia, M., Hogan, A., & Seibert, J. (2003). *A manual for the abridged Early Social Communication Scales (ESCS).* Coral Gables, FL: University of Miami, Department of Psychology.

Mundy, P., Kasari, C., Sigman, M., & Ruskin, E. (1995). Nonverbal communication and early language in children with Down syndrome or normal development. *Journal of Speech and Hearing Research, 38,* 157–167.

Mundy, P., Sigman, M., & Kasari, C. (1994). Joint attention, developmental level, and symptom presentation in autism. *Development and Psychopathology, 6,* 389–401.

Perucchini, P., & Camaioni, L. (1993). *When intentional communication emerges? Developmental dissociations between declarative and imperative functions of pointing gesture.* Poster presented at the British Psychological Society Annual Conference, Developmental Section, Birmingham.

Prutting, C., & Kirchner, D. (1987). A clinical appraisal of the pragmatic aspects of language. *Journal of Speech and Hearing Disorders, 52,* 105–119.

Reichle, J., Beukelman, D.R., & Light, J.C. (Vol. Eds.). (2002). *AAC Series: Exemplary practices for beginning communicators: Implications for AAC.* Baltimore: Paul H. Brookes Publishing Co.

Reichle, J., Drager, K., & Davis, C. (2002). Using requests for assistance to obtain desired items and to gain release from non-preferred activities: Implications for assessment and intervention. *Education and Treatment of Children, 25,* 47–66.

Reichle, J., & Johnston, S.S. (1999). Teaching the conditional use of communicative requests to two school-age children with severe developmental disabilities. *Language, Speech, and Hearing Services in Schools, 10,* 324–334.

Reichle, J., Rogers, N., & Barrett, C. (1984). Establishing pragmatic discriminations among the communicative functions of requesting, rejecting, and commenting in an adolescent. *Journal of The Association for Severely Handicapped, 9,* 31–36.

Reichle, J., York, J., & Sigafoos, J. (1991). *Implementing augmentative and alternative communica-*

tion: Strategies for learners with severe disabilities. Baltimore: Paul H. Brookes Publishing Co.

Rheingold, H., Gewirtz, J., & Ross, H. (1959). Social conditioning of vocalization in the infant. *Journal of Comparative Psychology, 52,* 68–73.

Sack, S.H., McLean, L.S., McLean, J.E., & Spradlin, J.E. (1992). Effects of increased opportunities within scripted activities on communication rates of individuals with severe retardation. *Behavioral Residential Treatment, 7,* 235–257.

Salmon, D.J., Pear, J.J., & Kuhn, B.A. (1986). Generalization of object naming after training with picture cards and with objects. *Journal of Applied Behavior Analysis, 19,* 53–58.

Sarokoff, R.A., Taylor B.A., & Poulson, C.L. (2001). Teaching children with autism to engage in conversational exchanges: Script fading with embedded textual stimuli. *Journal of Applied Behavior Analysis, 34,* 81–84.

Sherer, M., Pierce, K.L., Paredes, S., Kisacky, K.L., Ingersoll, B., & Schreibman, L. (2001). Enhancing conversation skills in children with autism via video technology: Which is better—"self" or "other" as a model? *Behavior Modification, 25,* 140–158.

Short-Meyerson, K.J., & Abbeduto, L.J. (1997). Preschoolers' communication during scripted interactions. *Journal of Child Language, 24,* 469–493.

Sigafoos, J., Drasgow, E., Reichle, J., O'Reilly, M., Green, V., & Tait, K. (2004). Teaching communicative rejecting to children with severe disabilities. *American Journal of Speech-Language Pathology, 13,* 31–42.

Stillman, R., Alymer, J., & Vandivort, J. (1983). *The functions of signaling behaviors in profoundly impaired deaf-blind children and adolescents.* Paper presented at the 107th annual meeting of the American Association on Mental Deficiency, Dallas, TX.

Thiemann, K., & Goldstein, H. (2004). Effects of peer training and written text cueing on social communication of school-age children with pervasive developmental disorder. *Journal of Speech, Language, and Hearing Research, 47,* 126–145.

Tomasello, M., & Farrar, J. (1986). Joint attention and early language. *Child Development, 57,* 1454–1463.

Tomasello, M., & Todd, J. (1983). Joint attention and lexical acquisition style. *First Language, 4,* 197–212.

Warren, S.F., & Rogers-Warren, A. (1980). The assessment and facilitation of language generalization. In W. Sailor, B. Wilcox, & L. Brown (Eds.), *Methods of instruction for severely handicapped students* (pp. 1–58). Baltimore: Paul H. Brookes Publishing Co.

Watson, J. (1978). Perception of contingency as a determinant of social responsiveness. In S. Trotter & E. Thoman (Eds.), *Social responsiveness of infants* (pp. 33–64). New York: Johnson & Johnson.

Weiner, J. (2005). Peer-mediated conversational repair in students with moderate and severe disabilities. *Research and Practices for Persons with Severe Disabilities, 30,* 26–37.

Wetherby, A.M., Alexander, D.G., & Prizant, B.M. (1998). The ontogeny and role of repair strategies. In S.F. Warren & M.E. Fey (Series Eds.) & A. Wetherby, S.F. Warren, & J. Reichle (Vol. Eds.), *Communication and language intervention series: Vol. 7. Transitions in prelinguistic communication* (pp. 135–160). Baltimore: Paul H. Brookes Publishing Co.

Wetherby, A., & Prizant, B. (1989). The expression of communicative intent: Assessment guidelines. *Seminars in Speech and Language, 10,* 77–91.

Wetherby, A.M., & Prizant, B.M. (2003). *CSBS™ manual: Communication and Symbolic Behavior Scales™ manual—Normed edition.* Baltimore: Paul H. Brookes Publishing Co.

Wetherby, A., & Prutting, C. (1984). Profiles of communicative and cognitive-social abilities in austistic children. *Journal of Speech and Hearing Research, 27,* 364–377.

Whalen, C., & Schreibman, L. (2003). Joint attention training for children with autism using behavior modification procedures. *Journal of Child Psychology and Psychiatry and Allied Disciplines, 44,* 456–468.

Winborn, L., Wacker, D., Richman, D., Asmus, J., & Greir, D. (2002). Assessment of mand selection for functional communication training packages. *Journal of Applied Behavior Analysis, 35,* 295–298.

Building Blocks of a Beginning Communication System

Communicative Modes

Susan S. Johnston and Joanna Cosbey

▷ CHAPTER OVERVIEW

Acquiring effective and efficient speech-language and communication skills is a significant achievement. Some individuals, however, have disabilities that make acquiring functional speech-language skills difficult. Augmentative and alternative communication (AAC) is one way parents, teachers, and other caregivers can assist children in compensating for these difficulties. AAC refers to using aids or techniques that supplement or replace an individual's vocal or verbal communication skills (Mustonen, Locke, Reichle, Solbrack, & Lindgren, 1991). Individuals with severe disabilities who have significant communication limitations have benefitted from AAC (Johnston, McDonnell, Nelson, & Magnavito, 2003; Johnston, Nelson, Evans, & Palazolo, 2003; Marcus, Garfinkle, & Wolery, 2001; Mirenda & Erickson, 2000; Rowland & Schweigert, 2000). It is important to identify which communication modes will be used (e.g., vocal, graphic, gestural) when addressing the needs of AAC users. Developing an understanding of the issues involved in selecting communicative modes will enable interventionists to create an individualized communication system for the learner being served.

▷ CHAPTER OBJECTIVES

After studying this chapter, readers will be able to

- Identify available communication modes
- Understand the research related to graphic and gestural communication modes
- Understand the variables to consider when selecting an augmentative communication mode
- Recognize the impact of graphic and/or gestural communication on the use of spoken communication

▷ KEY TERMS

- ▸ aided communication mode
- ▸ complementary gesture
- ▸ declarative
- ▸ deictic gesture
- ▸ duplicated mode
- ▸ gestural communication

- ▸ graphic symbol
- ▸ illocutionary communicators
- ▸ imperative
- ▸ locutionary communicators

- ▸ mixed mode
- ▸ nonsymbolic gesture
- ▸ Picture Exchange Communication System (PECS)
- ▸ protodeclarative

▶ protoimperative
▶ representational
  gesture
▶ symbol

▶ symbolic gesture
▶ translucency
▶ transparency

▶ unaided communication
  mode
▶ visual matching

DIFFERENT COMMUNICATION MODES THAT ARE AVAILABLE TO AAC USERS

AAC includes **aided communication modes** as well as **unaided communication modes.** Aided communication modes use additional materials or equipment and can involve a continuum of devices ranging from low-tech systems (e.g., picture communication boards) to high-tech systems (e.g., speech-generating devices [SGDs]). Unaided communication modes refer to methods of communication that do not involve additional equipment (e.g., speech, facial expressions, body language, gestures, sign language, sign systems).

Both aided and unaided communication modes can include the use of symbols. A **symbol** is "something that stands for or represents something else" (Vanderheiden & Yoder, 1986, p. 15). The symbols used in aided and unaided communication modes differ in that aided communication modes utilize **graphic symbols,** whereas unaided communication modes utilize verbal or gestural symbols. It is important to note that the decision regarding which mode(s) of communication to use is based on specific factors related to the AAC user and his or her environment. It is necessary to have an understanding of the relevant research and collect individualized assessment information comparing the efficiency and effectiveness of different modes for any given learner in order to identify the most appropriate communication mode(s) for an individual.

Graphic Mode

Graphic symbols are two- or three-dimensional representations of objects and concepts. There are a variety of symbols within the graphic mode of communication, including traditional orthography, line drawings, photographs, product logos, parts of objects, miniature objects, and real objects. Figure 2.1 provides descriptions and examples of several types of graphic symbols that have been used by individuals with disabilities.

Lloyd and Karlan (1984) identified numerous considerations that should be addressed when selecting symbols, including the cognitive and linguistic demands that are associated with any particular system. A number of researchers have compared the relative differences in cognitive and linguistic demands between existing graphic symbol systems by examining the **translucency** and/or **transparency** of symbols (e.g., Clark, 1981; Hurlburt, Iwata, & Green, 1982; Luftig & Bersani, 1985; Mirenda & Locke, 1989; Mizuko, 1987; Mizuko & Reichle, 1989; Musselwhite & Ruscello, 1984; Sevcik & Romski, 1986).

- *Translucency* describes the degree to which a symbol is similar to its referent. Two tasks are frequently used to measure translucency:

  The first task involves an interval scale asking an individual to rate the strength of the relationship between a symbol and its referent. This task has been mostly used with typically developing participants.

  The second task involves assessing the ability of participants to learn and/or recall particular symbols. This task has been successfully implemented with young typically developing learners and with learners who have developmental disabilities.

- *Transparency* refers to the guessability of a particular symbol to an untrained viewer.

  Asking an individual to match a symbol to its referent (i.e., the actual object, action, or person) without prior inter-

Symbol	Description	Example
Real objects	Real objects are used as symbols.	An empty milk carton is used to represent a full carton of milk.
Partial objects	Parts of objects are used as symbols.	A gum wrapper is used to represent "gum."
Photographs	Photographs serve as symbols. (Mirenda and Locke [1989] found that color photographs were more easily recognized than black-and-white photographs.)	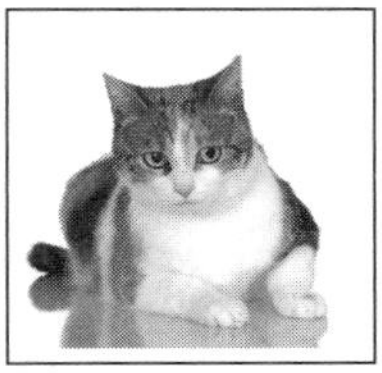
Product logos	Color reproductions of product logos and product packages are used as symbols. (The reproductions can be made and then reduced/enlarged as needed.)	A logo is used to represent a preferred beverage.
Nonidentical miniature objects	Miniature objects are used as symbols.	A doll's coat is used to represent "coat."
Picture Communication Symbols (PCSs)	Color and black-and-white drawings that were originally developed by Mayer-Johnson for use in low- or high-tech augmentative and alternative communication (AAC) systems are used as symbols. PCSs are often referred to as BoardMaker symbols because the symbols are available through the BoardMaker software program, which features more than 4,500 PCSs in 44 languages.	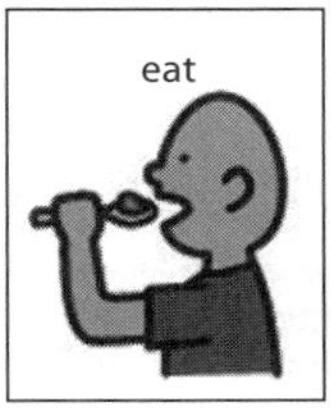 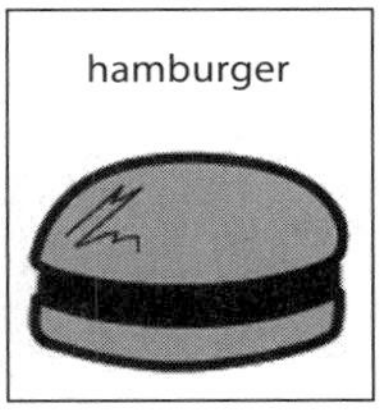 eat hamburger
Picsyms and DynaSyms	Line drawings that were originally developed by Carlson (1984) are used as symbols. These symbols are now a proprietary symbol set used on DynaVox speech-generating devices (SGDs) and are available for use with BoardMaker software.	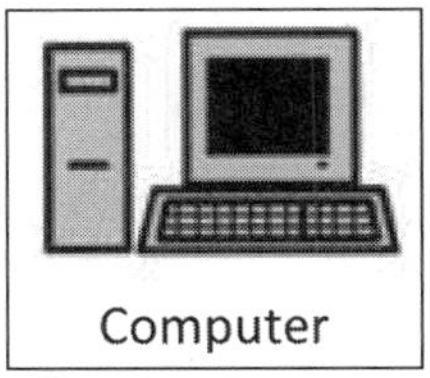 Computer
Pictograms	White line drawings on a black background are used as symbols. (May be useful for some individuals with visual impairments.)	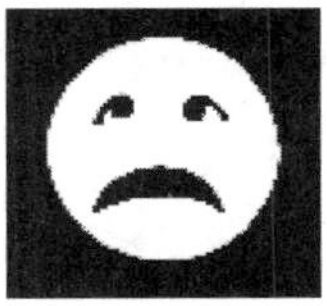 Sad
Rebus	Line-drawn pictures representing a sound or syllable are used as symbols.	A picture of a bee can be used to represent the verb be because both words sound the same.

Figure 2.1. Descriptions and examples of graphic symbol sets/systems that have been used with individuals with disabilities.

(continued)

Figure 2.1.   *(continued)*

Symbol	Description	Example
Blissymbols	A symbol set consisting of approximately 100 meaning-based shapes that can be combined into black and white line drawings to create messages.	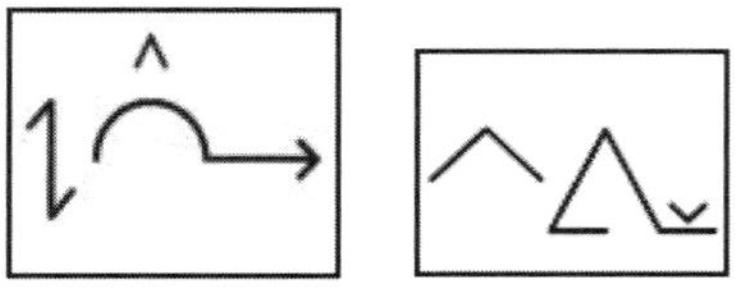 To Follow Shoes
Lexigrams	A 2-dimensional symbol set consisting of 9 design elements that can be used alone or in combination to produce 225 different symbols.	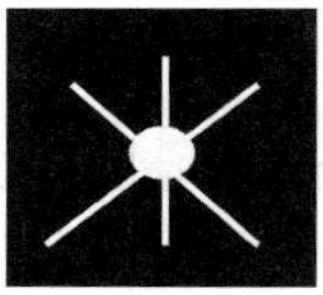 Hot Dog
Unity software with Minspeak symbols	A set of iconic picture symbols that provide a means for coding language in which combinations of multimeaning symbols result in specific messages. The symbols typically incorporate a variety of details to allow for multiple meanings to be assigned to each symbol. (Software that uses Minspeak concepts is available on SGDs manufactured by Prentke Romich.)	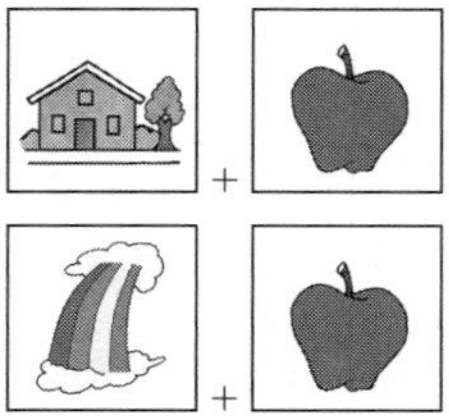 + = Grocery + = Red
Traditional orthography	Printed letters, words, or phrases. (Using traditional orthography is desirable if the AAC user can read because it enables the learner to create an unlimited number of messages.)	The printed word *dog* is used to represent "dog."

vention is the task most often used to measure transparency. This matching task has been implemented with individuals with and without disabilities.

Studies comparing symbol systems are in basic agreement on a general hierarchy that exists with regard to both the transparency and translucency of symbol systems. Although there are some inconsistencies in outcomes across investigations, the hierarchy starts with objects as most translucent/transparent, progressing to traditional orthography as the least translucent/transparent (see Table 2.1; Mirenda & Locke, 1989).

The general agreement across studies regarding a relative hierarchy is interesting considering that the symbols chosen from any particular system varied across investigators. For example, Luftig and Bersani's (1985) 20-item symbol set did not have any items in common with Clark's (1981) 15-item symbol set. It is important to note, however, that inconsistencies in the hierarchical relationship do exist. In addition, one must consider that the majority of studies have been completed with learners who do not have cognitive delays. Inconsistencies may be attributed to population differences (e.g., age of participants, disability) as well as the

Table 2.1.   Quasi-hierarchy for translucency and transparency of symbol system

Objects
Color photographs
Black-and-white photographs
Miniature objects
Black-and-white line drawings
Blissymbols
Traditional orthography

syntactic characteristics of the symbols across studies. Language comprehension (e.g., Romski & Sevcik, 1996), cultural factors (Huer, 2000), features of the referent (e.g., Stephenson, 2009a), color cues (e.g., Thistle & Wilkinson, 2009), symbol animation (Jagaroo & Wilkinson, 2008), and visual-perceptual skills (see Wilkinson, Carlin, & Thistle, 2008, for a review) are additional variables that may influence symbol translucency and transparency.

It is important for interventionists to exercise caution in attempting to use more arbitrary criteria in selecting graphic symbols while designing AAC systems for individuals with severe disabilities, given the differences across studies with regard to the relative translucency/transparency of symbol systems and research exploring additional variables that may affect graphic symbol use. Although symbol hierarchies offer some guidance to interventionists when choosing one type of graphic symbol over another, information collected informally (through interviews with caregivers as well as observation of the AAC user in his or her environment) and formally (through structured opportunities designed to assess the AAC user's existing skills/abilities) can be useful in selecting initial symbol representations.

Consider Casey, an 8-year-old child with severe cognitive delays. During an interview with Casey's parents, her teacher discovered that she was able to independently locate her favorite candy bar from an array of different candies when in the candy aisle of her local grocery store and at the counter of a gas station. This information suggests that Casey recognizes color logos that could potentially serve as symbols within an AAC system. Also, consider Adam, a 3-year-old boy with autism. While observing an interaction between Adam and his older sibling, interventionists noted that Adam identified various family members in a photograph album, which suggests that he recognizes color photographs that could potentially serve as symbols within an AAC system.

Information obtained through interviews and observation can be used to create hypotheses that can then be tested via structured opportunities. **Visual matching** is one commonly used assessment strategy that is particularly useful in working with individuals with severe disabilities. When conducting a visual matching assessment, the interventionist presents the AAC user with an object and then places two or more graphic symbols (e.g., photographs, line drawings) in front of the AAC user. The interventionist then asks the learner to match the object with its corresponding symbol. After conducting multiple trials with a variety of objects and symbols, the inteventionist is able to discern the AAC user's understanding of the relationship between a specific type of graphic symbol and its referent.

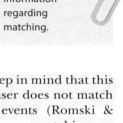

Chapter 8 provides additional information regarding matching.

It is important to keep in mind that this skill can be taught if a user does not match symbols to items and events (Romski & Sevcik, 1996). Furthermore, matching assessments can be implemented in a flexible manner based on the needs of the AAC user. For example, several sessions can be implemented to teach the relationship between a symbol and an object prior to assessing the individual's ability to demonstrate that skill (Beukelman & Mirenda, 2005). When implementing and interpreting the information obtained from a matching assessment

• Vary the placement of the symbols during the assessment in order to ensure that an AAC user is not engaging in a position bias response (i.e., making selections based on the location of the symbol in the array).

• Recognize that an AAC user's ability to identify the relationship between symbols (e.g., line drawings, traditional orthography) and their referents may change over time (e.g., through incidental learning, through systematic instruction), resulting in the need for ongoing assessment and attention.

- In addition to assessing the cognitive and linguistic demands across various symbol sets, the cognitive and linguistic demands for individuals within a given symbol set should also be examined. For example, Stephenson (2009b) found that verbal comprehension of the names of objects and pictures had an impact on individual results among participants with severe intellectual disabilities when examining the impact of color and outline shape on recognizing and using line drawings. Specifically, participants who scored highest on verbal comprehension tasks performed better on matching tasks with both pictures and objects as samples. Conversely, participants who scored lowest on verbal comprehension tasks did not perform as well on matching tasks.

- Preliminary research has revealed that individuals from different cultural/ethnic groups perceive graphic symbols differently. For example, Huer (2000) found that adults without disabilities from different cultural/ethnic communities assigned different translucency ratings to symbols. This suggests that graphic symbols should be selected in consultation with AAC users and their families, particularly when an AAC user's cultural/ethnic background differs from the interventionist's background.

Research suggests that individuals with a wide range of disabilities (developmental delay, cognitive delay, vision impairment, hearing impairment, autism, orthopedic impairment, seizure disorder) can learn to use graphic symbols. Furthermore, over time, AAC users can use more transparent and translucent symbol systems as a bridge to learning more abstract symbol systems (Rowland & Schweigert, 2000). Understanding the research regarding choosing graphic symbols along with understanding how to conduct within-learner comparative assessments of graphic symbols enables interventionists to make informed decisions regarding their use. This same understanding is important as it relates to **gestural communication** modes.

Gestural Mode

People use different types of gestures in their daily lives (e.g., nodding, pointing, waving). Gestures can vary in their form (involving the hands or arms, face, or whole body) and in their function (e.g., requesting, commenting, refusing), but they have one thing in common—they can be used for communication. Both children and adults use gestures to convey information not found in speech (Iverson & Goldin-Meadow, 2005), and research suggests that not only are gestures used to communicate information to listeners (Goodwyn, Acredolo, & Brown, 2000), but they also serve a function for the speakers by providing a means of expressing thoughts and facilitating problem solving (Iverson & Goldin-Meadow, 2005; Özçalişkan & Goldin-Meadow, 2005). Infants begin using gestures at a very early age (see Chapter 1). These gestures are nonintentional; that is, they are perlocutionary and are not used with the intent of communicating to other people (Iverson & Thal, 1998). These gestures may take different forms in an individual, including reaching toward a cup (without expecting someone to hand it to him or her), pointing at pictures in a book while reading alone (without commenting on the pictures or expecting someone to interact with him or her), or pushing something away. These earliest gestures generally appear in infants at approximately 6 months but can appear even earlier (Crais, Douglas, & Campbell, 2004).

Infants and children begin to use communicative gestures after these early, noncommunicative gestures emerge. Communicative gestures can be classified into two main types based on their function: those used to establish reference (**deictic** or **nonsymbolic**) and those used to represent something (**representational** or **symbolic**) (Bates, 1976; Goodwyn et al., 2000; Iverson & Thal, 1998). Both of these types of communicative gestures can be used in isolation by individuals who are not yet using spoken communication (**illocutionary communicators**) or can be combined with words by individu-

Table 2.2. Descriptions and examples of the various types of gestures used in communication

Gesture type and subtype	Description	Examples
Intentionality of gestures		
Nonintentional	Used during the perlocutionary stage of language development but are not intended to communicate meaning to others	Looking at a toy; pushing away a cup
Intentional	Used during the illocutionary and locutionary stages of language development and are intended to communicate meaning	Pointing at an object to draw another person's attention to it; waving good-bye
Function of gestures		
Deictic	Nonsymbolic gestures used to refer to objects or people present in the environment; they establish reference but do not carry any semantic content; interpretation of them depends heavily on context	Pointing at a book to show it to another person; showing an item to request help using it
• Imperative deictic gesture	A type of deictic gesture used to satisfy a need or want	Giving a shoe to someone as a request for help in putting it on
• Declarative deictic gesture	A type of deictic gesture used to establish joint attention	Pointing at a car to draw other people's attention to the car
Representational	Symbolic gestures that are used to refer to objects, people, or events; they both establish reference and carry semantic content and usually can be interpreted out of context	Waving good-bye; bringing a cup to one's mouth to request a drink
• Object related	A type of representational gesture that relates to specific objects, people, and so forth	Moving a finger back and forth by one's mouth to represent brushing teeth
• Conventional	A type of representational gesture that is more abstract and reflects culturally specific gestures to convey particular semantic content	Shrugging shoulders for "I don't know"
Relationship of gestures with verbal language		
Complementary	Gestures that are paired with words and convey the same meaning as the word	Pointing at a cat while saying, "Cat"; making a drinking motion while requesting a drink
Supplemental	Gestures that are paired with words and convey additional meaning	Pointing at a cat while saying, "Mine" to indicate who the cat belongs to; making a drinking motion while saying, "Orange soda" to request a specific drink

als who use spoken communication (**locutionary communicators**). See Table 2.2 for descriptions and examples of different types of gestures and how they are used.

Deictic, or nonsymbolic, gestures function to establish reference and include behaviors such as showing or giving an object to another person (form) to draw attention (function), reaching toward an object (form) to indicate a request (function), and pointing at an object (form) to refer to it (function). Deictic gestures can be further classified by function into **imperative** and **declarative** gestures (also called **protoimperative** and **protodeclarative** gestures for individuals who are not yet using spoken language). The same gesture (form) could be classified as imperative or declarative depending on the function. For example, if a child pointed at a dog in the park (form), then it would be considered imperative if the child was requesting to play with the dog (function) and declarative if the child was simply drawing an adult's attention to the presence of the dog (function). In addition, deictic gestures can be used alone by individuals who do not use spoken language or can be paired with spoken language to supplement or comple-

Table 2.3. Examples of the uses of various types of intentional communicative gestures across language development stages

Gesture type	Function	Possible gesture (and word) use at different language development stages		
			Locutionary	
		Illocutionary	Complementary	Supplementary
Deictic (imperative)	Request for something to eat	Pointing at kitchen cupboard	Pointing at kitchen cupboard and saying, "That."	Pointing at kitchen cupboard and saying, "Cereal."
Deictic (declarative)	Sharing excitement	Showing picture of self in a photograph album	Showing picture of self in a photograph album and saying, "Me."	Showing picture of self in a photograph album and saying, "Long time ago."
Representational (object related)	Request for help turning on music	Dancing	Dancing and saying, "Music on."	Dancing and saying, "I can't reach."
Representational (conventional)	Refusal	Shaking head when offered an item	Shaking head when offered an item and saying, "No."	Shaking head when offered an item and saying, "I'm allergic to that."

ment a spoken message (see Table 2.3 for examples of different uses of deictic gestures across language development stages).

Deictic gestures can only be interpreted within a specific context because their meanings can change depending on the specific referent. In other words, the *point* gesture, by itself, is meaningless. It is necessary to visually follow the direction of the point gesture to understand the meaning and identify the referent. This means that deictic gestures are relatively concrete because they can only be used to reference something that is currently present in the environment.

Representational gestures, as the name implies, are used to represent specific objects, concepts, places, and so forth and can be further classified into object-related gestures and conventional gestures (Iverson & Thal, 1998). Object-related gestures include actions such as making a drinking motion (with or without a cup) to refer to the act of drinking, sniffing to represent a flower, and moving a finger back and forth along teeth to represent brushing teeth (Goodwyn et al., 2000; Iverson & Thal, 1998). An example of a conventional gesture is nodding the head to indicate agreement. Representational gestures can be used alone or with other gestures by indi-

viduals who are not using spoken language or paired with spoken language to supplement or complement a message. See Table 2.3 for examples of different uses of representational gestures in different forms across language development stages. Representational gestures carry specific information and can generally be interpreted with consistency across contexts. In other words, the representational gesture *drink* can be reliably interpreted as *drink* regardless of where it takes place (e.g., home, school) and whether a cup or drink is present in the room at the time. Representational gestures, then, are used in a more abstract manner than deictic gestures, and the gestures themselves carry content.

How Do Gestures Develop?

As discussed in Chapter 1, developing gestures appears to precede developing spoken language, with gestures following a specific pattern of development that mirrors spoken language. Children appear to be able to use gestures expressively before they are able to understand them as communication (Iverson & Thal, 1998). For example, most 12-month-old children are able to point to objects to focus a communication partner's attention but are unable to follow a communication partner's point until several months later (Iverson & Thal, 1998). In addition, although children can use symbolic gestures around their first birthday, they do not consistently understand them until after their second birthday (Iverson & Thal, 1998).

When it comes to producing gestures, the earliest communicative gestures are deictic (nonsymbolic) gestures and generally appear between 9 and 12 months of age (Bates & Dick, 2002; Crais et al., 2004; Iverson & Goldin-Meadow, 2005; Iverson & Thal, 1998). Children usually begin by using *showing, giving,* and *reaching* gestures, followed by *pointing to comment* and *pointing to request*. At this time, most children also begin to use culturally specific gestural routines, such as waving good-bye. Symbolic gestures emerge after deictic gestures, at approximately 10–16 months of age (Bates & Dick, 2002; Crais et al., 2004; Goodwyn et al., 2000). The first symbolic gestures are concrete and often require the referent to be physically held by the child, such as an infant who moves a cup to his or her mouth in a drinking motion or brings a toy telephone to his or her ear. Gradually, these symbolic gestures become more abstract and less context bound, and children can generate the symbolic gesture regardless of whether the referent is present in the environment. This ability to use gestures in increasingly abstract ways continues to develop until children are preschool age (Goodwyn et al., 2000).

Children begin to pair their gestures with words early in the development of gestures. Children as young as 14–16 months of age begin to pair the two communication modes, primarily by using gestures to reinforce their spoken language (Crais et al., 2004; Iverson & Thal, 1998; Özçalişkan & Goldin-Meadow, 2005). For example, they will point at a shoe while simultaneously saying, "Shoe," which is called a **complementary gesture**. Some children at this age also start to use gestures to supplement their spoken language by conveying different content in the two communication modes, such as pointing at a shoe while simultane-

ously saying, "Mine," to indicate ownership of the shoe.

Children with severe developmental disabilities can be taught gestures concurrent with attempts at spoken language. Gestures need not be considered solely as a replacement for spoken language. Although most typically developing children rely extensively on gestures during the first 18 months of life, they vary in their preference for the verbal versus gestural mode of communication (Iverson, Capirci, & Caselli, 1994; Iverson & Thal, 1998). Iverson et al. found that 75% of the 16-month-old children in their study demonstrated a preference for the use of gestures over spoken communication, even though only 50% of the children in the study had more gestures than words in their vocabulary.

In general, gestures and words operate as a coordinated communication system for typically developing children after approximately 1 year of age, with little overlap in vocabulary in the two modes. If a child has the ability to use a word to refer to an object or event, then it is unlikely that he or she will have a consistent gesture to represent the same thing. In fact, Iverson et al. (1994) found the degree of overlap between spoken language vocabulary and gestural vocabulary to be less than 10%. Using symbolic gestures tends to decrease as children develop their spoken language vocabularies (Iverson et al., 1994; Iverson & Thal, 1998; Namy, Acredolo, & Goodwyn, 2000), with older children relying more on their spoken language and using deictic gestures than on using symbolic gestures.

What Can the Use of Gestures by Typically Developing Children Say About the Relationship Between Gestures and Spoken Language?

The change in gesture use as children develop spoken language raises the question of the nature of the relationship between the two. Insight into the nature of this relationship is especially relevant for interventionists working with individuals with severe cognitive disabilities because interventions need to be designed to target an individual's specific strengths and needs. Understanding how gestures relate to spoken language can provide interventionists with guidance regarding the potential impact of teaching an individual to use gestural language as well as determining the appropriateness of teaching spoken language for an individual.

Although individuals with developmental disabilities may use and develop gestures differently than typically developing children, the information about the relationship between gestures and spoken language can be used as a foundation to better recognize appropriate interventions for individuals with disabilities. Examining bilingual and monolingual children leads to a better understanding about how the two main types of gestures (deictic and representational) relate to spoken language for typically developing children.

There are three theories about the relationship between gestures and spoken language:

1. Gestures are used to substitute for spoken language until verbal skills develop.

2. Both gesture and spoken language development are related to overall cognitive development more than they are related to each other.

3. The use of gestures is closely linked to developmental changes in spoken language itself (Mayberry & Nicoladis, 2000).

Research on young bilingual children provides some insight into this relationship. Researchers can track a child's use of gestures in each language to examine the relationship between language and gestures because language development is typically uneven across the two languages in bilingual children. Each theory regarding these relationships may lead to different outcomes (Mayberry & Nicoladis, 2000). For example, if gestures are used simply as a substitute for spoken language, then bilingual children would be expected to use more gestures in their less developed language to compensate for the lack of spoken language skills. If

gestures and spoken language are related to the same underlying cognitive development, then bilingual children's use of gestures should be virtually identical in both languages. Finally, if the use of gestures is closely related to the development of spoken language itself, then it would be expected that bilingual children would use gestures differently when speaking in each language (i.e., would demonstrate a higher level of gesture development in their more developed spoken language). Knowing this information is essential when developing assessments and interventions to promote intentional communication for individuals with disabilities because an intervention based on the assumption that gestures are a substitute for spoken language might look different from an intervention based on the assumption that both gestures and spoken language are related to underlying cognitive development.

Although there is little research on very young bilingual children (i.e., younger than age 2) using symbolic gestures, the research that has been done on bilingual preschoolers (2–5 years) suggests that the third theory may be the most accurate, at least in relationship to developing symbolic gestures (Mayberry & Nicoladis, 2000; Nicoladis, 2002). By tracking the spoken language and gesture use of children who were bilingual in English and French, researchers found that the children used symbolic gestures in their more developed language before they used them in their less developed language (i.e., if the child was more proficient in French than in English, then he or she was observed to use symbolic gestures when speaking in French before he or she used them while speaking in English). The children in these studies were not observed using symbolic gestures to compensate in their less developed language. This indicates that the ability of preschool-age bilingual children to use gestures in conjunction with speech is strongly related to language development itself, not to general cognitive development, and not simply as a compensatory strategy, suggesting that when teaching gestures to an individual with a developmental disability, it may be more appropriate to link the gestures taught to his or her overall level of language development, rather than to his or her cognitive skill level.

Do Children with Disabilities Use Gestures Differently than Typically Developing Children?

Typically developing children appear to use gestures before they are able to understand them, which provides rich information regarding the general time line and sequence of developing expressive and receptive gestural communication for children who are typically developing. Additional information about developing gestures and the relationship between gestures and spoken language, however, can be found by examining how gestures are used by children with a variety of disabilities, including sensory impairments, autism spectrum disorder (ASD), and cognitive impairments (e.g., Down syndrome, Williams syndrome).

How Do Children with Sensory Impairments Use Gestures? Looking at how children who are deaf or hard of hearing use gestures, as well as looking at hearing children who are intensively exposed to sign systems (because of deaf parents), can determine if there is a natural advantage to a gestural mode of communication (i.e., if children find it easier to use gestures than spoken language). Examining the gesture use of children who are blind can determine if gestures are learned through modeling from adults or if there is some internal process for gesture use that develops independent of the input that a child receives.

Many of the early studies on children who are exposed to American Sign Language suggested that they reach certain vocabulary milestones 1–2 months earlier than children exposed to spoken language alone. The way these authors defined signs and spoken words, however, may lead to some incorrect conclusions (see Volterra & Iverson, 1995). For example, spoken words were only considered true words if they were spoken spontaneously. Signs, however, were included in the analyses even if they were imitated following an adult model (Bonvillian & Folven, 1987, as cited by Volterra & Iverson, 1995). In addition, studies involving children who were simultaneously learning sign and spoken languages often counted spontaneous representational gestures as signs, which would naturally increase the number of signs that children produce because these same gestures cannot ever be counted as words. After accounting for these methodological problems, it was concluded that there is not an inherent advantage for sign language over spoken language in terms of age of symbol acquisition or the rate or size of vocabulary. Instead, it appears that gestures seem to represent a useful mode of communication for most children, particularly early on in their language development, and that the early use of communicative gestures is similar for children exposed to spoken language and those exposed to sign language (Volterra & Iverson, 1995).

Children who are blind are not able to use traditional gestures (pointing, nodding, waving) to help them understand what their communication partners are talking about (i.e., receptively). How, then, do children who are blind develop and use gestures? A study of the use of gestures by toddlers who were blind and sighted (ages 14–28 months) provided interesting insight (Iverson, Tencer, Lany, & Goldin-Meadow, 2000). Children who were blind and children who were sighted used the same types of gestures (deictic and representational), although the children who were blind used fewer gestures than their sighted peers. The children who were blind produced a higher proportion of conventional gestures than their peers, including gestures such as shaking their heads to indicate "no" and waving good-bye. The other difference between the two groups was in the referent of their gestures. As would be expected, the children who were blind were less likely to use gestures to refer to distant items than their peers.

Iverson and Goldin-Meadow (1997) suggested that children who are blind from birth use gestures in much the same way as their sighted peers. They studied a small group of school-age children (10–12 years) and found that the blind and sighted children used gestures to convey the same content, and the form of gestures (hand shape and movement patterns) used by children who were blind was similar to the form of gestures produced by their sighted peers. The primary difference in gesture use was that the children who were blind tended not to point at distant objects, which is the same outcome as the study by Iverson et al. (2000). This was most evident during a task that required the children to give directions on how to navigate within an environment. The sighted children tended to view the environment as a whole and used pointing gestures to supplement their spoken directions ("Go that way" with a *point* gesture). Not surprising, the children who were blind tended to break the environment into smaller parts and use landmarks, rather than pointing gestures, to provide directions. The sighted children who gave spoken directions in a similar manner as the children who were blind (i.e., breaking the environment into parts rather than viewing the environment as a whole) were less likely to use pointing gestures; thus, their gesture use resembled that of their blind peers. In addition, when the children who were blind did refer to the environment as a whole, they also tended to point. This led the researchers to suggest that the difference in use between the two groups may be more related to a way of conceptualizing the environment (whole versus part) than to being blind versus sighted and supports the idea that gestures and spoken language work together as a single communication system, even for children who are not exposed to visual models for gesture use.

The information about how children who are deaf or hard of hearing and blind learn and use gestures provides valuable information to use when developing interventions for individuals with developmental disabilities. It reinforces the link between gestures and language development, illustrating that the use of gestures is a natural step in learning language. Although there does not appear to be an advantage for ges-

tural communication over spoken language, gestures do appear to serve an important communicative function for children with and without disabilities. This suggests that interventions developed for individuals with developmental disabilities should include systematic ways to model and promote gestural development using a variety of forms for a variety of functions.

How Do Children with Developmental Delays and Intellectual Disabilities Use Gestures?   Children with developmental delays and intellectual disabilities with delayed spoken language skills may also demonstrate difficulty with using communicative gestures. Brady, Marquis, Fleming, and McLean (2004) found that 3- to 6-year-olds with developmental delays had problems using gestures. The children who demonstrated a higher level of overall development were also the children who were more likely to use gestures, such as pointing. The authors suggested that a child's ability to point at items that are at a distance is a strong predictor of future expressive language development.

Children with Down syndrome develop gestures in much the same way as typically developing children (Chan & Iacono, 2001; see Capone & McGregor, 2004, for discussion), although they do demonstrate a relative impairment in using gestures to request assistance compared with using requesting gestures during social routines (e.g., continuation of tickling; Fidler, Philofsky, Hepburn, & Rogers, 2005). Chan and Iacono (2001) found that young children with Down syndrome (17- to 19-month-olds) used gestures as forms of intentional communication, and using gestures preceded their use of spoken language. The children with Down syndrome used gestures for a variety of purposes, including commenting, requesting, and naming objects. Chan and Iacono also found that the children with Down syndrome used a gestural mode of communication to compensate for difficulties with spoken language that were related to issues such as difficulty making the sounds required for speaking. Caselli and colleagues' (1998) research suggested that children with Down syndrome may end up developing gestural communication beyond what would be expected, given their production and comprehension of spoken language. Children with Down syndrome produced more symbolic gestures and engaged in more pretending than typically developing children after reaching a mental age of approximately 17–18 months. They reasoned that children with Down syndrome have had a longer time to be exposed to gestural communication because of their increased chronological age and essentially become specialists in gestural communication.

Iverson, Longobardi, and Caselli (2003) suggested that this apparent gestural advantage may be a manifestation of the research methods used but acknowledged the possibility that older toddlers and preschool-age children with Down syndrome may demonstrate gestural development that does not parallel that of their typically developing peers. It is important to remember that these studies do not utilize all components of a formal sign language.

Research addressing children with Down syndrome may not apply to the wider group of children with intellectual disabilities because individuals with intellectual disabilities encompass a wide variety of strengths and weaknesses. For example, children with Williams syndrome demonstrate significantly more difficulty with the use of pointing gestures (both for requesting objects and for initiating joint attention) than their typically developing peers and children with Down syndrome (Laing et al., 2002; Singer Harris, Bellugi, Bates, Jones, & Rossen, 1997). This emphasizes the need for more research on the use of gestures by children with a variety of intellectual disabilities and the need for educators and other professionals to examine the strengths and needs of their particular students when developing intervention plans.

How Do Children with Autism Spectrum Disorder Use Gestures?

A number of investigators have examined gestural use among children with ASD. Although children with ASD demonstrate difficulty with using and understanding gestures in general, they have more difficulty using gestures for social purposes (e.g., initiating joint attention) than for imperative purposes (e.g., requesting objects or assistance). Specifically, 12- and 18-month-old infants with ASD use pointing and showing gestures less than their typically developing peers, and they have more difficulty using gestures for social purposes (Mitchell et al., 2006; Osterling & Dawson, 1994). Osterling and Dawson conducted a retrospective study of gestures of children later diagnosed with autism. They examined home videos of the first birthday parties of children later diagnosed with autism and children who were typically developing. In addition to differences in behaviors such as eye contact, Osterling and Dawson found that the 12-month-olds later diagnosed with ASD used few gestures to initiate joint attention, including pointing and showing gestures, when compared with their peers. Mitchell et al. used a different methodology to see if the use of gestures (and other communicative behaviors) could be used to predict ASD in children. They collected data at 12 and 18 months of age on the gesture use of children who were at higher risk for ASD (based on having a sibling already diagnosed with ASD) and those who were at low risk for ASD. They then analyzed the results based on the children's status at 24 months of age (by 24 months, some of the children who were at high risk had received a diagnosis of ASD, but none of the children who were at low risk had). They found that the children with an early ASD diagnosis used significantly fewer gestures during social routines at both 12 months and 18 months than did either group of children who did not receive a later diagnosis of ASD. This finding has been supported by many other research studies, with the overall finding that children with ASD have impaired use of gestures, particularly showing, pointing, and waving gestures that are used for social communication purposes such as initiating joint attention (Charman, Drew, Baird, & Baird, 2003; see Bruinsma, Koegel, & Koegel, 2004, for a review). In addition to the differences in using gestures, a prospective study of children later diagnosed with ASD conducted by Landa, Holman, and Garrett-Mayer (2007) found that these children had a significantly smaller gestural vocabulary than their peers (children who were typically developing or who later demonstrated features similar to ASD but who did not meet diagnostic criteria for ASD). These differences were evident as early as 14 months of age. Children with ASD were further divided into two groups: those who received an early diagnosis of ASD (14 months) and those who received a later diagnosis (after 14 months). They found that the children who received the later diagnosis of ASD demonstrated a decrease in their gesture vocabulary between the ages of 14 and 24 months, suggesting some children with ASD may experience regression in their ability to use communicative gestures.

In addition to this information about the gestural production among children with ASD, there has been a significant amount of research examining gestural comprehension. As previously mentioned, typically developing children begin to understand gestures soon after their first birthday (Iverson & Thal, 1998). Limited gestural comprehension, particularly in responding to bids for joint attention, may be an important early indicator of autism for children who are not yet diagnosed (Dawson et al., 2004; Landa et al., 2007; Presmanes, Walden, Stone, & Yoder, 2007; Toth, Munson, Meltzoff, & Dawson, 2006). Much of the research addressing the responsiveness of children with ASD to bids for joint attention has used prompts that range from providing limited cues (silent eye gaze or eye gaze and a gasping sound) to more explicit cues (eye gaze, point, and spoken instructions) in an attempt to direct the children's attention. Most investigations have used redundant cues, such as gaining a child's attention and then looking and pointing at a target (Dawson et al., 2004; Landa et al., 2007; Sullivan et al., 2007). These researchers have found that 14-month-old children who were later diagnosed with

ASD responded to these gestures at the same level as their peers who were not later diagnosed with ASD (Landa et al., 2007; Sullivan et al., 2007), but there were some early indications that they struggled with these tasks (Sullivan et al., 2007). By the age of 24 months, children who were later diagnosed with ASD had significantly more difficulty with these tasks than their peers, meaning that they were not able to consistently and accurately establish joint attention initiated by another person (Dawson et al., 2004; Landa et al., 2007; Sullivan et al., 2007). There are two main limitations to these studies: 1) generally, experiments have occurred in relatively controlled environments with few distractions, and 2) experimenters gained the child's attention prior to attempting to elicit a response to the joint attention task (Dawson et al., 2004; Landa et al., 2007; Sullivan et al., 2007). Features of experimental contexts may mask some of the difficulties with responding to joint attention tasks that children with ASD may experience in natural situations (Presmanes et al., 2007). To address these concerns, Presmanes et al. measured the ability of siblings of children with ASD and siblings of typically developing children to respond to joint attention bids in a busy environment (with a variety of engaging toys present) without first gaining the child's attention. They also measured the children's responses to a variety of different prompts, ranging from silent eye gaze to a combination of eye gaze, pointing, and spoken prompts. Although virtually all children performed better on tasks with more explicit cues, there was a striking difference between the response patterns of the siblings of children with ASD and the siblings of children who were typically developing. The siblings of children with ASD had difficulty understanding and following moderately explicit cues (eye gaze paired with the verbal directive "look") when compared with the performance of their peers. This difference has not been found by other researchers but may be linked to the children's ability to respond correctly to bids for joint attention without first establishing eye contact with the examiner (Presmanes et al., 2007). Although researchers have found some slightly different patterns of responses to gestures by children who are deemed to be at risk for ASD and those later diagnosed with ASD, a consistent pattern across the research is that children with ASD have difficulty comprehending gestures, particularly those gestures that serve a more social function related to establishing joint attention, and these differences can be seen at an early age.

WHEN SHOULD GRAPHIC AND/OR GESTURAL MODES OF COMMUNICATION BE TAUGHT?

A thorough understanding of graphic and gestural communication modes enables interventionists to recognize the relative advantages and disadvantages of each. It is important to note that decisions regarding which mode(s) of communication should be used is based on specific factors related to the AAC user and his or her environment. Table 2.4 provides examples of AAC users and environmental features and implications.

All communication modes that can be functional for an individual learner should be used, given the wide array of variables that may influence the choice of mode of communication for a specific AAC user in a specific environment. Verbal, gestural, and graphic communication modes can be used in different combinations. For example, a learner can be taught to simultaneously use two or more modes, mix two or more communication modes, and/or duplicate communication modes.

Using a natural gesture with existing spoken language abilities is an example of the simultaneous use of two or more communication modes. Consider Anna, a 5-year-old girl with cerebral palsy who emits a spoken approximation of the word *eat* while simultaneously emitting a gesture for *eat* by bringing her hand toward her mouth. A potential benefit of a simultaneous mode of communication is that it can help a communication partner comprehend a message if one or more communication modes emitted by a learner are unclear. Furthermore, some researchers have found that teaching the same vocabulary in two different modes (e.g.,

Table 2.4.   "If . . . then" recommendations regarding communication modes

If	Then
Communication partners do not know sign language	Consider graphic modes and/or gestures that may be more universally understood
An augmentative and alternative communication (AAC) user has significant motor difficulties	Consider graphic modes because one motor movement (e.g., point, switch activation, eye gaze) can be used to access multiple symbols
An AAC user has difficulty memorizing or recalling symbols	Consider graphic modes because the symbol is constantly displayed
Portability of the AAC system is critical	Consider gestural modes that do not require the use of any additional materials/equipment
Immediate communication is critical	Consider gestural modes because the AAC user does not need to "prepare" for communication (e.g., turn on a device, find a page/symbol on a communication board)
An AAC user is unable to imitate verbal language	Consider gestural and/or graphic modes that can be prompted and do not require imitation skills
An AAC user's existing gestures are unconventional or difficult to interpret	Consider pairing or replacing the gestures with a mode that is more easily understood
An AAC user uses natural gestures that are easily interpreted by strangers	Continue to reinforce the use of those gestures
An AAC user needs to obtain the attention of a communication partner who is not in close proximity	Consider a mode of communication that will solicit the partner's attention, such as a natural gesture (e.g., raising his or her hand) or a system that provides voice output (e.g., a speech-generating device)

vocal, gestural) is more effective in establishing initial repertoires of expressive and receptive communication skills than when teaching in only one mode (e.g., Barrera, Lobato-Barrera, & Sulzer-Azaroff, 1980). Carr, Binkoff, Kologinsky, and Eddy (1978) noted, however, that when vocal and gestural modes were combined during instruction, young children with autism were more likely to attend to the gestural component than to the vocal component. Thus, it is critical for interventionists to carefully attend to the impact of simultaneous mode intervention strategies on a learner's communication skills in order to ensure that intervention outcomes are meeting the needs of both the learner and his or her communication partners.

Communicating some vocabulary using gestures while communicating other vocabulary using graphic symbols is an example of the **mixed mode** of communication. Consider Manuel, an 18-year-old with severe cognitive disabilities who is able to use gestures to greet customers as they enter a store (e.g., wave his hand "hi" and smile), but he needs a more explicit way of communicating what he would like to eat during his break (e.g., product logos representing an array of preferred candy bars). A potential benefit of the mixed mode of communication is that it allows a learner to use the most efficient and effective communicative behavior for a given environment. Advocates of mixed communication modes assert that 1) the use of a mixed mode allows learners and interventionists to maximize the relative advantages of gestural and graphic communication modes, and 2) vocabulary can still be represented in both graphic and gestural communication modes at a later date, if needed (Mustonen et al., 1991).

The **duplicated mode** of communication involves teaching individuals to represent the same vocabulary in both graphic and gestural modes. Consider Ben, an 8-year-old boy with severe disabilities. He uses a gestural mode (i.e., pointing to the swing set on the playground) to comment about his favorite activity during recess, but he uses a graphic mode (i.e., touching a symbol representing "swings") to make the same comment when interacting with family members during dinnertime at home. A potential benefit of the duplicated mode of communication is that a learner has more than one way to express him- or herself and can choose the most appropriate mode of communication based on the communicative environment. Mustonen et al. (1991) noted that introducing a duplicated mode of communication often occurs sequentially. For example, a learner who communicates primarily in sign language in his or her early childhood special education setting (where the special education teachers are fluent in sign language) may need to duplicate his or her skills by learning the same vocabulary in the graphic mode when he or she moves into a kindergarten class (where the teachers and peers do not know sign language).

Understanding research related to graphic and gestural modes is critical when meeting the needs of AAC users with severe disabilities. When educators and parents are developing intervention targets for children with communication difficulties, however, there is often discussion about whether it is appropriate to introduce an alternative mode of communication (e.g., gestures, graphic symbols) or if it would be more appropriate to focus solely on spoken language development. It is necessary to examine the impact of the various communicative modes on each other in order to make informed decisions about the most appropriate course of action. The following sections discuss the impact of graphic and gestural modes on spoken language development to help guide teams in developing educational programs.

If a Student Is Taught to Use Gestures or Signs, Will He or She Learn to Talk?

Parents and teachers are often reluctant to teach a child gestures or signing out of fear that he or she will then become so comfortable and dependent on the gestural mode of communication that he or she will not learn to talk. Most of the research, however, suggests that gestural and spoken language develop together as a single communication system, with gestural communication acting as a transition or a "bridge" to spoken language (e.g., Goodwyn et al., 2000; Iverson & Goldin-Meadow, 2005; Iverson & Thal, 1998). Research has not found that using gestural communication or teaching sign language to children who have difficulty with spoken language is detrimental to their speech development. In fact, Goodwyn et al. suggested that using symbolic gestures may actually increase spoken language skills, including vocabulary. Other studies have suggested that children who are systematically trained to use gestures demonstrate earlier vocabulary development and make the transition to two-word phrases faster than children who are not encouraged to use gestures (Goodwyn & Acredelo, 1998).

Millar, Light, and Schlosser (2006) conducted a systematic review of the literature related to the impact of alternative communication modes (e.g., gestural, graphic) on spoken language. Their review focused on research involving individuals with developmental disabilities and isolated the studies with the strongest methodology to help identify the impact of alternative communication modes on spoken language. They reported that 13 of the 15 participants involved in the studies related to the impact of gestural communication demonstrated increases in their speech production. According to Millar et al., the other two participants demonstrated no change in their use of spoken language during the time that they were taught to use gestural communication, so none of the participants demonstrated a loss of spoken language ability during their participation in the research studies. Although this research alone is not adequate to say conclusively that introducing gestural communication will not affect spoken language development, the evidence does suggest that gestural communication likely will not hinder spoken language development, and may, in fact, promote it (Millar et al., 2006).

What Does the Research Say?
Gestural Communication and Speech

More than 85% of participants demonstrated an increase in their verbal language while being taught to use gestural communication in studies examining the impact of gestural communication on verbal language development (Millar et al., 2006).

The presentation of simultaneous sign and speech, as in total/simultaneous communication, has been demonstrated to enhance speech among people with severe disabilities. Total/simultaneous communication involves the communication partner simultaneously speaking and signing to the learner with a developmental disability (Carr, 1979) and is often successful in establishing sign production among intervention recipients (e.g., Barrera et al., 1980; Carr & Dores, 1981; Konstantareas, Oxman, & Webster, 1977; Kouri, 1988, 1989). It also results in comprehension of spoken language for some learners (e.g., Carr & Dores, 1981). Total/simultaneous communication is also associated with improvements in speech production (e.g., Barrera et al., 1980; Barrera & Sulzer-Azaroff, 1983; Barrett & Sisson, 1987; Carbone et al., 2006; Kouri, 1988, 1989; Sisson & Barrett, 1984; Tincani, 2004; Wells, 1981).

Teaching sign through total/simultaneous communication has been demonstrated to positively affect speech production. For example, Kouri (1988, 1989) found improvements in speech production following use of a simultaneous communication approach to teach sign language to young children (2–4 years) with delays and diagnoses of autism, Down syndrome, or Klinefelter's syndrome.

Barrera and Sulzer-Azaroff (1983) found total communication was more successful than oral training alone in teaching expressive vocal labels to three children with autism (6–9 years) who showed echolalia and little functional speech. Sisson and Barrett (1984) even found this when teaching multiword sentences. Carbone et al. (2006) compared a total communication approach (providing models of both sign and vocalization to prompt a response) with vocal-only instruction (providing only a verbal model to prompt a response) to teach a 7-year-old child with autism to label an item in response to the question "What is it?" The participant already imitated and used vocalizations to request items, though she had acquired a limited number of labels over a long period of intervention. The participant showed more use of spoken labels in the total communication condition than vocal-only instruction and,

(continued)

in fact, required fewer trials to reach criterion. Of interest, Wells (1981) found greater improvement in articulation with a total communication approach than more traditional vocal imitation and oral motor training for three adult women with intellectual disabilities (18–26 years).

There is variability in the effect of total/simultaneous communication on participant outcomes for speech production (e.g., Kouri, 1988). Specifically, the effect of total/simultaneous communication on speech production is influenced by learner verbal imitation ability (Carr, 1979; Clarke, Remington, & Light, 1986, 1988; Layton, 1988). For example, Yoder and Layton (1988) compared speech, sign, alternating speech and sign, and the simultaneous presentation of speech and sign to teach comprehension and productive use of new vocabulary to children with autism. They concluded that, except for the sign-only intervention, the interventions were associated with increases in speech production, although reanalysis did not indicate such differences among the conditions (Schlosser & Wendt, 2008). Participants' increases in spontaneous speech were highly related to existing verbal imitation abilities, however.

There are several reasons why children may use gestural communication over spoken communication early in their development, and these theories provide information on some of the reasons why gestural communication may facilitate the development of spoken language. First, gestures may be easier to remember and produce than spoken language for many children. Developmentally, children appear "ready" to use their hands, faces, and bodies to gesture before they have the coordination to produce the complex sounds required for speech (Iverson & Goldin-Meadow, 2005; Iverson & Thal, 1998; Özçalışkan & Goldin-Meadow, 2005). Some have hypothesized that gestures are easier to remember than words, particularly when the gesture is linked to the action or characteristics of the object it represents (e.g., a throwing motion to represent "ball"; Iverson & Goldin-Meadow, 2005; Özçalışkan & Goldin-Meadow, 2005). Second, gestures appear to support successful communication. Although the exact mechanisms are unknown, gestures may facilitate the recall of spoken language because researchers have

found that adults are able to more easily recall words if they are gesturing while they are talking than if they are not (see Özçalışkan & Goldin-Meadow, 2005). Third, communication partners appear to be more responsive to children who are using symbolic communication than those who are not, so children who use early symbolic gestures generally receive more spoken language input from their caregivers than those who do not (Goodwyn et al., 2000). In addition, the ability to communicate a topic of interest allows for the caregiver to more clearly identify objects and activities that capture the child's interest, which allows for more child-led interactions and learning opportunities (Goodwyn et al., 2000). Finally, using symbolic gestures may help children learn the nature of symbolism and the concept of symbolic communication (Goodwyn et al., 2000; Iverson & Thal, 1998). Caregivers are able to scaffold the child's learning and help teach the child the importance of communication and how to use symbols.

In addition, there is also evidence that children will not get "stuck" using the gestural mode of communication once their spoken language abilities develop. Studies of children with and without disabilities have found that gestures support spoken language and that children make the transition from using symbolic gestures to the spoken word once they have learned to produce the spoken word (Chan & Iacono, 2001; Iverson & Thal, 1998). This information should provide reassurance to parents and educators who are considering teaching the use of gestural communication. It is important, however, to ask whether these same patterns hold true for children exposed to a graphic mode.

If an Individual Is Taught to Use a Graphic Mode, Will He or She Learn to Talk?

Concerns and reservations are often voiced by parents, teachers, and caregivers about introducing a graphic mode of communication and speech. They fear that the individual may rely so heavily on the graphic communication that he or she will never develop spoken language skills (see Millar et al., 2006, for discussion). Much like the research on gestural communication modes, however, the research on graphic modes suggests that the alternative mode may actually facilitate spoken language. The systematic review of the literature conducted by Millar et al. discussed earlier also examined the impact of graphic communication modes on spoken language. They only identified one research study related to the use of graphic communication that met their criteria for strong methodology. That study found that all three participants demonstrated increases in their spoken language use (Charlop-Christy et al., 2002, as cited by Millar et al., 2006). Because of the limited number of participants in this analysis, it is useful to look at all of the studies that Millar et al. identified, although these studies had methodological limitations that make it somewhat harder to make firm conclusions about the impact of graphic communication on spoken language development. They identified nine research studies (spanning from 1998 to 2003) that included information on the spoken language development of individuals taught to use graphic communication modes and found that the majority of the participants demonstrated increases in their spoken language (80%), with 8% demonstrating no change, and 12% demonstrating decreases (Millar et al., 2006).

Schlosser and Wendt (2008) conducted a similar review of AAC and speech that focused on learners with autism. They analyzed mean percentage of nonoverlapping data (PND) across the single-subject design studies reviewed. PND involves calculating the highest baseline data point and the percentage of data points in intervention that exceed this. Criteria to evaluate PND are set so that a PND more than 90% would indicate an effective intervention; 70%–90% a fairly effective intervention; 50%–70% a questionable intervention; and less than 50% an ineffective intervention (Scruggs, Mastropieri, & Castro, 1987; Scruggs, Mastropieri, Cook, & Escobar, 1986). Schlosser and Wendt's analysis revealed that, although

there were gains in speech, mean PND for many of the studies was less than 50% (although there was substantial variability), indicating a less than robust effect. Both Millar et al. (2006) and Schlosser and Wendt concluded that the fear that introducing AAC will impede speech production was not founded. Their reviews also suggested that evaluating the impact of AAC on speech production requires examining differences in learner characteristics as well as mode.

The **Picture Exchange Communication System** (**PECS**; Bondy & Frost, 1994) is one application of AAC that has been shown to increase speech production in learners with severe disabilities. The PECS involves the learner selecting drawings and sequencing them on a sentence strip that the learner then hands to his or her partner in a communicative exchange. With the PECS, the communication partner speaks the corresponding words. This modeling may be one explanation for increases in speech production associated with AAC. Bondy and Frost conducted follow-up observations of children 5 years or younger who used the PECS for more than 1 year. Although many continued to experience language delays, results revealed that 59% of the children developed independent speech and discontinued using the PECS as their sole mode of communication. Furthermore, an additional 30% of the children spoke while using the PECS. An increase in spoken language was also noted by Schwartz, Garfinkle, and Bauer (1998), whose research revealed a positive correlation between the use of the PECS and the development of speech with preschool-age children with communication delays/disorders. The PECS is discussed in more detail in Chapter 11.

What Does the Research Say?

**Graphic Communication
Systems and Speech Production**

More than 85% of the participants demonstrated an increase or no change in their verbal language while being

(continued)

taught to use graphic communication modes in studies examining the impact of graphic communication modes on verbal language development (Millar et al., 2006).

Johnston, Nelson, Evans, and Palazolo (2003) taught three preschoolers with ASDs to use a graphic symbol for "Can I play?" to initiate joining a play activity. The naturalistic intervention involved modeling use of the symbol in conjunction with the spoken request when learners expressed interest in an activity (by looking at it). Following intervention, two participants largely used both the graphic symbol and spoken language, and the third participant largely used speech to join play activities.

Garrison-Harrell, Kamps, and Kravits (1997) examined the introduction of a communication board (consisting of icons, words, and phrases) to three children (6–7 years) with autism in the context of creating and training peer networks. Not only did the participants use the AAC system, but the two participants who were verbal prior to the study (speaking in two- to four-word utterances, though there were problems with intelligibility) also showed increases in verbal communication (in contrast to the one participant who emitted only simple sounds when prompted prior to intervention). All three demonstrated decreases in their unintelligible speech.

There have been several reports of increases in speech production associated with the PECS (Bondy & Frost, 1994; Carr & Felce, 2007; Charlop-Christy, Carpenter, Le, LeBlanc, & Kellet, 2002; Ganz & Simpson, 2004; Schwartz et al., 1998; Tincani, 2004; Yoder & Stone, 2006), although not for all participants.

Graphic symbols have also been used in "scripts" to prompt specific vocalizations in learners who might otherwise refrain from talking or engage in inappropriate behavior (e.g., Charlop-Christy & Kelso, 2003; Krantz & McClannahan, 1998; Sarokoff, Taylor, & Poulson, 2001). For example, Ganz, Kaylor, Bourgeois, and Hadden (2008) examined using scripts with text and line drawings to increase reciprocal communication in three children with ASDs. Although only one showed increases in unscripted statements, the scripts resulted in an increase in participants' statements. Scripts are discussed in more detail in Chapter 12.

What Does the Research Say?
Effect of Speech-Generating Devices on Speech Production

Using SGDs may increase speech skills, though this varies across participants. Parsons and LaSorte (1993) found that the introduction of speech output increased spontaneous speech in young children with autism (4–6 years) who had limited speech prior to intervention. Blischak (1999) compared children's use of graphic symbols versus graphic symbols paired with synthetic speech output during rhyming instruction in nine preschool- and elementary-age children with varying diagnoses (e.g., Down syndrome, autism, cerebral palsy) and severe speech impairments (limited and largely unintelligible speech). Individual instruction focused on rhyming—while reading a story, the interventionist asked rhyming questions (e.g., "What rhymes with ____?"). Four children received instruction using graphic symbols with which they were prompted to answer the rhyming questions; the remaining children received instruction using an SGD with which they were prompted to answer the questions. The group receiving instruction using the SGD showed increases in their own speech production compared with the group using graphic symbols. There was individual variability, however. In the graphic symbol group, two children showed increases in speech, but the other two experienced decreases in speech production. Only one participant in the SGD group showed decreased speech production; the other four demonstrated increases in their speech production.

Increases in speech production may occur for only a subset of participants who are exposed to voice output (e.g., Blischak, 1999; Olive et al., 2007; Romski & Sevcik, 1996; Schlosser et al., 2007; Sigafoos, Didden, & O'Reilly, 2003). In Sevcik and Romski's (2005) work, learners' existing speech comprehension influenced speech acquisition. Several studies also suggested that verbal imitation may be related to the effects of voice output on natural speech production (Olive et al., 2007; Schlosser et al., 2007).

SGDs expose learners to both the graphic symbol and the consistent model of the spoken words from the device itself. SGDs may have a specific and positive effect on speech production because of the voice output (e.g., Romski & Sevcik, 1993).

Findings related to the impact of graphic modes of communication on speech are important because there are practitioners who believe that graphic communication modes should be considered as a "last resort" and should only be utilized when interventions designed to increase spoken language fail. There are a variety of reasons why graphic communication may facilitate spoken language. One explanation is that communication via a graphic mode involves a simultaneous discrimination between graphic symbols and, therefore, functions much like a multiple-choice task. This is in contrast to verbal and gestural communication modes that involve temporal discriminations and may, therefore, place a greater burden on memory recall (see Millar et al., 2006, for a discussion). There are also learner characteristics that are likely related to the effects of a graphic mode of communication on speech production (Carr, 1979; Schlosser & Wendt, 2008). Much more research is needed to examine this issue (Blischak, Lombardino, & Dyson, 2003; Millar et al., 2006; Schlosser & Wendt, 2008); however, preexisting verbal imitation skills (Clarke et al., 1988; Ganz & Simpson, 2004; Layton, 1988; Olive et al., 2007; Schlosser et al., 2007; Yoder & Layton, 1988) and preexisting speech comprehension skills (Romski & Sevcik, 1992; Sevcik & Romski, 2005) have been suggested by the research literature. Additional learner characteristics could logically influence the effect of AAC on speech production, such as oral motor functioning and existing sound and speech production (Blischak et al., 2003).

Although the reason for the relationship between alternative communication modes and the development of spoken language is not currently well understood, it does appear that these alternative modes do not negatively affect spoken language development. That information should help teachers and parents feel more confident in their decisions to introduce alternative modes to facilitate communication in general and perhaps have the added benefit of facilitating spoken language development along the way.

SUMMARY

It is critical to identify which mode or communication modes (vocal, graphic, gestural) will be used in any given situation in order to effectively address the communicative needs of AAC users. The issues discussed in this chapter provide interventionists with an understanding of the issues involved in making decisions regarding communication modes. This information will increase an interventionist's ability to effectively and efficiently meet the needs of individual AAC users.

REFERENCES

Barrera, R.D., Lobato-Barrera, D., & Sulzer-Azaroff, E. (1980). A simultaneous treatment comparison of three expressive language training programs with a mute autistic child. *Journal of Autism and Developmental Disorders, 10,* 21–37.

Barrera, R.D., & Sulzer-Azaroff, B. (1983). An alternating treatment comparison of oral and total communication training programs with echolalic autistic children. *Journal of Applied Behavior Analysis, 16,* 379–394.

Barrett, R.P., & Sisson, L.A. (1987). Use of the alternating treatments design as a strategy for empirically determining language training approaches with mentally retarded children. *Research in Developmental Disabilities, 8,* 401–412.

Bates, E. (1976). *Language and context.* San Diego: Academic Press.

Bates, E., & Dick, F. (2002). Language, gesture, and the developing brain. *Developmental Psychobiology, 40,* 293–310.

Beukelman, D., & Mirenda, M. (2005). *Augmentative communication: Supporting children and adults with complex communication needs* (3rd ed.). Baltimore: Paul H. Brookes Publishing Co.

Blischak, D.M. (1999). Increases in natural speech production following experience with synthetic speech. *Journal of Special Education Technology, 14,* 44–53.

Blischak, D.M., Lombardino, L.J., & Dyson, A.T. (2003). Use of speech-generating devices: In support of natural speech. *Augmentative and Alternative Communication, 19,* 29–35.

Bondy, A., & Frost, L. (1994). The Picture Exchange Communication System. *Focus on Autistic Behavior, 9,* 1–19.

Brady, N.C., Marquis, J., Fleming, K., & McLean, L. (2004). Prelinguistic predictors of language growth in children with developmental disabilities. *Journal of Speech, Language, and Hearing Research, 47,* 663–677.

Bruinsma, Y., Koegel, R.L., & Koegel, L.K. (2004). Joint attention and children with autism: A review of the literature. *Mental Retardation and Developmental Disabilities, 10,* 169–175.

Capone, N.C., & McGregor, K.K. (2004). Gesture development: A review for clinical and research practices. *Journal of Speech, Language, and Hearing Research, 47,* 173–186.

Carbone, V.J., Lewis, L., Sweeney-Kerwin, E.J., Dixon, J., Louden, R., & Quinn, S. (2006). A comparison of two approaches for teaching VB functions: Total communication vs. vocal-alone. *Journal of Speech Language Pathology-Applied Behavior Analysis, 1,* 181–191.

Carlson, F. (1984). *Picsyms categorical dictionary.* Lawrence, KS: Baggeboda Press.

Carr, E.G. (1979). Teaching autistic children to use sign language: Some research issues. *Journal of Autism and Developmental Disabilities, 9,* 345–359.

Carr, E.G., Binkoff, J.A., Kologinsky, E., & Eddy, M. (1978). Acquisition of sign language by autistic children: Expressive labeling. *Journal of Applied Behavior Analysis, 11,* 489–501.

Carr, E.G., & Dores, P.A. (1981). Patterns of language acquisition following simultaneous communication with autistic children. *Analysis and Intervention in Developmental Disabilities, 1,* 347–361.

Carr, D., & Felce, J. (2007). The effects of PECS teaching to phase III on the communicative interactions between children with autism and their teachers. *Journal of Autism and Developmental Disabilities, 37,* 724–737.

Caselli, M.C., Vicari, S., Longobardi, E., Lami, L., Pizzoli, C., & Stella, G. (1998). Gestures and words in early development of children with Down syndrome. *Journal of Speech, Language, and Hearing Research, 41,* 1125–1135.

Chan, J.B., & Iacono, T. (2001). Gesture and word production in children with Down syndrome. *AAC: Augmentative and Alternative Communication, 17,* 73–87.

Charlop-Christy, M.H., Carpenter, M., Le, L., LeBlanc, L.A., & Kellet, K. (2002). Using the Picture Exchange Communication System (PECS) with children with autism: Assessment of PECS acquisition, speech, social-communicative behavior, and problem behavior. *Journal of Applied Behavior Analysis, 35,* 213–231.

Charlop-Christy, M.H., & Kelso, S.E. (2003). Teaching children with autism conversational speech using a cue card/written script program. *Education and Treatment of Children, 26,* 108–127.

Charman, T., Drew, A., Baird, C., & Baird, G. (2003). Measuring early language development in preschool children with autism spectrum disorder using the MacArthur Communicative Development Inventory (infant form). *Journal of Child Language, 30,* 213–236.

Clark, C.R. (1981). A close look at the standard Rebus system and Blissymbolics. *Journal of The Association for Persons with Severe Handicaps, 9,* 37–48.

Clarke, S., Remington, B., & Light, P. (1986). An evaluation of the relationship between receptive speech skills and expressive signing. *Journal of Applied Behavior Analysis, 19,* 231–239.

Clarke, S., Remington, B., & Light, P. (1988). The role of referential speech in sign learning by mentally retarded children: A comparison of total communication and sign-alone training. *Journal of Applied Behavior Analysis, 21,* 419–426.

Crais, E., Douglas, D.D., & Campbell, C.C. (2004). The intersection of the development of gestures and intentionality. *Journal of Speech, Language, and Hearing Research, 47,* 678–694.

Dawson, G., Toth, K., Abbott, R., Osterling, J., Munson, J., Estes, A., et al. (2004). Early social attention impairments in autism: Social orienting, joint attention, and attention to distress. *Developmental Psychology, 40,* 271–283.

Fidler, D.J., Philofsky, A., Hepburn, S.L., & Rogers, S.J. (2005). Nonverbal requesting and problem-solving by toddlers with Down syndrome. *American Journal on Mental Retardation, 110,* 312–322.

Ganz, J.B., Kaylor, M., Bourgeois, B., & Hadden, K. (2008). The impact of social scripts and visual cues on verbal communication in three children with autism spectrum disorders. *Focus on Autism and Other Developmental Disabilities, 23,* 79–94

Ganz, J.B., & Simpson, R.L. (2004). Effects on communicative requesting and speech development of the Picture Exchange Communication System in children with characteristics of autism. *Journal of Autism and Developmental Disabilities, 34,* 395–409.

Garrison-Harrell, L., Kamps, D., & Kravits, T. (1997). The effects of peer networks on social-communicative behaviors for students with autism. *Focus on Autism and Other Developmental Disabilities, 12,* 241–254.

Goodwyn, S.W., & Acredolo, L.P. (1998). Encouraging symbolic gestures: Effects on the relationship between gesture and speech. In J. Iverson & S. Goldin-Meadows (Eds.), *The nature and functions of gesture in children's communication* (pp. 61–73). San Francisco: Jossey-Bass.

Goodwyn, S.W., Acredolo, L.P., & Brown, C.A. (2000). Impact of symbolic gesturing on early language development. *Journal of Nonverbal Behavior, 24,* 81–103.

Huer, M.B. (2000). Examining perceptions of graphic symbols across cultures: Preliminary study of the impact of culture/ethnicity. *Augmentative and Alternative Communication, 16,* 180–185.

Hurlburt, B.I., Iwata, B.A., & Green, J.D. (1982). Non-vocal language acquisition in adolescents with severe physical disabilities: Blissymbol versus iconic stimulus formats. *Journal of Applied Behavior Analysis, 15,* 241–258.

Iverson, J.M., Capirci, O., & Caselli, M.C. (1994). From communication to language in two modalities. *Cognitive Development, 9,* 23–43.

Iverson, J.M., & Goldin-Meadow, S. (1997). What's communication got to do with it? Gesture in children blind from birth. *Developmental Psychology, 33,* 453–467.

Iverson, J.M., & Goldin-Meadow, S. (2005). Gesture paves the way for language development. *Psychological Science, 16,* 367–371.

Iverson, J.M., Longobardi, E., & Caselli, M.C. (2003). Relationship between gestures and words in children with Down's syndrome and typically developing children in the early stages of communicative development. *International Journal of Language and Communication Disorders, 38,* 179–197.

Iverson, J.M., Tencer, H.L., Lany, J., & Goldin-Meadow, S. (2000). The relation between gesture and speech in congenitally blind and sighted language-learners. *Journal of Nonverbal Behavior, 24,* 105–130.

Iverson, J.M., & Thal, D.J. (1998). Communicative transitions: There's more to the hand than meets the eye. In S.F. Warren & M.E. Fey (Series Eds.) & A. Wetherby, S. Warren, & J. Reichle (Vol. Eds.), *Communication and language intervention series: Vol. 7. Transitions to prelinguistic communication: Pre-intentional to intentional and pre-symbolic to symbolic* (pp. 59–86). Baltimore: Paul H. Brookes Publishing Co.

Jagaroo, V., & Wilkinson, K.M. (2008). Further considerations of visual cognitive neuroscience for aided AAC: The potential role of motion perception systems in maximizing design display. *Augmentative and Alternative Communication, 24,* 29–42.

Johnston, S., McDonnell, A., Nelson, C., & Magnavito, A. (2003). Implementing augmentative and alternative communication intervention in inclusive preschool settings. *Journal of Early Intervention, 25,* 263–280.

Johnston, S., Nelson, C., Evans, J., & Palazolo, K. (2003). The use of visual supports in teaching young children with autism spectrum disorders to initiate interactions. *Augmentative and Alternative Communication, 19*(2), 86–103.

Konstantareas, M.M., Oxman, J., & Webster, C.D. (1977). Simultaneous communication with autistic and other severely dysfunctional nonverbal children. *Journal of Communication Disorders, 10,* 267–282.

Kouri, T.A. (1988). Effects of simultaneous communication in a child-directed treatment approach with preschoolers with severe disabilities. *Augmentative and Alternative Communication, 4,* 222–232.

Kouri, T. (1989). How manual sign acquisition relates to the development of spoken language: A case study. *Language, Speech, and Hearing Services in Schools, 20,* 50–62.

Krantz, P.J., & McClannahan, L.E. (1998). Social interaction skills for children with autism: A script-fading procedure for beginning readers. *Journal of Applied Behavior Analysis, 31,* 191–202.

Laing, E., Butterworth, G., Ansari, D., Gsödl, M., Longhi, E., Panagiotaki, G., et al. (2002). Atypical development of language and social communication in toddlers with Williams syndrome. *Developmental Science, 5,* 233–246.

Landa, R.J., Holman, K.C., & Garrett-Mayer, E. (2007). Social and communication development in toddlers with early and later diagnosis of autism spectrum disorder. *Archives of General Psychiatry, 64,* 853–864.

Layton, T.L. (1988). Language training with autistic children using four different modes of presentation. *Journal of Communication Disorders, 21,* 333–350.

Lloyd, L.L., & Karlan, G. (1984). Nonspeech communication symbols and systems: Where have we been and where are we going? *Journal of Mental Deficiency Research, 28,* 3–20.

Luftig, R.L., & Bersani, H.G. (1985). An investigation of the efficiency of Blissymbolic vs. print in symbol learning by nonreading preschool pupils. *Journal of Communication Disorders, 18,* 285–294.

Marcus, L., Garfinkle, A., & Wolery, M. (2001). Issues in early diagnosis and interventions with young children with autism. In E. Schopler, N. Yirmiya, C. Schulman, & L.M. Marcus (Eds.), *The research basis for autism intervention* (pp. 171–183). New York: Kluwer Academic Plenum.

Mayberry, R., & Nicoladis, E. (2000). Gesture reflects language development: Evidence from bilingual children. *Current Directions in Psychological Science, 9,* 192–196.

Millar, D., Light, J.C., & Schlosser, R.W. (2006). The impact of augmentative and alternative communication on the speech production of individuals with developmental disabilities: A research review. *Journal of Speech, Language, and Hearing Research, 49,* 248–264.

Mirenda, P., & Erickson, K. (2000). Augmentative communication and literacy. In A.M. Wetherby & B.M. Prizant (Eds.), *Autism spectrum disorders: A transactional developmental perspective* (pp. 333–369). Baltimore: Paul H. Brookes Publishing Co.

Mirenda, P., & Locke, P.A. (1989). A comparison of symbol transparency in nonspeaking persons with intellectual disabilities. *Journal of Speech and Hearing Disorders, 54,* 131–140.

Mitchell, S., Brian, J., Zwaigenbaum, L., Roberts, W., Szatmari, P., Smith, I., et al. (2006). Early language and communication development of infants later diagnosed with autism spectrum disorder. *Journal of Developmental and Behavioral Pediatrics, 27,* S69–S78.

Mizuko, M. (1987). Transparency and ease of learning symbols represented by Blissymbols, PCS, and Picsysms. *Augmentative and Alternative Communication, 3,* 129–136.

Mizuko, M., & Reichle, J. (1989). Transparency and recall of symbols among intellectually handicapped adults. *Journal of Speech and Hearing Disorders, 54,* 627–633.

Musselwhite, C.R., & Ruscello, D.M. (1984). Transparency of three communication symbol systems. *Journal of Speech and Hearing Research, 27,* 436–443.

Mustonen, T., Locke, P., Reichle, J., Solbrack, M., & Lindgren, A. (1991). An overview of augmentative and alternative communication systems. In J. Reichle, J. York, & J. Sigafoos (Eds.), *Implementing augmentative and alternative communication: Strategies for learners with severe disabilities.* Baltimore: Paul H. Brookes Publishing Co.

Namy, L.L., Acredolo, L., & Goodwyn, S. (2000). Verbal labels and gestural routines in parental communication with young children. *Journal of Nonverbal Behavior, 24,* 63–79.

Nicoladis, E. (2002). Some gestures develop in conjunction with spoken language development and others don't: Evidence from bilingual preschoolers. *Journal of Nonverbal Behavior, 26,* 241–266.

Olive, M.L., de la Cruz, B., Davis, T.N., Chan, J.M., Lang, R.B., O'Reilly, M.F., et al. (2007). The effects of enhanced milieu teaching and a voice output communication aid on the requesting of three children with autism. *Journal of Autism and Developmental Disabilities, 37,* 1505–1513.

Osterling, J., & Dawson, G. (1994). Early recognition of children with autism: A study of first birthday home videotapes. *Journal of Autism and Developmental Disorders, 24,* 247–257.

Özçalişkan, S., & Goldin-Meadow, S. (2005). Gesture is at the cutting edge of early language development. *Cognition, 96,* B101–B113.

Parsons, C.L., & LaSorte, D. (1993). The effect of computers with synthesized speech and no speech on the spontaneous communication of children with autism. *Australian Journal of Human Communication Disorders, 21,* 12–31.

Presmanes, A.G., Walden, T.A., Stone, W.L., & Yoder, P.J. (2007). Effects of different attentional cues on responding to joint attention in younger siblings of children with autism spectrum disorders. *Journal of Autism and Developmental Disorders, 37,* 133–144.

Romski, M.A., & Sevcik, R.A. (1992). Developing augmented language in children with severe mental retardation. In S.F. Warren & J. Reichle (Series & Vol. Eds.), *Communication and language intervention series: Vol. 1. Causes and effects in communication and language intervention* (pp. 113–130). Baltimore: Paul H. Brookes Publishing Co.

Romski, M.A., & Sevcik, R.A. (1993). Language comprehension: Considerations for augmentative and alternative communication. *Augmentative and Alternative Communication, 9,* 281–285.

Romski, M.A., & Sevcik, R.A. (1996). *Breaking the speech barrier: Language development through augmented means.* Baltimore: Paul H. Brookes Publishing Co.

Rowland, C., & Schweigert, P. (2000). Tangible symbols, tangible outcomes. *Augmentative and Alternative Communication, 16,* 61–78.

Sarokoff, R.A., Taylor, B.A., & Poulson, C.L. (2001). Teaching children with autism to engage in conversational exchanges: Script fading with embedded textual stimuli. *Journal of Applied Behavior Analysis, 34,* 81–84.

Schlosser, R.W., Sigafoos, J., Luiselli, J.K., Angermeier, K., Harasymowyz, U., Schooley, K., et al. (2007). Effects of synthetic speech output on requesting and natural speech production in children with autism: A preliminary study. *Research in Autism Spectrum Disorders, 1,* 139–163.

Schlosser, R.W., & Wendt, O. (2008). Effects of augmentative and alternative communication intervention on speech production in children with autism: A systematic review. *American Journal of Speech-Language Pathology, 17,* 212–230.

Schwartz, I.S., Garfinkle, A.N., & Bauer, J. (1998). The Picture Exchange Communication System: Communicative outcomes for young children with disabilities. *Topics in Early Childhood Special Education, 18,* 144–159.

Scruggs, T.E., Mastropieri, M.A., & Castro, G. (1987). The quantitative synthesis of single subject methodology: Methodology and validation. *Remedial and Special Education, 8,* 24–33.

Scruggs, T.E., Mastropieri, M.A., Cook, S.B., & Escobar, C. (1986). Early intervention for children with conduct disorders: A quantitative synthesis of single-subject research. *Behavioral Disorders, 11,* 260–275.

Sevcik, R.A., & Romski, M.A. (1986). Representational matching skills of persons with severe retardation. *Augmentative and Alternative Communication, 2,* 160–164.

Sevcik, R.A., & Romski, M.A. (2005). Early visual-graphic symbol acquisition by children with developmental disabilities. In L.L. Namy (Ed.), *Symbol use and symbolic representation: Developmental and comparative perspectives* (pp. 155–170). Mahwah, NJ: Lawrence Erlbaum Associates.

Sigafoos, J., Didden, R., & O'Reilly, M. (2003). Effects of speech output on maintenance of requesting and frequency of vocalizations in three children with developmental disabilities.

Augmentative and Alternative Communication, 19, 37–47.

Singer Harris, N.G., Bellugi, U., Bates, E., Jones, W., & Rossen, M. (1997). Contrasting profiles of language development in children with Williams and Down syndromes. *Developmental Neuropsychology, 13,* 345–370.

Sisson, L.A., & Barrett, R.P. (1984). An alternating treatments comparison of oral and total communication training with minimally verbal retarded children. *Journal of Applied Behavior Analysis, 17,* 559–566.

Stephenson, J. (2009a). Iconicity in the development of picture skills: Typical development and implications for individuals with severe intellectual disabilities. *Augmentative and Alternative Communication, 25,* 187–201.

Stephenson, J. (2009b). Recognition and use of line drawings by children with severe intellectual disabilities: The effects of color and outline shape. *Augmentative and Alternative Communication, 25,* 55–67.

Sullivan, M., Finelli, J., Marvin, A., Garrett-Mayer, E., Bauman, M., & Landa, R. (2007). Response to joint attention in toddlers at risk for autism spectrum disorder: A prospective study. *Journal of Autism and Developmental Disorders, 37,* 37–48.

Thistle, J., & Wilkinson, K.M. (2009). The effects of color cues on typically developing preschoolers' speed of locating a target line drawing: Implications for AAC display design. *American Journal of Speech-Language Pathology, 18,* 231–240.

Tincani, M. (2004). Comparing the Picture Exchange Communication System and sign language training for children with autism. *Focus on Autism and Other Developmental Disabilities, 19,* 152–163.

Toth, K., Munson, J., Meltzoff, A.N., & Dawson, G. (2006). Early predictors of communication development in young children with autism spectrum disorder: Joint attention, imitations, and toy play. *Journal of Autism and Developmental Disorders, 36,* 933–1005.

Vanderheiden, G.C., & Yoder, D.E. (1986). Overview. In S.W. Blackstone (Ed.), *Augmentative communication: An introduction* (pp. 1–28). Rockville, MD: American Speech-Language-Hearing Association.

Volterra, V., & Iverson, J.M. (1995). When do modality factors affect the course of language acquisition? In K. Emmorey & J.S. Reilly (Eds.), *Language, gesture, and space* (pp. 371–390). Mahwah, NJ: Lawrence Erlbaum Associates.

Wells, M.E. (1981). The effects of total communication training versus traditional speech training on word articulation in severely mentally retarded individuals. *Applied Research in Mental Retardation, 2,* 323–333.

Wilkinson, K.M., Carlin, M., & Thistle, J. (2008). The role of color cues in facilitating accurate and rapid location of aided symbols by children with and without Down Syndrome. *American Journal of Speech-Language Pathology, 17,* 179–193.

Yoder, P.J., & Layton, T.L. (1988). Speech following sign language training in autistic children with minimal verbal language. *Journal of Autism and Developmental Disabilities, 18,* 217–229.

Yoder, P., & Stone, W.L. (2006). A randomized comparison of the effect of two prelinguistic communication interventions on the acquisition of spoken communication in preschoolers with ASD. *Journal of Speech, Language, and Hearing Research, 49,* 698–711.

AAC System Features

3

Susan S. Johnston and Kathleen M. Feeley

▷ CHAPTER OVERVIEW

Augmentative and alternative communication (AAC) systems enable individuals with severe disabilities to more clearly communicate and engage in home, school, and community activities in ways that were previously unthinkable. Unaided AAC modes (e.g., gestures, sign languages/ systems) and aided AAC modes (e.g., line drawings on a communication board, written words on paper, laptop computers with speech output, dedicated AAC devices) offer individuals at any communicative level an opportunity to enhance their existing skills. It is important to understand AAC system features and how each may enhance communication to ensure that AAC systems meet the learners' needs and the needs of their communication partners. This chapter provides an overview of aided AAC system features particularly relevant for individuals with severe disabilities (see Chapter 2 for information on unaided AAC modes).

▷ CHAPTER OBJECTIVES

After studying this chapter, readers will be able to

- Identify different features of aided AAC systems
- Explain how individual features may enhance communication
- Understand how research related to AAC system features can be used to support evidence-based practice

▷ KEY TERMS

- ▶ activation feedback
- ▶ active dynamic display
- ▶ alphanumeric encoding
- ▶ auditory scanning
- ▶ circular scanning
- ▶ digitized speech output
- ▶ direct selection
- ▶ directed scanning
- ▶ dynamic display
- ▶ encoding
- ▶ electronic eye gaze
- ▶ fixed display
- ▶ grid displays
- ▶ group item scanning
- ▶ group row column scanning

- ▶ iconic codes
- ▶ indirect selection
- ▶ infrared technology
- ▶ integrated visual scene display
- ▶ inverse scanning
- ▶ keypad sensitivity
- ▶ letter category codes
- ▶ light/laser pointing
- ▶ linear scanning
- ▶ message output
- ▶ message prediction
- ▶ nonelectronic auditory scanning
- ▶ nonelectronic eye gaze

- ▶ passive dynamic display
- ▶ phrase/sentence prediction
- ▶ scanning patterns
- ▶ scanning speed
- ▶ scrolling
- ▶ single letter prediction
- ▶ slots
- ▶ speech output
- ▶ symbol display
- ▶ synthesized speech output
- ▶ visual output
- ▶ visual scanning
- ▶ word prediction

Advances in technology enable interventionists to consider a range of options when selecting the most appropriate communication system. These options can be viewed on a continuum ranging from no tech, to light tech, to high tech.

No-Tech Communication Systems

No-tech communication systems do not involve technology and can utilize a variety of graphic symbols (e.g., photographs, line drawings, written words) that can be displayed on a key chain, within a book, or on a communication board. The left-hand column of Figure 3.1 provides examples of no-tech communication systems.

Light-Tech Communication Systems

Light-tech communication systems utilize technology that is relatively simple in form (e.g., simple battery-operated devices) and include speech-generating devices (SGDs) such as tape recorded messages and single-switch voice output communication aids. The middle column of Figure 3.1 provides examples of light-tech communication systems.

High-Tech Communication Systems

High-tech communication systems consist of SGDs containing more advanced technology, which allows for expansive speech output, environmental control, e-mail access, and so forth. There are two types of SGDs—dedicated and nondedicated. Dedicated SGDs are used solely for communication purposes by the AAC user (e.g., Eco by Prentke Romitch). Nondedicated SGDs are not used solely for communication purposes and have the capacity to run software for other purposes. Nondedicated SGDs include laptop/desktop computers, personal digital assistants, and cell phones. Software

A list of AAC device manufacturers and distributors is included on the accompanying CD-ROM.

(e.g., Proloquo2Go) can be downloaded onto these nondedicated devices for use as AAC systems.

Some devices such as the DynaVox Vmax can have both a computer operating system and dedicated software. Both dedicated and nondedicated SGDs have the potential for more advanced forms of technology and may provide features such as message storage, retrieval, and output (either voice or printed) as well as environmental controls. The right-hand column of Figure 3.1 provides examples of SGDs.

Interventionists should understand the features available on aided AAC systems in order to identify and procure a system that meets the needs and communicative potential of the AAC user. The next section provides an overview of several features of aided AAC systems.

FEATURES OF AUGMENTATIVE AND ALTERNATIVE COMMUNICATION SYSTEMS

Each AAC system can be described in terms of its features. Although multiple features are available, the features described in the following sections are most relevant for individuals with severe disabilities.

Output

AAC systems can have visual and/or auditory output. Higher tech devices tend to have multiple output options, whereas light-tech options, tend to have more limited output capabilities.

Visual Output

Virtually all high-tech AAC systems incorporate visual **message output** that enables the message to be displayed for the benefit of the AAC user and his or her communicative partner. **Visual output** can be presented temporarily on a message window screen until the next message is selected or can be presented on a permanent product (e.g., printed on paper).

No-tech AAC systems	Light-tech AAC systems	High-tech AAC systems
Communication wallet—Symbols are stored in the photograph holders within a wallet. 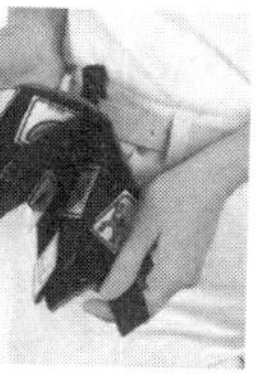	*Simple scanning systems*—These items are scanned via cursor. 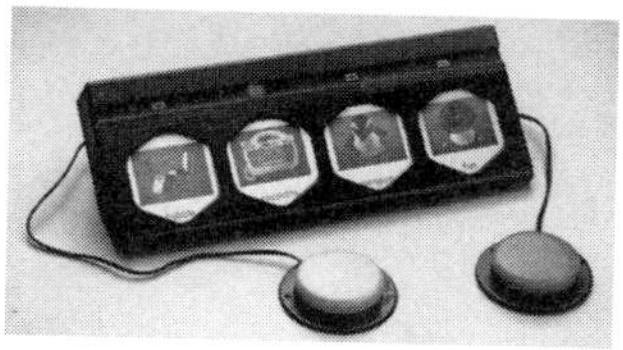	*The Chat Box (by Saltillo)*—This dedicated speech-generating device (SGD) has digitized speech. 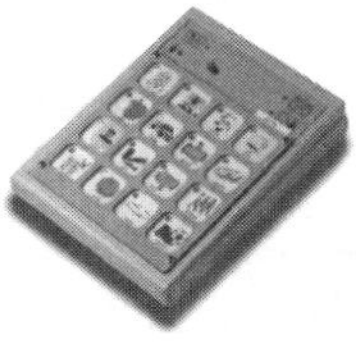
Communication board—Symbols are stored on a board that can be mounted on a wheelchair tray, wall, or desk. 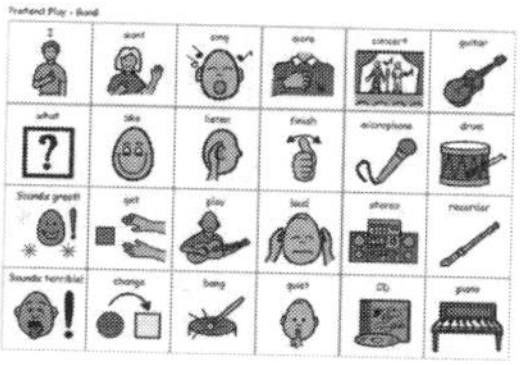	*Single-switch SGD[a]*—A single message is emitted when switch is selected. 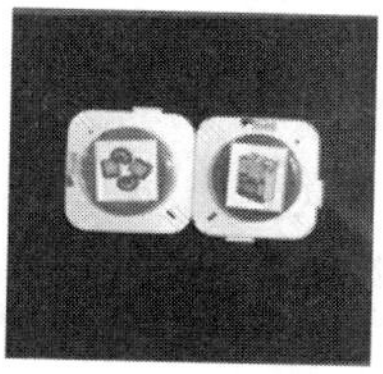	*Eco (by Prentke Romich)[b]*—This dedicated SGD has text-to-speech capability, scanning, and computer access. 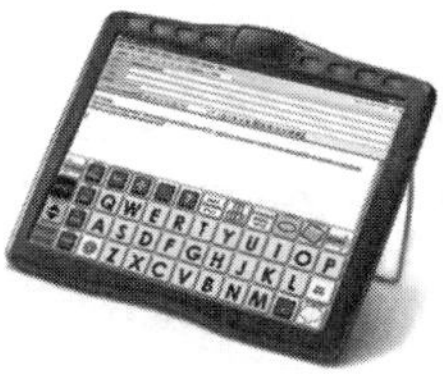
Communication book—Symbols are mounted in a book, which can be of various sizes.	*Tape recorded messages (by Enabling Devices)*—A switch that is connected to a tape recorder activates a recorded message when selected. (Switch not included)	*The Vmax (by DynaVox Technologies)[c]*—This dedicated SGD has text-to-speech capability, dynamic display, scanning, and computer access.
		iPAD/iPhone (by Apple) with Proloquo2Go Assistiveware software—This nondedicated SGD is a tablet computer/cell phone with software that allows for text to speech and displaying symbols.

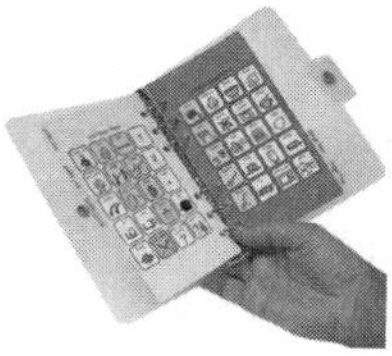

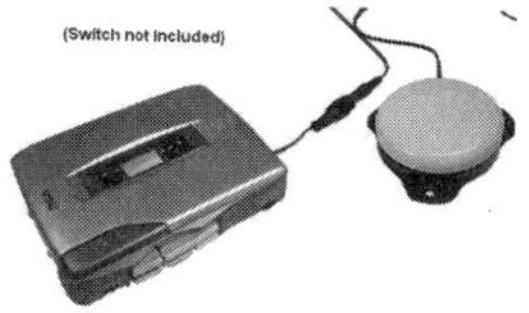

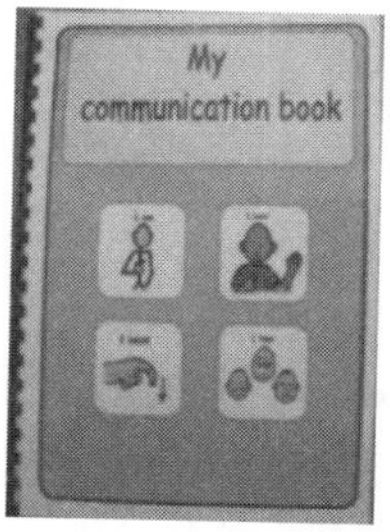

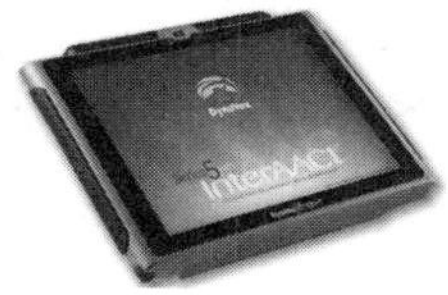

Figure 3.1. Examples of no-tech, light-tech, and high-tech augmentative and alternative communication (AAC) systems. ([a]Photo © 1985–2011 AbleNet, Inc. All Rights Reserved. Used with permission. [b]Photo courtesy of PRC at prentrom.com. [c]Photo of Vmax courtesy of DynaVox Technologies, Pittsburgh, PA [www.dynavoxtech.com].)

The message window in most devices faces the AAC user. Some devices, however, have one message window facing the AAC user and another facing the communicative part- ner (e.g., LightWriter by Toby Churchill). This is useful in environments where the voice output might be disruptive (e.g., class- room, religious service) or when the communicative partner cannot understand the message, by allowing him or her to read, rather than hear, the message. Consider the following to determine whether temporary visual output will meet the needs of an AAC user:

- The extent to which the visual output can be seen across environments

- Whether the visual output can and/or needs to be positioned so that the AAC user and communicative partner can see it

- The size of the visual output and number of characters that can appear at one time

Some AAC systems allow for permanent visual output of the AAC user's message. Many AAC systems have the capability of interfacing directly (or through a computer) to a printer. Consider the speed with which the message needs to be communicated (e.g., ordering a meal at a restaurant by presenting the cashier with the message on paper) and the extent to which the message needs to be efficiently conveyed to determine whether permanent visual output will meet the needs of an AAC user. In addition to visual output, most light- and high-tech AAC systems provide speech output.

Speech Output

SGDs provide **speech output** capabilities and provide the AAC user with a means of communicating messages across a range of communicative partners within a range of environments. There are two types of speech output available—digitized speech and synthesized speech.

Digitized Speech   **Digitized speech output** consists of actual recordings of a human voice or environmental event. For an AAC user to use recorded speech, the interventionist must 1) identify messages the AAC user would like to communicate, 2) have someone who is verbal record the message, and 3) store the message so that the AAC user can locate and access it (i.e., assign the message to a specific location and affix a corresponding symbol).

The amount of memory for digitized speech within a device can range from 16 seconds (e.g., Voicemate by TASH), to several minutes (e.g., SideKick by Prentke Romich; SuperTalker by Ablenet), to 1 hour (Vantage Lite by Prentke Romich) or 2 hours of memory (e.g., e-Talk by Synapsis Adaptive), or more (DynaVox Vmax; Eco2 by Prentke Romich; Blue Bird II by Saltillo).

Synthesized Speech   Synthesized speech is computer-generated voice output that is comprised of speech sounds individually recorded and then pulled together electronically to formulate speech (e.g., AT&T Natural Voices). Systems with **synthesized speech output** have text-to-speech capability, allowing AAC users to generate novel voice messages by typing in letters to create words/phrases. Messages can be spoken immediately, or the AAC user can store the message behind one or more keys/symbols to quickly retrieve at a later time. If the AAC user is unable to type the message, then someone else can type the message and assign it to a specific symbol. The message is spoken when the AAC user selects that symbol.

The relative advantages and disadvantages of digitized and synthesized speech output can be found in Table 3.1. Although some devices have only digitized or synthesized speech output, other devices contain both.

Why Is Output Important?

Temporary visual output is important to consider because it allows the AAC user to construct and check a message before it is sent. The AAC user can also share a message in private (i.e., the partner can read the message without it being spoken). Permanent visual output (print display) allows for the creation of a permanent record (which may be particularly important for AAC users who are in environments where written text is required). Speech output is important to consider because it does not require visual orientation on the part of the communication partner and, thus, can be used if the AAC user is at a distance from his or her

Table 3.1. Features of digitized and synthesized speech

Digitized speech output	Synthesized speech output
Advantages	*Advantages*
More closely resembles natural speech (retaining voice quality, intonation, and dialectical characteristics) and can be matched to age/gender of the augmentative and alternative communication (AAC) user	Requires less memory
	Can generate novel utterances for AAC users who have text-to-speech capability
More intelligible than synthesized speech, with older children performing better than younger children and intelligibility increasing with increased length of messages (Drager, Clark-Serpentine, Johnson, & Roeser, 2006)	
Allows for the recording of nonspeech sounds (e.g., horn beeping)	
Disadvantages	*Disadvantages*
Only prerecorded vocabulary available (no novel messages)	Limited intelligibility and lack of voice quality and intonation patterns for some synthesized speech
More memory required than for synthesized speech; limited memory means limited number of stored messages	

communication partner (even over the telephone). Consistently pairing spoken output with symbol selection may assist beginning communicators in acquiring collateral behavior, including comprehending graphic symbols (Schlosser, Belfiore, Nigam, Blischak, & Hetzroni, 1995), comprehending speech, and producing speech (although available evidence suggests that imitation represents a critical competence among those who acquire speech [Millar, Light, & Schlosser, 2006; Schlosser & Wendt, 2008]).

What Does the Research Say?

Researchers have compared the effectiveness of SGDs with other modes of AAC. Iacono, Mirenda, and Beukelman (1993) compared using speech and signs with using speech, signs, and an SGD on the ability of two learners with intellectual disabilities to express two-word combinations. Although both children learned to use two-word utterances, one learner relied on the SGD, and the other, on speech and sign alone.

Iacono and Duncum (1995) used an alternating treatments design and compared using sign and speech with using the DynaVox Vmax SGD (dynamic display with voice output) and speech on the number of words/word combinations and the number of imitated productions and modalities used for each. The participant was a girl who was slightly older than 2½-years-old with Down syndrome. Interventions were implemented within two scripted rou-

tines (cooking and dress-up), and each routine was assigned 19 different vocabulary words. Using the SGD in combination with sign language resulted in more single-word productions as well as more two- and three-word combinations.

Romski, Sevcik, and Adamson (1999) observed experienced AAC users with severe disabilities (13–28 years) interacting with unfamiliar adults with and without their SGD within a scripted routine. In the SGD condition, there was an increase in appropriate conversational events for 10 of 13 participants, as well as more messages produced by 9 of 13 participants.

Several researchers have compared using SGDs with using low-tech graphic communication systems. Son, Sigafoos, O'Reilly, and Lancioni (2006) examined acquisition rates of requesting in three preschoolers with autism, finding little difference between the Picture Exchange Communication System (PECS; Bondy & Frost, 1994) and the SGD. Two children demonstrated a preference for the SGD and one for the PECS, however. Soto, Belfiore, Schlosser, and Haynes (1993) found no difference between the performance of a 22-year-old man with severe disabilities when using a communication board versus an SGD; however, he did display a preference for the SGD. Sigafoos, Didden, and O'Reilly (2003) also found no difference in the frequency of requesting in three children with developmental disabilities (3–13 years) when the SGD's speech output was on versus when it was off. Dyches, Davis, Lucido, and Young (2002) used an alternating treatments

(continued)

design and examined the performance of a 17-year-old girl with multiple disabilities using 11 line-drawn symbols (e.g., requests, food items, THANK YOU) and an identical display attached to an SGD. The participant produced generalized communication (across individuals and settings) using both systems with similar rates of comprehensibility on the part of the communicative partner. Bock, Stoner, Beck, Hanley, and Prochnow (2005), however, found faster acquisition rates using the PECS in three of six preschoolers with disabilities. These latter findings were replicated by Beck, Stoner, Bock, and Parton (2008), who found that acquisition rates were faster in the PECS versus the SGD condition in four preschoolers with disabilities. They attributed inferior acquisition with the SGD to difficulty in physically manipulating the device, however.

Symbol Displays

It is important to consider how a large and/or expanding symbol set will be displayed for efficient access by the AAC user. Symbols should be displayed in a manner that is maximally transparent to the AAC user so that the time, effort, and energy involved in learning the location of a vocabulary item is low, whereas the efficiency and effectiveness of the AAC user's communicative interactions is high (Light, 1997). Options related to **symbol display** include permanence of the display (e.g., static, dynamic) and layout (e.g., **grid displays,** integrated scenes). See Light, Wilkinson, and Drager (2008) for a more in-depth review of these options.

Static or Dynamic Displays

A static (or **fixed**) **display** occurs when all of the available symbols are simultaneously displayed on one page (Beukelman & Mirenda, 2005). The primary advantage of a static display is that a learner may view all available symbols during a communicative opportunity and engage in a simultaneous discrimination in which he or she can compare the symbols concurrently with the referent. This discrimination may be easier for learners with severe disabilities than discriminations

during which the symbol array cannot be viewed in its entirety (see Chapter 8). The number of symbols that can be displayed at one time on a static display tends to be limited, however. When an AAC user acquires more symbols than can be displayed, symbols must be made smaller, the display must be made larger, the learner must combine symbols to create new messages (**encoding,** discussed later in this chapter), or symbols must be spread across multiple pages, resulting in a **dynamic display**.

When using a dynamic display, the learner is not able to view his or her symbols simultaneously with a dynamic display. For example, if the learner selects a symbol of a house, then the display can be programmed to change so that a set of symbols representing household vocabulary is immediately displayed. The AAC user must then "travel" within or across pages on the AAC system. Traveling within pages can be accomplished through **scrolling**.

What Does the Research Say?

Research investigating issues related to static and dynamic displays is increasing.

- The majority of research validating the use of aided AAC systems with individuals with severe disabilities has involved the use of static/fixed-symbol displays (e.g., Dyches et al., 2002; Sigafoos et al., 2003.

- Dudek, Beck, and Thompson (2006) found that there was no significant difference in the attitudes of participants (60 typically developing children in third and fifth grades) after viewing a videotape of AAC users when using dynamic displays versus fixed displays.

- Reichle, Dettling, Drager, and Leiter (2000) examined the relative efficiency of three different symbol displays for a 16-year-old experienced AAC user with severe disabilities. The three symbol displays were 1) fixed, 2) dynamic display with direct links, and 3) dynamic display with levels. Results revealed that response time was fastest and accuracy was greatest for the fixed and dynamic display with direct links. Differences between the displays were more evident when more symbols were added to the displays.

Traveling within Pages on an AAC System

Scrolling involves sliding the presentation of content (e.g., AAC system symbols) across a screen or display window to reveal new content as old content disappears. The word *scroll* is derived from the way in which people read scrolls of paper, by rolling up the top of the page and allowing objects lower on the page to move into view. Some SGDs allow the scrolling feature to be individualized for each AAC user. For example, the AAC system can be set so that a predetermined amount of content (e.g., one line of symbols on a grid display) is scrolled each time the scroll symbol is accessed. Or, the speed at which the content is scrolled can be preset. In this case, the AAC user must access a button to stop the scrolling. Alternatively, a device could be configured to allow the learner to scroll using a release switch activation strategy in which he or she places his or her hand on a symbol and drags to scroll. Pausing his or her hand would stop the scrolling. IntelliPoint (by Microsoft) is an example of a computer mouse software that supports scrolling. When activated, a special icon appears on the screen where the cursor was blinking. The cursor can be moved above or below the icon to scroll up or down. The further the cursor moves from the icon, the faster the resulting scroll action. Using this type of scrolling may be particularly helpful to users who access their AAC systems and/or computers using head pointers because it will allow a user to scroll a large page by simply moving the head up and down (instead of having to continuously click on a scroll button).

Traveling Across Pages on an AAC System

Traveling across pages can be accomplished through the use of levels. Levels provide an opportunity for interventionists to 1) organize symbols in a manner that is more transparent to the AAC user and/or 2) teach skills related to organizing and classifying communicative utterances. For example, consider a situation when a learner is out with friends. Symbols related to activities that are done with friends (e.g., LET'S GO TO A MOVIE; LET'S GO TO THE MALL; LET'S GO OUT TO EAT) are provided on one page. When the learner selects one of these symbols (e.g., LET'S GO OUT TO EAT), he or she will travel to a page consisting of restaurant logos. Then, the learner will travel to a page containing a menu from the restaurant he or she selected from the logos.

Traveling through pages can occur nonelectronically (e.g., turning pages of a communication book) or electronically. Traveling across pages using an SGD with a static display may be accomplished by turning a knob on the back of the device to select the desired page/level. Alternatively, traveling across pages may involve physically replacing one page of symbols, sometimes referred to as an overlay, with another page of symbols. In many cases, turning knobs on the back of the device and/or changing overlays will require the assistance of a communication partner, which may limit the learner's independence.

SGDs with dynamic displays are often categorized as either passive or active (Reichle, Halle, & Drasgow, 1988). An SGD with a passive dynamic display might have one page that contains vocabulary related to getting ready for school as well as a GO TO symbol that, when pressed, results in a page containing vocabulary related to the next activity—riding the school bus. An advantage of a **passive dynamic display** is that it provides an opportunity for interventionists to teach a learner to search within as well as across pages. For example, a learner can be taught to look at the symbols on a page. If the desired symbol is on the page, then the learner is taught to select the symbol. If the desired symbol is not on the page, however, then the learner is taught to turn the page.

An SGD with an **active dynamic display** allows the learner to link from any symbol on a page to another page of symbols. For example, when a learner selects a symbol representing I WANT TO DRAW, the device can be programmed to automatically display a new page containing questions, answers, and vocabulary that may typically be used in this context (e.g., DO YOU WANT TO DRAW WITH ME?; I LIKE THAT). The visual relationship between the new page and the original page and what happens when a symbol is selected on the new page are two critical areas to consider when the new page appears.

Visual Relationship Between Pages   When a learner selects a symbol that is linked to a new page, the new page can either be displayed so that the learner is unable to see the original page (e.g., similar to turning a page in a book) or it can be displayed in a smaller window so that the original page is still partially visible to the learner (e.g., similar to a "pop-up" window). Presenting the new page as a pop-up window may result in symbols that are too small and/or too visually distracting (because the symbols from the original page are still visible) for some learners. Other learners, however, may benefit from a pop-up window because it visually shows the connection between the original window and the pop-up window. What happens when a symbol is selected on the new page is the second issue to consider.

Influence of Symbol Selection on the Page
When a learner selects a symbol on the new page, the new page can either close automatically or remain open. If the new page remains open following a symbol selection, then the device can be programmed with a GO BACK symbol that allows the user to return to a master page or a preceding page. Having the new page close automatically may be helpful if the learner will only be selecting one symbol on the new page because it will allow the learner to return quickly to the original page without any additional symbol selections (e.g., the GO BACK symbol). If the learner is likely to make more than one symbol selection on the new page, however, it may be beneficial for the new page to remain open until the GO BACK symbol is selected. This will provide the learner with more flexibility with regard to selecting additional symbols or returning to the original page.

Grid and Integrated Visual Scene Displays

Grid displays occur when the symbols are organized into rows and columns, forming a grid. Typically, there is no or extremely limited context in the background of the symbols and the symbols on a grid display do not maintain relative perspective (e.g., an apple symbol may be the same size as a house symbol; Light & Drager, 2007). The symbols on a grid display can be organized according to semantics/syntax, taxonomy, or schematics (Beukelman & Mirenda, 2005). Semantic/syntactic grids display symbols in terms of spoken word order or usage. The Fitzgerald Key (McDonald & Schultz, 1973) is the basis for one frequently used format for organizing symbols in this manner. The Fitzgerald Key format arranges symbols from left to right based on the word order used in spoken English sentences. This format can be used to encourage AAC users to move from left to right across the display as they search for and select symbols to form a sentence. Taxonomic grids display groups of symbols according to categories, such as people, places, activities, feelings, and foods. Schematic grids display symbols according to specific events/situations, including items that are related to an activity (e.g., eating lunch at school) or routines within that activity (e.g., going through the lunch line, sitting at a table with friends).

Grid displays can also be arranged based on motor skills/abilities. For example, if a child is able to access symbols on the right side of a display more efficiently, then more frequently used and/or more important symbols can be placed on that side. Finally, it is important to note that the different types of grid displays are not necessarily mutually exclusive. For example, the items within a schematic grid display could be grouped taxonomically (e.g., all nouns in one area of the display).

An **integrated visual scene display**, in which symbols are embedded into contextual scenes, is an alternative to a grid display. Digital photographs or high-quality line drawings of scenes (e.g., storefronts of preferred fast food restaurants) are taken and stored in the AAC system. Selecting one of the photographs (e.g., McDonald's) links to a page containing additional symbols for communication (e.g., a McDonald's counter with a picture menu of food/drink choies).

▷ Helpful Hint

Dietz, McKelvey, and Beukelman (2006) suggested four criteria influencing the efficacy of visual scene displays: 1) environmental context (e.g., a scene that includes information regarding the relevant setting, people, objects, activities), 2) interactional context (e.g., a scene that depicts people performing the relevant actions), 3) personal relevancy (e.g., a scene that includes photographs of the learner participating in the relevant activity/event), and 4) clarity regarding the relationship between relevant elements of the visual scene.

What Does the Research Say?

Research investigating issues related to grid and visual scene displays is increasing.

- Drager, Light, Curran Speltz, Fallon, and Jeffries (2003) examined the performance of 30 typically developing 2½-year-olds in locating symbols on dynamic displays presented in three different formats (two were organized in a grid array, and the third was organized in an integrated scene format). Results revealed that the children had great difficulty locating target vocabulary in all conditions and were not able to generalize their learning to new vocabulary items. The children learning to locate vocabulary items in the integrated scene condition, however, performed significantly better than the children learning to use either of the grid formats.

- Drager et al. (2004) examined the performance of 30 typically developing 3-year-olds in locating symbols on dynamic displays that differed in system layout and menu page approaches. Two approaches to layout were investigated (grid display and integrated scene display), and two approaches to menu page representation were investigated (options on a menu page represented by a single symbol and options on a menu page represented by smaller versions, or screen shots, of the actual page of vocabulary). Results revealed that the children had difficulty with all of the approaches

on initial exposure. After the initial learning session, however, children performed slightly better in an integrated scene/screen shot format than in either of the two grid formats. Some limited generalization to new vocabulary was observed.

- Light and Drager (2005) examined the use of visual scene displays on the language development of 10 children (15–40 months) with significant intellectual disabilities. Results revealed that participants used the visual scene display in social interactions, increased turntaking following their introduction, sustained gains in turntaking across time, and learned to use other display types (e.g., grid displays) following instruction with visual scene displays.

- Drager et al. (2005) examined the use of visual scene displays combined with instructional strategies to support communication (e.g., providing opportunities, modeling) on the communication development of four children (3–5 years) with autism and pervasive development disorder-not otherwise specified. Results revealed significant increases in rates of turntaking and range of semantic relations that were expressed.

Translating Research to Practice

Traditional grids and/or visual scenes have inherent advantages and disadvantages to consider when making decisions regarding which to use with a given learner. For example,

- Typically, there is no context in the background of the symbols in grid displays, and the symbols on a page do not maintain relative perspective (e.g., an apple symbol may be the same size as a house symbol). Beginning communicators with severe disabilities, therefore, may have difficulty acquiring symbols (Light & Drager, 2007; Olin, Reichle, Johnson, & Monn, 2010).

- Some have theorized that visual scene displays reduce metalinguistic demands and facilitate early language learning because the symbols include contextual information (Drager et al., 2003).

- Personalized visual scenes (e.g., scenes that are familiar to the learner with regard to setting and referents) may be easier for young children and individuals with severe cognitive disabilities than nonpersonalized scenes (Light & Drager, 2005).

- Some learners with autism may have difficulty with visual scene displays because of a tendency to focus on nonrelated components of the scene (Light & Drager, 2005).

- Embedding symbols into visual scene displays may compromise the ability of learners with severe disabilities to generalize symbol use to other activities.

SELECTION TECHNIQUES

Selection techniques refer to the manner in which the AAC user accesses a symbol to communicate his or her message. Dowden and Cook (2002) described selection techniques in terms of *direct* and *indirect*. **Direct selection** refers to the act of the AAC user "specifically indicating the desired item in the selection set" (Dowden & Cook, 2002, p. 395). Thus, the AAC user comes into direct contact with the selected symbol with a body part (e.g., a finger) or the use of eye gaze, a stick (handheld or attached to one's head), or an optical pointer. **Indirect selection** involves the learner waiting for one or more intermediary steps by a device or a communication partner to occur before making a selection (Cook & Hussy, 1995). Both types of selection techniques are discussed in the following section.

Direct Selection Techniques

There are several ways symbols can be directly selected by the AAC user (Buekelman & Mirenda, 2005).

- *Pointing with physical contact*: The AAC user contacts the symbol with a body part or assistive device (e.g., head stick).

This selection technique can be used with nonelectronic communication systems (e.g., books, boards) as well as with SGDs. Typing on a keyboard is an example of direct selection as well as a touch screen, an adapted interface that allows AAC users to make selections on a computer monitor.

- *Control interface (switch)*: A learner's physical impairments may warrant use of a control interface (e.g., an electronic switch) as a means of direct selection. The electronic switch converts movement into meaningful output, functioning as an interface between the learner and the AAC system (see Chapter 4). An SGD is started when a symbol that is placed directly on a switch is activated. Some devices allow several messages to be recorded, and each recording is selected when a different switch is activated. In addition, a touch screen is actually a switch that allows the discrete selection of a number of different symbols.

- *Pointing without physical contact*: An AAC user need not physically contact a symbol to directly select it. Selections may be made by

  Nonelectronic eye gaze *(eye pointing)*: Selections are presented, and the learner gazes at the desired symbol for a period of time to indicate the selection. This selection technique has been used by individuals of all ages who have extensive physical impairments (Beukelman & Mirenda, 2005) as well as with learners with Rett syndrome (Hetzroni & Rubin, 2006). Unique adaptations of eye gaze systems include symbols placed on a vest worn by the communicative partner, on the learner's lap tray, or on a transparent display (e.g., a frame) placed between the AAC user and the communicative partner (Goossens', 1989; Goossens' & Crain, 1987).

  Light/laser pointing: Symbols can be selected directly using a light or laser pointer held or affixed via the AAC user's headband or glasses and directed at the desired symbol. The pointer can be used with nonelectronic symbol displays (e.g., communication board) or with an SGD (some of which allow for adjustments in activation strategies discussed later in this chapter).

Electronic eye gaze: Infrared technology is used to allow a computer to interpret the AAC user's symbol selection. A sensor (e.g., worn on the forehead or attached to eyeglasses; e.g., Eyegaze Edge by LC Technologies) or fine movements made by the AAC user control a cursor, directing it to symbols on the computer screen (Beukelman & Mirenda, 2005). More advanced applications utilize remote cameras that measure eye movements. Such systems have advanced greatly, decreasing the use of traditional scanning selection techniques.

- *Speech commands to a computer*: Computer software is available that converts speech sounds into computer commands (e.g., Dragon Naturally Speaking, V6.0 Standard by Scansoft). An individual's distinct vocalizations are stored onto the computer, and each is assigned a specific command. The AAC user vocalizes to activate a command instead of making a selection with a body part (Lancione et al., 2005; Lancioni, Singh, O'Reilly, Oliva, et al., 2004; Lancioni, Singh, O'Reilly, Sigafoos, et al., 2004). Although systems recognize variations in utterances (Koester, 2004), individuals with severe developmental disabilities whose vocal skills are limited may find it challenging to produce distinctly different as well as sufficiently consistent vocalizations.

Why Is It Important to Explore Direct Selection as a Selection Strategy?

If the AAC user has sufficient motor control, then direct selection is the fastest method of selection; easy to learn; and, in many cases,

is already in the learner's repertoire because pointing is a common form of prelinguistic communication. Direct selection also imposes few cognitive demands (Dowden & Cook, 2002; Mizuko, Reichle, Ratcliff, & Esser, 1994). The primary disadvantage is it requires significant motor skills to reach all items in the selection set and requires fine resolution of movement to allow for the smallest amount of space between symbols so that several can be included in the display (Dowden & Cook, 2002). A number of interface adjustment options are available when designing direct selection systems, however, each of which are discussed in the following sections.

What Are the Options for Interface Adjustments?

The following paragraphs discuss areas of interface adjustments that include keypad sensitivity, activation feedback, acceptance time, and release time.

Keypad Sensitivity   Several SGDs allow the amount of pressure required to activate the keypad to be adjusted. **Keypad sensitivity** can be useful for AAC users who have limited motor control; thus, a very small amount of pressure can activate the device.

Activation Feedback   **Activation feedback** indicates that a symbol selection has been made. The feedback can be auditory (e.g., beep, click) or visual (e.g., a light flash, a change in the shade of the symbol on a dynamic display).

Acceptance Time   Some SGDs can be set so that the AAC user must come into contact with the symbol (applying pressure or selecting with a light pointer) for it to be activated (referred to as touch enter, input filtering, or sticky/filter keys [e.g., M3 by DynaVox]) and can be set for a prespecified amount of time (e.g., 4-second acceptance time) before the message is activated. This feature is helpful for learners who may inadvertently select other symbols while navigating to the desired symbol.

Release Time   Release time occurs when a message is activated by the AAC user who removes pressure or a light beam from the keypad (referred to as touch exit) instead of activating the message by selecting a symbol. Selections will not be made for a learner who makes unintentional selections through brief contact with the symbol until he or she stabilizes him- or herself on the device and then releases (Beukelman & Mirenda, 2005). This application is often used with learners with motor disabilities that involve tremors in which there may be a high level of inadvertent symbol activations.

What Does the Research Say?

A small number of studies have compared direct selection techniques. Battenberg and Merbler (1989) compared use of a touch screen with a traditional keyboard with 40 kindergarteners with developmental delays and 40 without delays. Each participated in matching and spelling tasks in both touch screen and traditional keyboard conditions. A repeated measures design indicated performance by both groups was enhanced (i.e., quicker response time and few errors) when using the touch screen. Durfee and Billingsley (1999) used an alternating treatments design to compare use of a touch screen with a mouse with an enlarged on-screen arrow by a 9-year-old boy with spastic quadriplegic cerebral palsy and cognitive and vision impairments. The task—matching uppercase letters—was performed with fewer errors using the mouse.

Indirect Selection Techniques

Indirect selection involves either a device or the communication partner performing an intermediary step prior to the AAC user making a selection (Dowden & Cook, 2002). Indirect selection techniques include scanning and directed/joystick scanning.

Scanning

Communication options are menued for the AAC user by a communication partner or via an SGD when using scanning. A discrete response (i.e., specific sound or movement) can be used to indicate to the communicative partner that the desired item has been menued. The learner can also be taught to select a switch (a mechanism that controls an electric circuit) to activate a buzzer or a recording to indicate his or her selection. Items are menued electronically and selected via a switch mechanism when using electronic applications.

Three issues must be contemplated when considering scanning: 1) the switch activation strategy (i.e., how the scanner is activated), 2) the scanning selection technique (visual or auditory), and 3) the scanning pattern (i.e., the way in which the items or groups of items are menued). Information regarding switch activation strategies is provided in Chapter 4. The following sections provide information regarding scanning selection techniques and scanning patterns.

Scanning Selection Technique   Items are visually or auditorially menued for the AAC user when scanning. Auditory scanning is discussed later in this chapter. The communicative partner menus (points to the items one at a time) the items or symbols for the AAC user with nonelectronic **visual scanning**. The AAC user emits a predetermined response (referred to as a *signaling response*) when the partner arrives at the desired item/symbol. Symbols are menued via an SGD with electronic visual scanning. The learner activates the scanning mechanism (via an electronic switch), and a cursor (or change in symbol shade) indicates the symbol/group being menued. The learner then selects (via an electronic switch) the desired item. Activation techniques are discussed later in this chapter.

Scanning Patterns   **Scanning patterns** refer to the way items in the array are systematically menued (electronically or nonelectronically). Items may be menued individually; however, menuing can take a long time when there are several communicative items. Therefore, menuing items in groups may be more efficient. Determining the number of "pulses" (Kulikowski, 1986) required to access a symbol is one way to measure the efficiency of a scanning pattern. A pulse consists of the actual menuing of a symbol. Thus, if there are four symbols in an array, it would require one pulse to access the first symbol, two pulses to access the second, and so forth (see Figure 3.2). There are several patterns from which to choose, and each has advantages and disadvantages with respect to cognitive effort and speed with which symbols are accessed.

Symbols are arranged in a circular fashion in **circular scanning,** and items are menued (usually clockwise) via a hand as on a clock (see Figure 3.3) or by individual lights close to each symbol. Circular scanning is considered to be less cognitively demanding than other scanning arrays (Beukelman & Mirenda, 2005) because it does not require the learner to reorient to the cursor once it moves from one row to the next (as in **linear scanning**).

Symbols are arranged in one or more rows in linear scanning and are menued one at a time, usually from left to right (see Figure 3.2). When the cursor reaches the end of the row, it moves to the first symbol (from the left) in the next row. Cognitive demands associated with linear scanning are relatively low because the learner is only required to follow the cursor and occasionally glance at the target symbol to coordinate

the impending arrival of the cursor with switch activation. The learner must orient to the cursor when it drops from one row to the next, however, which might be difficult. One disadvantage is that it is relatively slow.

Two or more groups of symbols are offered in **group item scanning.** The learner first selects the group containing the target symbol. Symbols within that group are then menued.

Row column scanning in which symbols are arranged in rows is a common group item scanning pattern (see Figure 3.4). The cursor menues each row. When the cursor arrives at the row containing the desired symbol, the learner produces a discrete response causing the cursor to offer individual symbols within that row, moving from left to right. When the desired symbol is offered, the learner again produces a discrete response to make the selection.

Variations of group item scanning can be combined. For example, two or more groups of symbols are offered in **group row column scanning,** which proceeds among the rows and then items in the selected group. Although this scanning pattern requires three selection responses (one for the group, one for the row, and one for the column), it can increase speed when there are many items in the selection set (Beukelman & Mirenda, 2005).

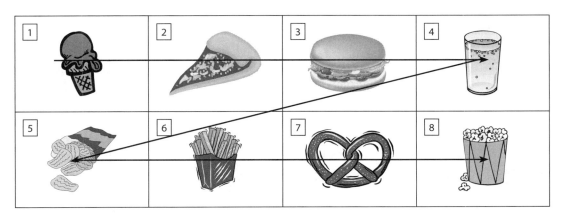

Figure 3.2.   Linear scanning pattern with number of pulses required to access each symbol.

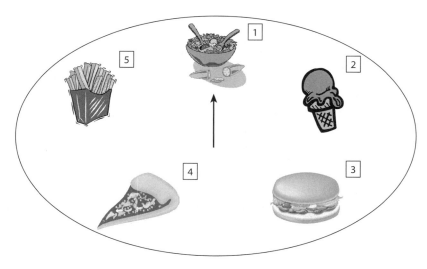

Figure 3.3. Circular scanning pattern in clockwise direction with corresponding number of pulses.

Symbols in visual scanning may be grouped by evenly dividing the display (e.g., one half, one third, one fourth) or arranged into semantic categories (e.g., nouns, verbs) or environments (e.g., rooms at home, classes). Groups of items can be assigned a label with **auditory scanning.** For example, FOOD, GAME, and WALK could be menued (electronically or nonelectronically), and items in the selected group are menued individually following a selection (e.g., CHIPS, COOKIE, PRETZEL).

The cognitive demands associated with group item scanning are greater than with circular or linear scanning. The learner must not only monitor the cursor but also must quickly scan the array to determine if the group being offered contains the de-

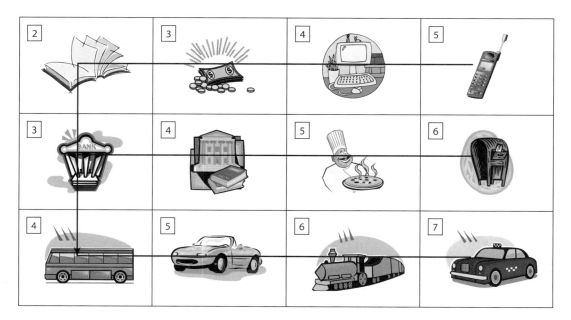

Figure 3.4. A group item scanning array (row column) with the number of pulses required to access each symbol.

sired symbol. Attention must continuously shift between the cursor and the group of symbols (row or column) more quickly and in a more coordinated fashion than during linear or circular scanning. The learner must also choose the group and then choose the item, requiring a chain of two signaling responses.

🐦 Helpful Hint

Symbols used in nonelectronic scanning can be placed on cards that are held up one at a time by the communication partner. The AAC user produces the signaling response when the card containing the desired symbol is menued. The communication partner then offers each item on that card. Symbols in a communication book can be offered in the same manner (i.e., first the pages of the book are offered, followed by groups of items and then individual items).

Directed/Joystick Scanning

Directed scanning can be considered a combination of direct selection and scanning because the learner directs the cursor to the desired symbol. The cursor typically begins in the center of the display in directed scanning (see the third display in Figure 3.5), requiring the use of a directional control switch (e.g., joystick, series of switches that control a different movement direction). Readers familiar with video games accessed via directional joysticks may be familiar with directed scanning. A computer mouse also functions in the same way because it directs the cursor on a computer.

An advantage of directed scanning is that it is faster than other scanning patterns because more symbols can be reached with fewer pulses when the cursor starts at the center. A disadvantage is that it requires the use of a multifunction switch, which might be difficult for some learners. It may also require a chain of signaling responses (change in direction of joystick or selection of multiple switches), resulting in cognitive demands that are greater than circular or linear scanning. It also requires the learner to identify the target symbol prior to initiat-

ing the cursor movement, again requiring a shift in attention between the cursor and symbol.

What Does the Research Say?

Petersen, Reichle, and Johnston (2000) compared preschoolers' (2–4 years) performance on linear and row column scanning patterns when selecting black-and-white line-drawn symbols on an SGD with a dynamic display. Although 23 children were recruited, only 12 met criteria (i. e., were able to successfully select symbols) during practice trials. No significant differences were found in the overall number of errors; however, there were differences in errors with respect to the number of cursor movements necessary to access a symbol as well as the number of times the cursor menued through the display.

McCarthy et al. (2006) conducted a study with 20 typically developing 2-year-olds randomly assigned to traditional or enhanced linear scanning of an array of three line-drawn animals. Items in the traditional scanning condition were offered by a red square moving across the array accompanied by a recorded voice labeling each item. The recorded voice labeled the item when it was selected. Items in the enhanced scanning condition were offered by appearing to move to the forefront of the screen increasing in size, and the recorded voice identified the choice with rising intonation (e.g., "Duck?"). The item moved in the same manner when the child made a selection, with the recorded voice labeling the item with flat intonation (e.g., "Duck."). After three instructional sessions, the children in the enhanced group were more than twice as accurate using enhanced scanning.

A handful of researchers have used a game format to teach scanning skills. For example, Light (1993) utilized a game of Tag to teach the relationship between the cursor and the target item in an array and between the switch activation and the selection of the item to a 4-year, 11-month-old girl who required more than thirty 20-minute instructional sessions to reach criterion. Horn, Jones, and Hamlett (1991) developed a video game in which children with speech and motor impairments were asked to "catch" a drawn animal by selecting the switch when the animal was in a drawing of a hand. One of three learners acquired scanning with three targets after approximately 10 instructional sessions. The others required 40 and 63 sessions, and their level of performance using an AAC device did not match that demonstrated when they were using the game.

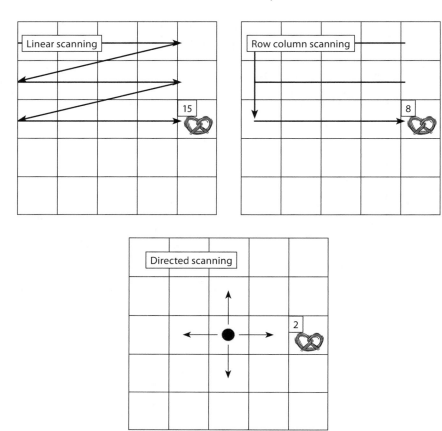

Figure 3.5. The number of pulses required to reach a symbol in the same location in each of three different 25-item displays.

USING EVIDENCE-BASED STRATEGIES TO TEACH VISUAL SCANNING

Visual scanning instruction can begin with the simple offering of actual items or symbols via pointing and can proceed through the electronic offering of sophisticated scanning patterns depending on the skill level of the AAC user. Procedural steps are as follows:

Step 1: *Identify teaching situations.* Start with requesting preferred items to enhance the learner's motivation to engage in the task. Actual items can be offered, or symbols can be used for learners discriminating between graphic representations.

Step 2: *Select a signaling response.* A signaling response is a discrete motor or vocal movement that is produced voluntarily (e.g., vocalization, motor response [raising hand, moving head to side], depressing a switch to activate a loop tape that says, "That's the one"). Be sure to choose a signaling response that can be easily prompted.

Step 3: *Teach the learner to use the signaling response conditionally (i.e., only when the communicative partner is pointing to the desired item).* Present the preferred item only, and then prompt the signaling response when the communicative partner points to the item. The communicative partner should delay pointing to the item on some occasions to ensure the learner only responds when the item has been offered. Vary the position of the item so that the learner continues to emit the signaling response regardless of its position.

Step 4: *Teach the learner to use the signaling response in the presence of multiple items.* Add items to the array once the learner consistently waits for the item to be offered before emitting the signaling response. Initially, a preferred item and an item of no particular interest should be displayed. Offer the target item first on some occasions, and offer the nontarget item first on other occasions. Continue to vary the positions of items to prevent the learner from selecting the signal based on where the item is located (position bias) rather than on which item is offered. More items can be added once the learner selects correctly from an array of two. Nontarget item(s) should still be used, however, to ensure the learner is discriminating between all of the items in the array.

MOVING FROM LINEAR TO ROW COLUMN SCANNING

Step 1: *Vary the scanning array.* Consider organizing some instructional opportunities with a vertical scanning array to prepare the learner to scan in the presence of more sophisticated arrays (e.g., row column). The symbol display can also be set up to facilitate acquisition. For example, if the learner has both general (e.g., *food, drinks, leisure items*) and specific vocabulary (e.g., *pretzel, burger, pizza; juice, milk, water*) within his or her repertoire, then the array can first be arranged so that general vocabulary are listed vertically as in Figure 3.6.

See Chapter 5 for more information on forward chaining procedures.

Step 2: *Expand the vertical display to a row column display.* Specific vocabulary can be added to each row depending on the skill level of the AAC user, with the symbol for the general category functioning as a label. Figure 3.7 illustrates an array that can be used during initial instruction. Notice there is only one choice for each row, and its position is varied across rows. After

the learner selects the symbol for DRINK, the cursor begins scanning the row. When it approaches JUICE, the learner can be prompted to select the more explicit symbol. Thus, a forward chain is used to teach the skill.

⮞ *Helpful Hint*

Some learners can benefit from using a game to teach scanning skills (Horn et al., 1991; Light 1993). A game using a row column scanning pattern can be used to determine a learner's readiness to move from linear to row column scanning. The interventionist asks, "Is this the row with the cheese?" while moving the mouse from row to row (see Figure 3.8). The learner should produce the signaling response when the mouse approaches the row with the cheese. The learner is likely ready to switch from linear to row column scanning when he or she successfully identifies the correct row.

TEACHING DIRECTED SCANNING

The symbol array can be divided into four quadrants to teach directed scanning, and instruction can take place within one quad-

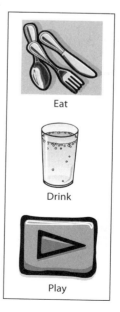

Figure 3.6. An example of a vertical display to prepare for instruction in row column scanning.

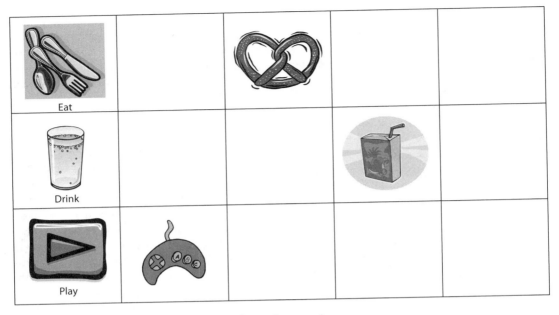

Figure 3.7. An example of an initial display used to teach row column scanning.

rant at a time. Figure 3.9 shows that the AAC user should be taught to move the cursor to the right to access some symbols in the upper right quadrant (X1 and X2) and up to access other symbols in the upper right quadrant (X3 and X4). Thus, instruction can proceed by teaching one direction at a time. The learner must combine upward and rightward cursor movements to access other symbols in the array, however.

If the learner is taught to access one symbol that requires the combined movements of up and right (e.g., X5), then he or she may be able to access (in the absence of instruction) the remaining symbols in that quadrant of the array (e.g., P1, P2, P3). If the learner fails to demonstrate generalization, then intervention should proceed by teaching additional examples prior to probing generalization within the quadrant.

Probes can be implemented at various positions in the remaining three quadrants once all symbols in the upper right quadrant have been accessed. If generalization has not occurred, then intervention should begin in either the upper left or the lower right quadrant because each of those quadrants requires one of the previous learned skills (e.g., moving the cursor up in the former, moving the cursor down in the latter). Intervention should then proceed in each of those quadrants in the same manner as described for the upper right quadrant.

What Are the Options for Switch Interface Adjustments?

Oftentimes, adjustments can be made to the switch interface in order to increase the accuracy of a learner's responses. Options for switch interface adjustments are discussed in the following sections.

Scanning Speed

Scanning speed refers to how quickly (or slowly) the cursor on an SGD (or communicative partner with nonelectronic scanning) moves from one symbol to the next. This feature is important for learners who require more time to produce the discrete response.

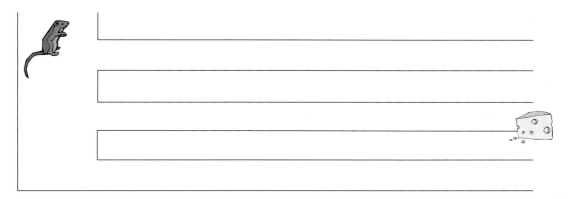

Figure 3.8. A maze game used to determine a learner's readiness to move from linear to row column scanning. (From Piche, L., & Reichle, J. [1991]. Teaching scanning selection techniques. In J. Reichle, J. York, & J. Sigafoos [Eds.], *Implementing augmentative and alternative communication: Strategies for learners with severe disabilities*. [p. 268]. Baltimore: Paul H. Brookes Publishing Co.; reprinted by permission.)

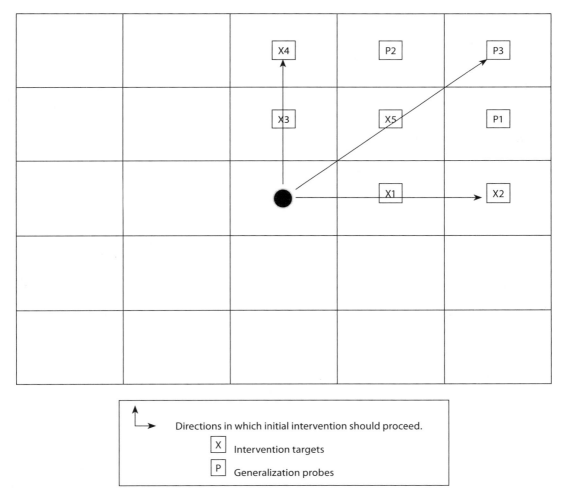

Figure 3.9. A directed scanning array indicating initial intervention strategies. (From Piche, L., & Reichle, J. [1991]. Teaching scanning selection techniques. In J. Reichle, J. York, & J. Sigafoos [Eds.], *Implementing augmentative and alternative communication: Strategies for learners with severe disabilities*. [p. 269]. Baltimore: Paul H. Brookes Publishing Co.; adapted by permission.)

Acceptance Time

Acceptance time is the amount of time that the AAC user maintains contact with the switch before the item is selected. Some SGDs allow for adjustment (e.g., set at 1 second, switch activation must be maintained for 1 second to select the item). This is appropriate for learners who may inadvertently activate their switch while unwanted items are offered.

Release Time

Release time is the amount of time following a switch activation in which any other activation of the same switch will not be accepted by the device (e.g., if a 2-second release time is set, then accidental selections will not be accepted for 2 seconds following a switch activation). This is particularly useful for learners who have limited motor control.

Switch Control Methods

Electronic scanning requires a switch activation to begin the scanning process, with the switch activated again to make a selection. Physical and cognitive capabilities should be considered, and learners should be given an opportunity to try each switch control technique (step, automatic, and inverse; Angelo, 1992).

Count or Step The cursor makes one movement through the array (from symbol to symbol in linear or circular scanning and from group to group, row to row, and item to item in group row item scanning) each time the learner activates the switch. The desired item is selected when the learner refrains from making another switch activation for a specified period of time. Alternatively, the learner can select a second switch to indicate the desired symbol. This technique is useful for learners beginning to acquire scanning skills because the correspondence

See Chapter 4 for a review of the research related to switch control methods.

between each switch activation and the movement of the cursor can be a salient feature. It is also useful for learners who have a tendency to "miss" opportunities to select the desired symbol during other control techniques. However, for learners with severe motor limitations, the required switch activations may result in fatigue (Beukelman & Mirenda, 2005).

Automatic The AAC user activates the switch to start the cursor, and the cursor moves through the array until the switch is activated a second time, resulting in the selection of the desired item. This switch control is useful for learners who can accurately activate the switch but who have difficulty maintaining activation (Beukelman & Mirenda, 2005).

Inverse The AAC user activates and maintains activation for the cursor to begin and continue menuing items. An item is selected when the learner releases the switch. This type of switch activation is appropriate for learners who can easily maintain switch activation.

What Does the Research Say?

Several studies compared the use of direct selection techniques with indirect selection techniques (e.g., scanning). Ratcliff (1994) compared direct selection with an optical head pointer to row column scanning with a single switch. One hundred typically developing elementary students were randomly assigned to either direct selection or scanning and asked to locate a single shape in an array of 128 shapes on a Prentke Romich Light Talker. Students using row column scanning had significantly more selection errors than those using direct selection via optical head pointer.

Mizuko and Esser (1991) investigated the effect of selection technique on visual sequential recall. They taught 12 typically developing 4-year-olds to select two- or three-symbol sequences using direct selection (via pointing) or circular scanning (via a single-switch **inverse scanning**). No significant differences between performance across the two groups were found. *(continued)*

Szeto, Allen, and Littrell (1993) compared the speed of using row column scanning with a single switch, directed scanning via joystick, and direct selection via a head mounted light pointer on four different devices with 16 typically developing college students. Direct selection using the head-mounted light pointer was the fastest of the methods across all four devices. The joystick was more rapid than single-switch row column scanning for some devices.

Mizuko et al. (1994) examined the effects of selection techniques and array size on short-term memory. Twenty-two typically developing 4-year-olds were randomly assigned to direct selection or row column scanning conditions, shown pairs of line drawings, and asked to find the same symbols in the same order on arrays of 10, 20, 30, and 40 items. The presence of the 40-item display was the only difference in performance between the groups; students assigned to the direct selection group performed better.

Horn and Jones (1996) taught a nonverbal 48-month-old child with cerebral palsy to select line-drawn symbols. Performance during direct selection via a head-mounted optical pointer versus scanning using an inverse circular scanning technique was compared. The child's frequency of correct responses using direct selection was higher, whereas his average response time was shorter. Thus, the optical pointer appeared to be the more appropriate selection technique.

Dropik and Reichle (2008) compared the performance of 13 typically developing preschoolers during directed scanning and group item scanning while selecting line-drawn symbols from a 36-symbol array. The children were more accurate using directed versus group item scanning. Although there were no time differences with respect to selection techniques, a greater number of cursor movements were required in the group item scanning condition.

Wagner and Jackson (2006) compared the cognitive demands of direct selection and visual linear scanning in 120 typically developing kindergarten, first-, and third-grade students. Children randomly assigned to direct selection or visual linear scanning were asked to recreate displays of line-drawn symbols by selecting identical symbols on fixed displays. Participants selected more corresponding line drawings during direct selection than scanning, with older children performing better than younger children. Differences were attributed to cognitive demands associated with scanning, engaging in anticipatory monitoring as the cursor menued items, and keeping the original display in working memory while waiting for the cursor to menu the items.

Auditory Scanning

Items in the form of words or even environmental sounds (e.g., beeping horn to represent an automobile, barking to represent a dog) are menued for the AAC user either nonelectronically or electronically when using auditory scanning.

Nonelectronic Auditory Scanning

A communication partner verbally menues the items in **nonelectronic auditory scanning.** For example, a teacher might offer activities (reading, math, computer), with the learner subsequently indicating his or her selection by emitting a predetermined response (e.g., vocalization, motor response) or activating a loop tape that says, "That's the one," when the desired item is mentioned.

Electronic Auditory Scanning

Items are menued by an SGD in electronic auditory scanning. Subsequently, when the desired item has been offered, the learner would activate a switch to signal a selection. A "pillow speaker" or earphones allow the items to be offered at a volume only the AAC user can hear. The selected message is produced at a volume loud enough for the communication partner to hear. SGDs also allow for an abbreviated message to be offered to the speaker (e.g., names can be menued, such as GRANDMA, EVE, KAREN), and a more elaborate message can be spoken when the desired message is selected for the benefit of the listener (e.g., I WANT TO GO TO EVE'S HOUSE).

A straightforward decision can be made about which scanning technique is most appropriate for a given learner. Specifically, if a learner has a visual impairment preventing him or her from seeing or discriminating among symbols, then texture symbols or auditory scanning might be more appropriate. Auditory scanning requires memory skills, however, because the learner must recall and compare the choices in the absence of a permanent display. If the same learner can benefit from voice output, then an electronic auditory scanning system might be appropriate. It would also allow him or her to independently access the scanning mechanism and, thus, not be dependent on a communicative partner to menu the items.

USING EVIDENCE-BASED STRATEGIES TO TEACH AUDITORY SCANNING

Auditory scanning can range from the use of a communicative partner for verbally listing a choice of items to the use of an SGD for menuing items. Following are procedural steps for auditory scanning instruction:

Step 1: Identify teaching situations. Beginning with situations in which the learner is requesting access to preferred items will likely enhance his or her motivation to engage in the task.

Step 2: Select a signaling response. A signaling response is one that is emitted voluntarily; for example, a vocalization, a motor response (e.g., raising a hand, moving head to the side), or depressing a switch that activates a loop tape that says, "That's the one." It is important to choose a signaling response that can be easily prompted.

Step 3: Teach the learner to use the signaling response conditionally (i.e., only when the communicative partner menus the desired item) by verbally menuing the preferred item and then immediately prompting the learner to emit the signaling response. If the partner touches a symbol representing an undesired item, the learner should refrain from responding.

Step 4: Teach the learner to use the signaling response. Teach the conditional use of a signaling response in the presence of multiple choices. Initially, one choice should be a neutral item that prevents the learner from using the signaling response when any item is offered and helps determine if the learner is using the signaling response conditionally. Learners may also have a tendency to select the last item named (i.e., order of mention selection strategy). If this happens, then initially

offer the desired item first and the nondesired item last. Randomize the order of the items when the learner is consistently signaling in response to the desired item. (Or, the desired item can be menued at a higher volume than the neutral item). More items can be be offered once the learner is selecting from a choice of two items.

☞ *Helpful Hint*

Learners with extensive communicative repertoires might benefit from group item auditory scanning. The communicative partner menus groups of items (e.g., SNACKS, MUSIC, PLACES). The communicative partner menus items within the group (e.g., CHIPS, PRETZELS, APPLE) when the learner makes his or her choice.

RATE ENHANCEMENT STRATEGIES

Individuals with severe disabilities who use AAC often have difficulty fully participating in communicative interactions (Harris, 1982; Light, Collier, & Parnes, 1985). The relatively slow rate of communication by AAC system users when compared with verbal language users is one variable that contributes to this difficulty. A variety of strategies can be used to enhance rate of communication, including encoding, slots, and message prediction.

Encoding refers to any strategy in which the user can use multiple signals (e.g., a sequence of symbols or keystrokes) that together specify a desired message. Encoding can increase the number of prestored messages on a fixed/static display because it uses one or more symbols to communicate a message. Consider a learner who uses a six-symbol display. The learner could only communicate six different prestored messages without encoding. The learner, however, could communicate these six different prestored messages plus any messages that are stored under combinations of those symbols with encoding. In addition, encoding allows a learner to use the same symbol in pragmatically different ways. For example, a symbol for ORANGE JUICE could activate the comment "orange juice," a symbol for WANT could activate the request "I want that," a symbol for LIKE could activate the comment "I like that," and a symbol for YOU could represent the request for information "Do you like that?" These four symbols could each be used in isolation or they could be combined with encoding to represent the following"

- "I'd like some orange juice, please." (WANT symbol and ORANGE JUICE symbol)

- "I like orange juice." (LIKE symbol and ORANGE JUICE symbol)

- "Do you like orange juice." (YOU symbol and ORANGE JUICE symbol)

A number of encoding techniques are available to AAC system users (see Beukelman & Mirenda, 2005, for a complete review). **Letter category codes** and **iconic codes** are among the more common techniques used by individuals with severe disabilities.

Letter Category Codes

Letter category codes typically involve two or more letters in which the first represents a category and the second represents a specific word or phrase within that category. For example, when letter category codes are used for single words, the letter S might represent the category "sports," then SF for football, SB for basketball, and SS for soccer. Similarly, if the letter M represents the category "movies," then MC for comedy, MD for drama, and MA for action. The first letter in a category code used for phrases might be H to represent the general category "requesting help or assistance." Then, the second letter would represent the specific message within that category (e.g., HB for "Help me move my body," HU for "Help me understand," HO for "Help me open this").

Iconic Codes

Iconic codes use icons (e.g., picture symbols) to represent words or phrases. A picture of a smiling face might represent "like," a picture of a house might represent "home," and a picture of a cup might represent "coffee." The smiling face and home symbols

used together would be "I'd like to go home now, please." The smiling face and cup symbols used together would be "I'd like some coffee, please." Semantic compaction or Minspeak (Baker, 1982) is one frequently encountered iconic coding technique. In this system, icons are selected based on their semantic associations (e.g., the sun icon might represent "weather, yellow, hot, outside"; the clock icon might represent "time, schedule, numbers"). The icons can be combined to form messages (e.g., clock combined with sun might represent "It's time to go outside").

What Does the Research Say?

Research investigating issues related to encoding techniques is limited. Yet, findings in this area include the following:

- Angelo (1992) examined learning curves and retrieval speed for three encoding methods (word truncation using the first three letters of each word; word contraction using the first letter, middle consonant, and last letter of each word; and random codes, which were two letters randomly chosen for each word) with 66 typically developing college students randomly assigned to one of the three methods. Results revealed that truncation was learned and retrieved faster than the other two methods.

- Beukelman and Yorkston (1984) found participants (10 literate adults without disabilities) performed most accurately and retrieved codes most quickly using encoding strategies that followed a logical pattern compared with codes that were arbitrary.

- Hinderscheit and Reichle (1987) taught an 18-year-old woman with severe cognitive delays and physical disabilities to encode to increase the available vocabulary on her fixed display communication board.

- Light, Lindsay, Siegel, and Parnes (1990) found that participants (six adults who were nonverbal, functionally literate, and had physical disabilities) recalled salient letter codes more accurately than letter category codes or iconic-based codes. Furthermore, the researchers found that recall was better for concrete than for abstract messages.

- Light and Lindsay (1992) found that participants (12 adults with severe speech impairments who had phys-

(continued)

ical disabilities) were more accurate in recalling codes using a two-letter encoding technique than when using an iconic coding technique, with no differences found between recall performance with personalized versus nonpersonalized codes. Code recall improved over time across all techniques, and accuracy was higher for recalling codes for concrete versus abstract messages, with no significant differences in rates of learning across encoding techniques.

- Light, Drager, McCarthy, et al. (2004) found that participants (80 typically developing 4- and 5-year-old children) were more accurate locating target vocabulary in the three dynamic display conditions (taxonomic grid, schematic grid, schematic scene) than in an iconic encoding condition.

- Hill, Holko, and Romich (2001) discussed that research based on individuals who rely on AAC revealed that communication rate using encoding can be up to 6 times that of spelling.

Slots are a second strategy related to rate enhancement. Slots allow learners to take advantage of sentence starters such as "I would like _____," "I am _____," and "After school, I am going _____" without requiring a separate symbol/button for each of the possible endings to the sentence starter. A choice of different slot fillers appears when a learner selects a symbol that functions as a slot (e.g., the place holder on the DynaVox Vmax is indicated by text that is blue and a symbol that is underlined). For example, if a learner selects the symbol with the sentence starter representing "After school, I am going _____," then slot fillers such as "home," "to grandma's," "to the doctor," "shopping," and so forth appear.

Message prediction techniques provide another strategy for increasing the overall rate of AAC users' communication. A list of options are suggested when letters, number, and symbols are entered. The user then completes the message by selecting the desired option. A number of message prediction techniques are available to AAC users, including icon prediction, **single letter prediction**,

word prediction, and **phrase/sentence prediction** (Beukelman & Mirenda, 2005).

What Does the Research Say?

- Koester and Levine (1998) examined the influence of word prediction on user performance during text entry tasks. Fourteen participants (eight participants were able-bodied and used mouth-stick typing, six participants had high-level spinal cord injury and used their typical method of keyboard access) transcribed text with and without a word prediction feature. Results revealed that word prediction significantly decreased text generation rate for the participants with spinal cord injury and only modestly enhanced it for the able-bodied participants. The authors indicated that the cognitive cost of using word prediction largely overwhelmed the benefit provided by keystroke savings under the conditions established in this experiment.

- Lanspa, Wood, and Beukelman (1997) compared the effect of word list order (length, alphabetic, and frequency of word use) on rate with target words identified from a word prompt list. Results revealed that participants (14 students without disabilities between 10 and 13 years of age, 14 students with language/learning disabilities between 8 and 15 years of age) identified target words more quickly when words were ordered by length.

- Tam, Reid, Naumann, and O'Keefe (2002) evaluated the effect of word prediction on the rate and accuracy of text entry when the location of the word prediction list was manipulated (e.g., upper right corner, following the cursor, lower middle border) with four children ages 10–12 years with spina bifida and hydrocephalus. Results revealed that word prediction did not improve rate but did improve accuracy of text entry. No statistical differences were found in rate or accuracy across the different locations of the word prediction list. Three participants had their lowest rate, and all participants had their lowest accuracy when the prediction list followed the cursor, however.

- Venkatagiri (1994) evaluated the effect of "window" size (the number of words displayed in a word selection menu) on the efficiency of communication for 21 adult female college students. Results revealed that a 15-word window produced roughly the same rate of

(continued)

communication (e.g., message preparation time) as a five-word window but with significantly less effort (keystrokes/switch activations).

- Higginbotham, Bisantz, Sunm, Adams, and Yik (2009) explored performance related to different word prediction techniques across two conditions for 24 pairs of adults without disabilities as they completed three tasks. In one condition, the SGD was primed with task-specific vocabulary. In the other condition, the SGD was not primed with task-specific vocabulary. Results revealed that context priming had a marginally significant effect on keystroke savings. Savings in number of keystrokes, however, did not translate into higher levels on communication or task performance measures. Based on these findings, the authors suggested that measures such as number of keystrokes may not predict SGD performance in communicative interactions.

- Drager and Light (2010) examined the impact of icon prediction on learning to locate and generalize vocabulary with 20 typically developing 5-year-old children. Results indicated children who used icon prediction did not perform more accurately than children who did not use icon prediction. Data did suggest, however, that icon prediction may help to facilitate generalization of the use of iconic encoding to novel vocabulary.

Translating Research to Practice

Rate enhancement techniques help a learner to more quickly access symbols/messages. Encoding, slots, and message prediction are three strategies to enhance the rate of communication. Being aware of the variety of encoding techniques available for AAC users is important. It is equally important to determine whether an individual might benefit from an encoding technique and, if yes, which encoding technique(s) should be considered for a specific individual. Issues to consider when making these decisions include the following:

- Can the individual use single symbols to communicate wants/needs? If no, then interventionists should teach single-symbol use before considering encoding, slots, and message prediction.

- Does the individual have sufficient symbols on his or her AAC system and/or communication needs to warrant encoding as a rate enhancement technique? If no, then encoding, slots, and message prediction may not be of benefit at this time. (It may be helpful to teach the AAC user to use these strategies now, however, so that he or she is able to use them in the future.)

- What symbol set(s)/feature(s) does the individual use (or may use in the future) as part of his or her AAC system? If the learner uses letters and numbers, then consider alpha encoding and/or **alphanumeric encoding.** If the learner uses icons, then consider using iconic encoding.

ENVIRONMENTAL CONTROLS

Many SGDs also provide control over other aspects of the environment, which may be useful for individuals who have physical challenges in addition to communication impairments. That is, many devices have the capability to act as an interface with televisions, CD players, video game devices, telephones (also cell phones), and so forth, allowing the AAC user who has limited mobility independent access to activities.

What Does the Research Say?

There are a limited number of studies that examined strategies for teaching individuals with severe disabilities to use environmental controls. Lancioni, O'Reilly, Oliva, and Coppa (2001) taught two children with multiple disabilities (7 and 9 years) to use vocal responses to activate a microswitch, which in turn activated recordings of preferred auditory stimuli (e.g., songs, animal calls, bells). Both participants increased their frequency of vocalization and, thus, their access to the recordings.

Lancioni, Singh, O'Reilly, and Oliva (2003) taught two participants (17 and 19 years) with multiple disabilities, including visual impairments, to activate multiple microswitches. Three messages were linked to each of three

(continued)

microswitches so that one of the three messages was emitted (e.g., activating a push-button switch resulted in the menuing of dance music, a second activation resulted in stories being menued, and a third activation resulted in voices being menued) each time a microswitch was activated. The participant emitted a vocal utterance when reaching the desired choice, and, in turn, a voice-detecting device activated the actual event (e.g., a story played, voices played). Four to six 20-minute instructional sessions were implemented daily by research assistants. A multiple probe design across microswitches indicated little to no switch activations in baseline and consistent use of the three switches as well as the choice activation switch following intervention. Probes conducted 1 and 2 months later revealed similar performance with parents and educational staff.

SUMMARY

Interventionists must be knowledgeable in the features of AAC systems as well as the ways in which individual features may enhance an AAC user's communication to ensure individuals with severe disabilities are provided with AAC systems that meet their needs as well as the needs of their communication partners. This chapter provided an overview of aided AAC system features, explained how specific features of AAC systems may enhance communicative efficiency and/or effectiveness, and discussed ways in which research related to AAC system features can be used to support evidence-based practice.

REFERENCES

Angelo, J. (1992). A comparison of three coding methods for abbreviation expansion in acceleration vocabularies. *International Journal of Rehabilitation Research, 13,* 161–166.

Baker, B. (1982). Minspeak: A semantic compaction system that makes self-expression easier for communicatively disabled individuals. *Byte, 7,* 186–202.

Battenberg, J.K., & Merbler, J.B. (1989). Touch screen versus keyboard: A comparison of task performance of young children. *Journal of Special Education Technology, 10,* 24–28.

Beck, A.R., Stoner, J.B., Bock, S.J., & Parton, T. (2008). Comparison of PECS and the use of a VOCA: A replication. *Education and Training in Developmental Disabilities, 43,* 198–216

Beukelman, D.R., & Mirenda, P. (2005). *Augmentative and alternative communication: Supporting children and adults with complex communication needs* (3rd ed.). Baltimore: Paul H. Brookes Publishing Co.

Beukelman, D., & Yorkston, K. (1984). Computer enhancement of message formulation and presentation for communication augmentation system users. *Seminars in Speech and Language, 5,* 1–10.

Bock, S.J., Stoner, J.B., Beck, A.R., Hanley, L., & Prochnow, J. (2005). Increasing functional communication in nonspeaking preschool children: Comparison of PECS and VOCA. *Education and Training in Developmental Disabilities, 40,* 264–278.

Bondy, A., & Frost, L. (1994). The Picture Exchange Communication System. *Focus on Autistic Behavior, 9,* 1–19.

Cook, A.M., & Hussey, S.M. (1995). *Assistive technologies: Principles and practice.* St. Louis: Mosby.

Dietz, A., McKelvey, M., & Beukelman, D. (2006). Visual scene displays (VSD): New AAC interfaces for persons with aphasia. *Perspectives on Augmentative and Alternative Communication, 15,* 13–17.

Dowden, P., & Cook, A.M. (2002). Choosing effective selection techniques for beginning communicators. In D. Beukelman & J. Reichle (Series Eds.) & J. Reichle, D.R. Beukelman, & J.C. Light (Vol. Eds.), *AAC series: Exemplary practices for beginning communicators: Implications for AAC* (pp. 395–429). Baltimore: Paul H. Brookes Publishing Co.

Drager, K.D.R., Clark-Serpentine, E.A., Johnson, K.E., & Roeser, J.L. (2006). Accuracy of repetition of digitized and synthesized speech for young children in background noise. *American Journal of Speech-Language Pathology, 15,* 155–164.

Drager, K., & Light, J. (2010). A comparison of the performance of 5-year-old children with typical development using iconic encoding in AAC systems with and without icon prediction on a fixed display. *Augmentative and Alternative Communication, 26*(1), 12–20.

Drager, K., Light, J., Angert, E., Finke, E., Larson, H., Venzon, L., & Johnson, J. (2005, November). AAC and interactive play: Language learning in children with autism. Seminar presented at the Annual Convention of the American Speech-Language-Hearing Association, San Diego, CA.

Drager, K., Light, J., Carlson, R., D'Silva, K., Larsson, B., Pitkin, L., et al. (2004). Learning of dynamic display AAC technologies by typically developing 3-year-olds: Effect of different layouts and menu approaches. *Journal of Speech, Language, and Hearing Research, 47*, 1133–1148.

Drager, K., Light, J., Curran Speltz, J., Fallon, K., & Jeffries, L. (2003). The performance of typically developing 2½-year-olds on dynamic display AAC technologies with different system layouts and language organizations. *Journal of Speech, Language, and Hearing Research, 46*, 298–312.

Dropik, P.L., & Reichle, J. (2008). Comparison of accuracy and efficiency of directed scanning and group-item scanning for augmentative communication selection techniques with typically developing preschoolers. *American Journal of Speech-Language Pathology, 17*, 35–47.

Dudek, K., Beck, A., & Thompson, J. (2006). The influence of AAC device type, dynamic vs. static screen, on peer attitudes. *Journal of Special Education Technology, 21*(1), 17–27.

Durfee, J.L., & Billingsley, F.F. (1999). Comparison of two computer input devices for uppercase letter matching. *American Journal of Occupational Therapy, 53*, 214–220.

Dyches, T.T., Davis, A., Lucido, B.R., & Young, J.R. (2002). Generalization of skills using pictographic and voice output communication devices. *Augmentative and Alternative Communication, 18*, 124–131.

Goossens', C. (1989). Aided communication intervention before assessment: A case study of a child with cerebral palsy. *Augmentative and Alternative Communication, 5*, 14–26.

Goossens', C., & Crain, S. (1987). Overview of nonelectronic eye-gaze communication devices. *Augmentative and Alternative Communication, 3*, 77–89.

Harris, D. (1982). Communicative interaction processes involving nonvocal physically handicapped children. *Topics in Language Disorders, 2*(2), 21–37.

Hetzroni, O.R., & Rubin, C. (2006). Identifying patterns of communicative behaviors in girls with Rett syndrome. *Augmentative and Alternative Communication, 22*, 48–61

Higginbotham, J., Bisantz, A., Sunm, M., Adams, K., & Yik, F. (2009). The effect of context priming and task type on augmentative communication performance. *Augmentative and Alternative Communication, 25*, 19–31.

Hill, K., Holko, R., & Romich, B. (2001, November). *AAC performance: The elements of communication rate.* Poster presented at the American-Speech-Language Hearing (ASHA) Annual Convention, New Orleans, LA.

Hinderscheit, L., & Reichle, J. (1987). Teaching direct select color encoding to an adolescent

with multiple handicaps. *Augmentative and Alternative Communication, 3*, 137–142.

Horn, E.M., & Jones, H.A. (1996). Comparison of two selection techniques used in augmentative and alternative communication. *Augmentative and Alternative Communication, 12*, 23–31.

Horn, E., Jones, H., & Hamlett, C. (1991). An investigation of the feasibility of a video game system for developing scanning and selection skills. *Journal of The Association for Persons with Severe Handicaps, 16*, 108–115.

Iacono, T., & Duncum, J. (1995). Comparison of sign alone and in combination with an electronic communication device in early language intervention: Case study. *Augmentative and Alternative Communication, 11*, 249–259.

Iacono, T., Mirenda, P., & Beukelman, D.R. (1993). Comparison of unimodal and multimodal AAC techniques for children with intellectual disabilities. *Augmentative and Alternative Communication, 9*, 83–94.

Koester, H. (2004). Usage, performance, and satisfaction outcomes for experienced users of automatic speech recognition. *Journal of Rehabilitation Research and Development, 41*, 739–754

Koester, H.H., & Levine, S.P. (1998). Model simulations of user performance with word prediction. *Augmentative and Alternative Communication, 14*, 25–35.

Kulikowski, S. (1986). *Scanning data types in nonvocal communication.* Paper presented at Closing the Gap Conference, Minneapolis, MN.

Lancioni, G.E., O'Reilly, M.F., Oliva, D., & Coppa, M.M. (2001). Using multiple microswitches to promote different responses in children with multiple disabilities. *Research in Developmental Disabilities, 22*, 309–318.

Lancioni., G.E., O'Reilly, M.F., Singh, N.N., Sigafoos, J., Oliva, D., Montironi, G., et al. (2005). Extending the evaluation of a computer system used as a microswitch for word utterances of persons with multiple disabilities. *Journal of Intellectual Disability Research, 49*, 639–646.

Lancioni, G.E., Singh, N.N., O'Reilly, M.F., & Oliva, D. (2003). Some recent research efforts on microswitches for persons with multiple disabilities. *Journal of Child and Family Studies, 12*, 251–256.

Lancioni, G.E., Singh, N., O'Reilly, M.F., Oliva, D., Montironi, G., Piazza, F., et al. (2004). Using computer systems as microswitches for vocal utterances of persons with multiple disabilities. *Research in Developmental Disabilities, 25*, 183–192.

Lancioni, G.E., Singh, N.N., O'Reilly, M.F., Sigafoos, J., Oliva, D., & Montironi, G. (2004). Evaluating a computer system used as a microswitch for word utterances of persons with multiple disabilities. *Disability and Rehabilitation, 26*, 1286–1290.

Lanspa, A., Wood, L., & Beukelman, D. (1997). Efficiency with which disabled and nondisabled students locate words in cue windows: Study of three organizational structures—frequency of word use, word length, and alphabetical order. *Augmentative and Alternative Communication, 13*, 117–125.

Light, J. (1993). Teaching automatic linear scanning for computer access: A case study of a preschooler with severe physical and communication disabilities. *Journal of Special Education Technology, 21*, 135–134.

Light, J. (1997). Communication is the essence of human life: Reflections on communication competence. *Augmentative and Alternative Communication, 13*, 61–70.

Light, J., Collier, B., & Parnes, P. (1985). Communicative interaction between young nonspeaking physically disabled children and their primary caregivers: Part I: Discourse patterns. *Augmentative and Alternative Communication, 1*, 74–83.

Light, J., & Drager, K. (2005, November). *Maximizing language development with young children who require AAC.* Seminar presented at the Annual Convention of the American Speech-Language-Hearing Association, San Diego, CA.

Light, J., & Drager, K. (2007). AAC technologies for young children with complex communication needs: State of the science and future research directions. *Augmentative and Alternative Communication, 23*, 204–216.

Light, J., Drager, K., McCarthy, J., Mellott, S., Parrish, C., Parsons, A., et al. (2004). Performance of typically developing four and five year old children with AAC systems using different language organization techniques. *Augmentative and Alternative Communication, 20*, 63–88.

Light, J., & Lindsay, P. (1992). Message-encoding techniques for augmentative communication systems: The recall performances of adults with severe speech impairments. *Journal of Speech and Hearing Research, 35*, 853–864.

Light, J., Lindsay, P., Siegel, L., & Parnes, P. (1990). The effects of message encoding techniques on recall by literate adults using AAC systems. *Augmentative and Alternative Communication, 6*, 184–201.

Light, J., Wilkinson, K., & Drager, K. (2008, November). *Designing effective AAC systems: Research evidence and implications for practice.* Paper presented at the Annual Conference of the American Speech-Language-Hearing Association, Chicago.

McCarthy, J., Light, J., Drager, K., McNaughton, D., Grodzicki, L., Jones, J., et al. (2006). Redesigning scanning to reduce learning demand: The performance of typically developing 2-year-olds. *Augmentative and Alternative Communication, 22*, 269–283.

McDonald, E., & Schultz, A. (1973). Communication boards for cerebral palsied children. *Journal of Speech and Hearing Disorders, 38*, 73–88.

Millar, D.C., Light, J.C., & Schlosser, R.W. (2006). The impact of augmentative and alternative communication intervention on the speech production of individuals with developmental disabilities: A research review. *Journal of Speech, Language, and Hearing Research, 49*, 248–264.

Mizuko, M., & Esser, J. (1991). The effect of direct selection and circular scanning on visual sequential recall. *Journal of Speech and Hearing Research, 34*, 43–48.

Mizuko, M., Reichle, J., Ratcliff, A., & Esser, J. (1994). Effects of selection techniques and array size on short-term visual memory. *Augmentative and Alternative Communication, 10*, 237–244.

Olin, A.R., Reichle, J., Johnson, L., & Monn, E. (2010). Examining dynamic visual scene displays: Implications for arranging and teaching symbol selection. *American Journal of Speech-Language Pathology, 19*, 284–297.

Petersen, K., Reichle, J., & Johnston, S.S. (2000). Examining preschoolers' performance in linear and row-column scanning techniques. *Augmentative and Alternative Communication, 16*, 27–36.

Ratcliff, A. (1994). Comparison of relative demands implicated in direct selection and scanning: Considerations from normal children. *Augmentative and Alternative Communication, 10*, 67–74.

Reichle, J., Dettling, E., Drager, K., & Leiter, A. (2000). Comparison of correct responses and response latency for fixed and dynamic displays: Performance of a learner with severe developmental disabilities. *Augmentative and Alternative Communication, 16*, 154–163.

Reichle, J., Halle, J., & Drasgow, E. (1998). Implementing augmentative communication systems. In S.F. Warren & M.E. Fey (Series Eds.) & A. Wetherby, S. Warren, & J. Reichle (Vol. Eds.), *Communication and language intervention series: Vol. 7. Transitions to prelinguistic communication: Pre-intentional to intentional and pre-symbolic to symbolic* (pp. 417–436). Baltimore: Paul H. Brookes Publishing Co.

Romski, M.A., Sevcik, R.A., & Adamson, L.B. (1999). Communication patterns of youth with and without their communication devices. *American Journal on Mental Retardation, 104*, 249–259.

Schlosser, R.W., Belfiore, P.J., Nigam, R., Blischak, D., & Hetzroni, O. (1995). The effects of speech output technology in the learning of graphic symbols. *Journal of Applied Behavior Analysis, 28*, 537–549.

Schlosser, R., & Wendt, O. (2008). Effects of augmentative and alternative communication intervention on speech production in children with autism: A systematic review. *American Journal of Speech-Language Pathology, 17*(3), 212–230.

Sigafoos, J., Didden, R., & O'Reilly, M. (2003). Effects of speech output on maintenance of requesting and frequency of vocalizations in three children with developmental disabilities. *Augmentative and Alternative Communication, 9,* 37–47.

Son, S., Sigafoos, J., O'Reilly, M., & Lancioni, G.E. (2006). Comparing two types of augmentative and alternative communication systems for children with autism. *Pediatric Rehabilitation, 9,* 389–395.

Soto, G., Belfiore, P.J., Schlosser, R.W., & Haynes, C. (1993). Teaching specific requests: A comparative analysis on skill acquisition and preference using two augmentative and alternative communication aids. *Education and Training in Mental Retardation, 28,* 169–178.

Szeto, A., Allen, E., & Littrell, M. (1993). Comparison of speed and accuracy for selected electronic communication devices and input methods. *Augmentative and Alternative Communication, 9,* 229–242.

Tam, C., Reid, D., Naumann, S., & O'Keefe, B. (2002). Effects of word *predication* and location of word prediction list on text entry with children with spina bifida and hydrocephalus. *Augmentative and Alternative Communication, 18,* 147–162.

Venkatagiri, H.S. (1994). Effect of window size on rate of communication in a lexical prediction AAC system. *Augmentative and Alternative Communication, 10,* 105–112.

Wagner, B.T., & Jackson, H.M. (2006). Developmental memory capacity resources of typical children retrieving picture communication symbols using direct selection and visual linear scanning with fixed communication displays. *Journal of Speech Language, and Hearing Research, 49,* 113–126.

Improving Communicative Competence Through Alternative Selection Methods

4

Patricia Dowden and Albert M. Cook

▷ CHAPTER OVERVIEW

This chapter addresses individuals with complex communication needs who require an alternative selection method because of their physical disabilities. The challenges can be immense in implementing aided communication with this population when a learner has not had previous experience with a more conventional communication system. Additional complications arise if the individual has sensory or cognitive limitations. The chapter also describes a myriad of technology-based tools, such as keyboards, switches, and joysticks, as well as no-tech strategies, such as letter, word, and symbol displays.

▷ CHAPTER OBJECTIVES

After studying this chapter, readers will be able to

- Develop interventions to address an alternative method of communication for individuals who do not yet have a means of symbolic communication
- Identify alternatives to direct selection for individuals with severe motor impairments
- Discuss uses of technology for early communicators who need alternative selection methods
- Develop interventions to make existing selection methods (scanning or other alternative methods) more efficient for individuals
- Improve the communicative competence of individuals who need alternative selection methods

▷ KEY TERMS

- acceptance time
- aided symbolic communication
- asymmetrical tonic neck reflex (ATNR)
- communicative competence
- communicative independence

- context-dependent communicator
- control interface
- control site
- direct selection
- dyadic eye gaze
- dynamic matrix rearrangement
- dysconjugate gaze

- emerging communicator
- independent communicator
- indirect selection
- latching switch
- linguistic competence
- Model of Communicative Independence
- momentary switch

- ▶ operational competence
- ▶ Partner-Assisted Scanning (PAS)
- ▶ potential communicative acts (PCAs)
- ▶ primitive reflexes

- ▶ rate enhancement
- ▶ resolution
- ▶ selection technique
- ▶ social competence
- ▶ strategic competence
- ▶ switch latch

- ▶ switch latch and timer
- ▶ tonic labyrinthine reflex (TLR)
- ▶ triadic eye gaze
- ▶ unaided symbolic communication
- ▶ volitional

ALTERNATIVES TO DIRECT SELECTION

Access to augmentative and alternative communication (AAC) is straightforward for many individuals who are able to touch keys on a device or point to symbols on visual displays. Individuals with severe motor disabilities have more difficulty accessing AAC systems, and it often becomes a primary limitation in the effectiveness of their communication. The term **direct selection** is used universally to describe one type of **selection technique** in which the individual points to the desired item directly, using fingers, hands, a headwand, a mouthwand, or a foot. All items in the selection set are available to the user at the same time with direct selection; there is no waiting for intermediary steps as in other selection methods (Cook & Polgar, 2008). There is less agreement regarding the term to use for all other methods of selection. We prefer the term **indirect selection** to highlight the fact that the individual can only make a selection after waiting for some intermediary steps by the device or the partner. Indirect techniques include (Dowden & Cook, 2002) the following:

- *Single- or dual-switch scanning*: Items are presented sequentially to the user.

- *Directed/joystick scanning*: The user directs the curser and waits for it to reach the target.

- *Morse code*: The sequence of dots and dashes are presented sequentially.

What Does the Research Say?
Direct and Indirect Selection

Horn and Jones (1996) compared direct selection via head pointer with single-switch circular scanning. They found 1) direct selection was more effective even though pre-assessment data indicated that scanning should be more appropriate, 2) behavioral concerns (e.g., attention, off task, fatigue) played a role in determining the most effective selection method, and 3) moving to indirect selection before exhausting all direct selection methods can limit possibilities for the child.

Ratcliff (1994) compared direct selection via an optical head pointer with row column scanning for 100 typically developing elementary students. Students across all grades using row column scanning made significantly more selection errors than students using direct selection.

Mizuko, Reichle, Ratcliff, and Esser (1994) examined differences in short-term memory requirements between selection techniques in 22 children who were approximately 4 years of age. Participants were shown pairs of line drawings and instructed to find the same symbols in the correct order on randomly arranged arrays of 10, 20, 30, and 40 items. Results showed no significant difference in the accuracy of the selection techniques, although the mean level of accuracy was significantly greater with direct selection than with scanning for the 40-item array.

Wagner and Jackson (2006) studied 120 kindergarten, first-, and third-grade typically developing students using direct selection and visual linear scanning in a memory recall task using line drawings. The students retrieved more symbols correctly using direct selection than scanning. The third graders retrieved more symbols than first graders or kindergartners.

Treviranus and Roberts (2003) summarized research on direct selection and indirect selection (i.e., scanning and coded access). Specifically, 1) direct selection is faster than indirect selection, 2) direct selection is less demanding cognitively than indirect selection, 3) direct selection to multiple targets requires more motor control than indirect selection, and 4) direct selection has less negative impact on short-term visual memory.

Two individuals will serve as case examples throughout this chapter to illustrate the process of developing alternatives to direct selection.

CASE EXAMPLES

Genna

Genna was 4 years old when we first met her. She had severe spastic cerebral palsy with quadriplegia, resulting in extremely limited control over her entire body. Genna lived with her mother and father, recent immigrants from Laos, and her 1-year-old brother. At our first appointment, Genna was most comfortable in her mother's arms or on the floor. She was clearly uncomfortable in her wheelchair, even though it had been custom designed with maximum supports for her torso, legs, arms, and head. Genna would arch her back and scream when being transferred into the wheelchair.

She was referred for an AAC evaluation to "find a way for her to communicate." It became clear that Genna used a number of communication modes, but they were all nonsymbolic in nature. She used subtle facial expressions, vocalizations, and a head turn/eye gaze combination in addition to the body posture (arched back) and crying described previously. Familiar partners reported that she smiled for "yes" and pursed her lips for "no" to accept or reject objects or actions offered to her. Less familiar partners said they could not trust those signals at all. This difference in perception may have contributed to extreme differences in perspective about Genna's abilities among members of her team. Her parents reported that she could understand everything said to her, whereas less familiar school personnel believed she did not understand even the simplest statements. School staff reported much of the day was spent soothing her crying to prevent screaming.

Victor

Victor was 13 years old when we met him. He was a handsome young teenager with moderate cerebral palsy affecting all four limbs. He was seated in a power wheelchair that he operated with a joystick in his right hand. His control of the chair was not flawless, but he was able to navigate safely through the environments within his daily routine.

Chapter 3 provides additional information regarding direct and indirect selection.

Victor was referred to us by his school team because they wanted a speech-generating device (SGD) to supplement his other modes of communication. He used a number of communication strategies effectively. His speech was severely unintelligible but could be understood by his most familiar partners if they knew the context. Beyond that, he used a set of 15 visual communication displays with 20–25 symbols each. Most displays were hung from the back of his wheelchair until retrieved and placed on his lap tray by his communication partners. He requested which display he wanted and pointed to items on each display by slamming his right arm onto the display and "walking" his fingers to the item of choice. The symbols on the displays represented primarily single words with a few short phrases. Victor had access to the alphabet for spelling, but it was provided on two separate displays, in other words, A–L and M–Z. Victor only used those displays for spelling practice, according to the school team.

Victor was extremely engaging with familiar and unfamiliar partners. He would move his chair right up to anyone to begin a dialogue. Although his speech was extremely unintelligible to unfamiliar people, his facial expressions, body language, and general demeanor kept everyone engaged long enough to learn how to present his visual displays for extended conversations. The upcoming prom, his date, his clothes, and the mischief he intended were his favorite topics when we first met.

DEVELOPING COMMUNICATIVE COMPETENCE AND INDEPENDENCE

It is critical that interventionists focus on communication and not become distracted too early by specific technological solutions when they work with learners such as Genna and Victor. It is tempting to dive into an assessment of seating and positioning and motor and sensory abilities and begin to search for technologies that match each learner's capabilities in these realms. Focusing on technology, however, may mean that other important modes of communication are neglected. Genna's case study will show that these other modes might be crucial in the long run. Therefore, it is important to begin by examining the individual's communication in all modes and then identifying those areas in which technological assistance might be required.

☞ *Helpful Hint*

Technology: Problem or Panacea?

It's not about the technology, it's about interaction or communication.

It is important to realize that the technology is neutral, neither the evil problem maker nor a panacea for all obstacles. How these tools are put to use and whether they match the needs and goals of the person who relies on them are the critical questions. They alone will determine whether technology is considered a solution or a new problem.

A broad perspective on communication helps focus the interventionist's attention on the most essential elements first—building competence and independence. The concepts of **communicative competence** and **communicative independence** are integral to our approach and are described next as background for the intervention approach selected for individuals with significant disabilities such as Genna and Victor.

Light used the term *communicative competence* to describe the ability "to express ideas, thoughts, and feelings freely" (2003, p. 3), a basic human right from her perspective. She suggested a framework of four competencies necessary for successful use of alternative communication: **linguistic, operational, social,** and **strategic competence** (Light, 1989, 1997, 2003). To benefit from a new or enhanced mode of communication, learners must be able to communicate what they wish (linguistic competence) with a system that they can access and run (operational competence) in a natural communicative context (social and strategic competence).

☞ *Helpful Hint*

These competencies ultimately have to be examined together because the goal is always overall communicative competence. Examining some components in isolation is important early on in decision making, however. For example, it is inappropriate to examine operational competence in a context with high linguistic, social, or strategic demands. Interventionists must be able to distinguish operational problems, such as accuracy, speed, and fatigue, from distractibility, memory limitations, or linguistic errors.

Examining operational competence in isolation does not mean the learner is given meaningless tasks. On the contrary, operational competence is best examined when the learner is fully engaged in an enjoyable interaction. Thus, the linguistic and strategic demands of a task should be minimized until operational competence is established when the focus is on the learner's ability to use a selection technique (e.g., visual scanning). Implementing this approach while engaging the learner is discussed throughout this chapter.

Attending to multiple types of competence helps interventionists avoid focusing too long on specific skills, such as operational control of a device, at the expense of other competencies, such as maintaining social interactions. Attention to multiple types of competence does not steer the actual intervention process, however (particularly with individuals such as Genna and Victor). The **Model of Communicative Independence** (Blackstone & Hunt Berg, 2003; Dowden, 1999; Dowden & Cook, 2002) may help move learners such as Genna and Victor into independent communication by focusing on the learner's existing expressive communication abilities at the time of intervention. This model identifies three types of communicators—**independent communica-**

tors, context-dependent communicators, and **emerging communicators.**

An independent communicator has full communicative competence and can freely express ideas, thoughts, and feelings. Typically, this requires multiple modes of communication, with or without technology, and sufficient spelling and composition ability so that the individual can generate any novel utterance he or she wishes to convey.

A context-dependent communicator does not have a means of communicating absolutely everything he or she may wish to express to everyone. He or she is dependent on others and the context in some crucial ways. The learner may

- Have access to a limited vocabulary selected by others (e.g., pictures or words in a book or device, the signs that someone has chosen to teach)

- Be able to communicate with only a limited number of partners because few partners understand his or her speech or know how to use complex systems such as eye gaze displays

Context-dependent communicators are limited by these factors, but there is a wide range of capabilities among these individuals. The most sophisticated learners in this category have a relatively large vocabulary available to them and, even more important, have strategies for conveying concepts for which they have no words, phrases, signs, or signals. These strategies (e.g., linguistic cues such as "It rhymes with. . . ." or "It starts with the letter. . . .") still require the partner to figure out the intended concept. They are great strategies when used by capable AAC users, but they are also dependent on a good communication partner. Unfortunately, most context-dependent communicators are not able to use these linguistic strategies to express concepts for which they have no vocabulary. Most are dependent on pointing or responding to the physical environment and relying on the shared knowledge of familiar partners.

It is clear that Victor was a context-dependent communicator when we first met.

He was confined to the limited vocabulary on his communication displays when interacting with unfamiliar partners who could not understand his speech. He had no way to generate utterances about novel topics. He had substantially more freedom communicating with familiar partners who understood his speech as long as the context was clear.

Emerging communicators are by far the most limited in their communication. They rely solely on nonsymbolic modes of expression, such as facial expressions, body postures, common gestures, vocalizations, and so forth. Emerging communicators do not yet have any demonstrably reliable means of **aided** or **unaided symbolic communication,** whether speech, signs, pictures, or voice output. Their nonsymbolic signals are important for communication with familiar partners, but they are unable to communicate beyond the "here and now" because they are not using representational symbols.

It is clear that Genna was limited to emerging communication when we met her. She had nonsymbolic methods of communication in her crying, vocalizing, body postures, and signals for acceptance and rejection. Yet, she had no demonstrably reliable method of symbolic communication by which she could communicate beyond the immediate physical context, even with familiar partners.

Context-dependent and emerging communication are not diagnostic categories that predict later communication; they only reflect the individual's current expressive abilities. A learner may be currently limited to nonsymbolic signals because he or she has not yet been provided reliable access to symbolic communication. Similarly, a learner showing context-dependent communication may be limited by his or her current system because he or she has not been provided with adequate vocabulary or a spelling selection set for producing novel utterances.

Although communicative competence and independence are the ultimate goals for learners showing either emerging or context-dependent communication, the initial approach is different for each type of communicator. This is particularly true for individuals with severe physical disabilities, the focus of this chapter.

LEARNERS WHO SHOW EMERGING COMMUNICATION

Learners showing emerging skills have no experience with reliable symbolic communication, resulting in extremely limited interactions. If learners also have severe motor impairments, then they likely have had little or no experience controlling their environment, whether directly, through technology, or indirectly, by communicating to other people. Interventionists begin by building on the learner's current communicative competence, beginning with two primary objectives:

1. Build on current communicative competence with existing nonsymbolic methods.

2. Explore new modes in order to enhance communicative independence. All modes of communication must be considered, whether technology enabled or not.

Building on Current Communicative Competence

With learners showing a limited communicative repertoire, it is particularly important to start by examining existing competencies to understand how the learners communicate and with whom. Then, we can expand and improve their communication.

Examine Current Competencies

Examining an individual's current competencies requires a careful consideration of each of the areas that are delineated below. Failing to consider these is apt to result in a less satisfactory outcome from intervention.

Step 1: Identify Primary Communication Partners
Identify individuals with whom the learner interacts most often in each relevant setting

(e.g., school, work, home). For Genna, we determined that she interacted primarily with two groups of people—her parents and grandmother at home and her instructional assistant, speech-language pathologist (SLP), and physical therapist (PT) at school.

Step 2: Inventory Potential Communicative Acts
Learners may show signals of communication, whether they are intentional or preintentional acts. Sigafoos, Arthur-Kelly, and Butterfield (2006) referred to such signals as **potential communicative acts (PCAs)** in order to acknowledge that such behaviors may be, or may become, intentional communicative signals, particularly if partners recognize and respond to them consistently. Sigafoos et al. developed an inventory to assess PCAs. Important information to obtain from an inventory of PCAs includes

- Behaviors that seem communicative to someone on the team
- The meanings (pragmatic functions) the partners ascribe to these acts in specific contexts
- Which partners best recognize which PCAs
- Whether any PCAs are unpleasant or disruptive to any partners, in any contexts

We were able to interview one of Genna's partners from home and one from school. The interview was structured around Genna's typical day. We followed up with questions about Genna's behaviors in each activity during the day. Her family reported they were able to rely on many signals, such as smiling and vocalizations. We could not know whether these signals were intentional communication by Genna or simply preintentional actions that the family interpreted as meaningful. These signals, such as the arched back during transfers, were important to the family.

Step 3: Identify Potential Pragmatic Functions of Those Acts Understanding the meaning attributed to those signals is important when identifying PCAs. The family clearly knew when Genna wanted to get out of her chair, wanted some interaction, and liked or disliked something they offered in different contexts. The SLP was less confident about any signals from Genna other than crying and screaming.

The information gained from an assessment of PCAs can be summarized to show the learner's signal repertoire and to highlight any gaps or inconsistencies. Table 4.1 contains information obtained from the interviews about Genna's signal repertoire. We could see there were some important differences in reporting by different partners, which is not uncommon for emerging communicators. Genna's most familiar partners reported the most signals and the most meanings attributed to those signals. They also reported relying on somewhat subtle signals, which only occasionally escalated into crying as a protest or squealing in delight. The SLP reported a smaller repertoire of signals, most of which were unpleasant, such as crying or screaming. Vocalizing in games of sound play was the only positive PCA on which there was agreement. It is often impossible to determine at this point whether the child's signals are intentional and the extent to which they are consistent (Sigafoos et al., 2006). However, it is clear that some signals were recognized by some partners and not by others, particularly the more subtle signals (e.g., vocalizing before she escalated to crying and screaming). Sigafoos et al. advocated building on the signals through consistent and predictable adult responses.

Genna's sensory and motor abilities were screened before we determined the consistency and persistence of her signals as well as the predictability of her partner's responses.

Table 4.1. Genna's repertoire of potentially communicative acts

Pragmatic function	Behavior reported by family	Behavior reported by school
Social conventions		
Greeting	Look at, smile, tense arms and legs	None
Response to name	Look at, smile	None
Attention to self		
Seeks social attention	Vocalization leads to squeal	Cry leads to scream
Seeks comfort	Vocalization leads to squeal	Cry leads to scream
Reject/protest		
Food offered	Pout, purse lips, head turns away	Pout leads to cry, which leads to scream
Current position	Tense body, arched back leads to cry	Cry leads to scream
Request/accept		
Visible object	Lean toward, smile	Cry leads to scream
Visible food	Lean toward, smile, mouth open	Cry leads to scream
Repeat action	Vocalization	Cry leads to scream
Repeat sound play	Vocalization	Vocalization
Comment		
Is happy	Smile, vocalization	None
Is excited	Vocalization leads to squeal	None
Feels pain	Pout leads to whine, which leads to cry	Cry leads to scream
Is angry	Pout leads to whine, which leads to cry	Cry leads to scream
Make choice from array	Function not reported	Function not reported
Answer	Function not reported	Function not reported
Request information	Function not reported	Function not reported

Source: Sigafoos, Arthur-Kelly, and Butterfield (2006).

Step 4: Screen Sensory and Motor Abilities   Play-based/leisure assessment is the best approach to examining hearing, vision, and motor abilities in emerging communicators (Casey, 1995; Dowden & Cook, 2002). Ideally, assessment activities should take place in a familiar environment, with familiar partners, while the learner is positioned (with or without support) for the greatest comfort and motor control. Play for young children may involve interacting with a parent in a favorite game such as Peekaboo, playing with toys, looking at books, or eating a snack. The activity for an older learner might focus on a special interest (e.g., a special collection of family photographs) or a pleasant daily activity (e.g., putting on makeup, playing cards).

The interventionist uses these activities to examine the learner's response to sensory input (auditory or visual) as well as motor control of the eyes, hands, arms, legs, and head. The tasks should provide some information about the following:

- Movement of learner's head from side to side as well as up and down

- Movement of learner's eyes independently of his or her head

- Learner's tracking of moving objects or locating of stationary items throughout his or her visual field

- Learner's reaching, grasping, and releasing items of interest

- Range of movement of the learner's arms (including across midline)

- Learner's ability to coordinate movement of both arms independently

- Identification of the smallest size targets that the learner can see, reach, and touch

- Identification of the greatest number of separate targets (**resolution**) that the learner can see, reach, and touch

Initially, information about leg control is less important if the learner has some ability to reach with his or her hands. It is essential, however, to examine the range and resolution of that control for some learners. Results

of these screening assessments should provide some information about both sensory and motor issues. A more systematic motor assessment (see Cook & Polgar, 2008) may be warranted, depending on the results.

It was very difficult to engage Genna in play in our setting because she cried loudly except when held by her mother or grandmother. She was not interested in any activities, whether with objects (e.g., toys, bubbles) or actions (e.g., singing, dancing). Her only play was in the context of two reciprocal interactions with her mother. The first was a "rocking" game in which Genna's mother would rock her, then stop, waiting for a vocalization. Genna's mother would rock her again when she vocalized. In the second game, Genna's mother sang and then paused until Genna vocalized to request more singing.

The interaction with Genna and her mother and grandmother provided some general information regarding her sensory and motor abilities:

- Genna displayed limited **volitional** control of her head, arms, and legs.

- She required head support in all positions.

- She leaned forward and tensed her torso and extremities in an apparent attempt to return to her mother's lap.

- She retained **primitive reflexes,** such as the **asymmetrical tonic neck reflex (ATNR)** resulting in involuntary movement and posturing of the head, arms, and, to some extent, legs.

- She vocalized frequently, with some variation in intonation (i.e., quiet vocalization to whining, crying, squealing, and screaming).

- She appeared able to hear vocalizations at a conversational level.

- She visually tracked people and objects, with head and eyes moving together.

- She had a **dysconjugate gaze**, making it appear as if her eyes were tracking in two different directions. Consequently, the interventionist would not be able to rely on eye gaze as a signal or on vision as the only way for Genna to find targets in communication tasks.

📖 Helpful Hint

Primitive reflexes are automatic movements performed at a subconscious level (Cook & Polgar, 2008). They are present at or soon after birth in typically developing infants but are gradually integrated or inhibited as the child develops. Neurological damage may result in the continued presence of these reactions long after infancy. The reflexes that have the greatest effect on AAC system use include the following:

- ATNR, in which the head is turned to one side and the arm on that side is extended outward while the opposite arm is flexed inward. This reduces the individual's ability to use hands or arms for switch control as well as to keep his or her trunk and head at midline facing a communication display.

- **Tonic labyrinthine reflex (TLR)** increases tone in the lower limbs and trunk causing the individual to slide forward in his or her chair. This disrupts the learner's ability to remain in an upright position, thus preventing him or her from accessing the display.

Step 5: Verify Consistency of Signals and Partners' Responses   Consistency and persistence do not ensure that signals are intentional but are two indicators of intentionality (Iacono, Carter, & Hook, 1998; McLean, McLean, Brady, & Etter, 1991). They increase the likelihood that signals will be recognized and reinforced by communication partners, which facilitates communicative intentionality (Sigafoos et al., 2006).

PCAs can be verified in both structured and naturalistic environments, focusing first on the most important and more observable signals (Sigafoos et al., 2006). In a sense, this is the establishment of operational competence of unaided signals. The interventionist should design activities so that he or she can examine several specific aspects of a learner's signals. Carefully document whether

the learner uses the same signals consistently in the same communicative context across opportunities. Also, record whether the learner is persistent when his or her original communicative signal does not receive a response. In addition to the learner's consistency and persistence in signal use, the partners' responses should be examined to determine whether they are relying on the signal or interpreting the learner's intentions from the context (e.g., knowing that he or she always likes crackers best).

Genna was reluctant to interact with us despite our efforts; therefore, we focused our attention on verifying Genna's signals for acceptance and rejection of objects/actions. With her mother and grandmother, she demonstrated some limited operational competence by using her nonsymbolic, unaided signals consistently. She demonstrated at least some rudimentary social competence by initiating interactions and by being persistent, even escalating at times until the partner responded. She may have shown some strategic competence as well by using slightly different signals with different partners. However, the extreme limitations in Genna's communication modes (operational competence) made it impossible for her to develop linguistic competence or demonstrate more sophisticated social competence.

We also examined the extent to which Genna's partners recognized and responded to her signals consistently. We arranged activities so that Genna's mother could offer objects or actions without her grandmother seeing or hearing the stimulus items. Her grandmother, seated behind an observation window, interpreted whether Genna accepted or rejected the objects or actions through facial expressions, body postures, and vocalizations. Signals were produced and interpreted consistently during 90% of opportunities. That is, signals for acceptance occurred for activities that were predicted to be positive (e.g., "Sing a song?"), and signals for rejection occurred with negative items (e.g., "Brush teeth?"). Genna was 90% accurate when the questions were posed in Laotian by her mother. Performance dropped to 50% (chance) in later assessments in which the questions were posed in English without the objects available as visible stimuli. We mistakenly expected similar performance in both languages because Genna had been in an English language preschool for several years. We set out to improve Genna's communicative competence using her existing signals with the information just described.

Improve Competencies with Existing Signals

Improve Unclear Signals Across All Partners All parties should consistently prompt the communicative behavior and then respond in a reinforcing manner for learners who exhibit some communicative behaviors (e.g., eye gaze) with some communicative partners (e.g., with parents but not educators).

For example, Genna's intervention focused on improving competence with existing signals, one of which was her eye gaze. Genna's parents reported that she looked at people in greeting and in response to her name (see Table 4.1). School personnel had not noticed eye contact of any kind. It is likely that the discrepancy was due to her dysconjugate gaze. It seemed important for the team to systematically reinforce a head turn/eye gaze combination as eye contact. Her team members were given the following instructions:

Step 1: Physically move close to, but not into, Genna's line of vision when beginning any interaction with her.

Step 2: Call Genna's name to encourage her to turn her head and make eye contact.

Step 3: Engage Genna in a preferred activity (e.g., sing her favorite song, stroke her arm) once eye contact is generally established.

Systematic instruction can lead to mastery of **dyadic eye gaze**—looking at an object or an adult. **Triadic eye gaze** (i.e., joint attention; discussed in Chapter 1)—looking back and forth between an object and an adult—for communicative purposes (Olswang & Pinder, 1995; Pinder & Olswang,

1995) could be systematically addressed by Genna's interventionists.

Replace an Unclear Signal with an Existing Signal
Some learners have unclear signals that can be improved or even replaced with a clearer signal. For example, some learners may gaze but not reach for a desired item. Another learner may make soft vocalizations instead of a head shake to reject nonpreferred activities. The systematic prompting of a more recognizable response in these instances may be necessary for a clearer understanding of communicative intent.

Step 1: Deliver the cue that should result in the communicative behavior (e.g., showing a preferred item, presenting a nonpreferred item).

Step 2: Immediately prompt the more recognizable response (i.e., physically prompt the learner to move a hand in the direction of the item, physically prompt the learner to move his or her head in the opposite direction from the item).

Step 3: Reinforce the behavior through a natural response (e.g., giving the item for a request, removing it for a rejection).

Genna's motor impairments limited us to more subtle signals: acceptance signaled by an open mouth and pleasant vocalization and rejection/protest associated with a closed mouth, lips pursed in a pout, and no vocalization (see Sigafoos et al., 2004; Tait, Sigafoos, Woodyatt, O'Reilly, & Lancioni, 2004). After we found that Genna could vocalize on demand, we taught Genna's mother and grandmother to elicit a sound each time they believed she intended acceptance. We also taught them to respond quickly to her pout for rejection/protest before she escalated to whining as described previously.

Develop a Signal Dictionary to Train New Partners
The partners of emerging communicators can benefit from information that systematically describes the learners' communicative behaviors. A dictionary listing signals/ behaviors, what each one means, and how

communicative partners should respond can be beneficial (see Beukelman & Mirenda, 2005). These dictionaries can be text based or consist of digital photograph albums, or even video clips on a web site. Although termed a dictionary, it is less likely to serve as a reference in an anxious moment than as a way for new partners to get to know learners with severe disabilities. The team and family should decide what type of dictionary would best fit their needs. Genna's team and family preferred a text-based dictionary describing her signals and what they meant.

Test Hearing and Vision to the Extent Possible
Vision impairments are reported to occur in 75%–90% of all individuals with severe motor impairments (Cress et al., 1981), and many may have unrecognized hearing impairments (Beukelman & Mirenda, 2005). Therefore, interventionists should examine the learner's hearing and vision abilities (Dowden & Cook, 2002; McCarthy, 1992) while also making a referral to specialists (e.g., audiologists, ophthalmologists).

Utley (2002) described both formal and informal procedures to assess vision, even in emerging communicators. Assessments included visual-motor skills, binocularity, and presentation distance as well as visually directed reach and touch and how the findings affected AAC intervention. Others have described hearing assessment procedures in similar detail (Beukelman & Mirenda, 2005; Bush, 2003; DeCoste, 1997).

Vision and hearing testing was recommended for Genna. Her family was willing to proceed but did not believe that such testing was necessary because they had no doubts about her vision or hearing at home. Results of the vision testing were unremarkable. The results of the hearing testing, however, showed that Genna had a bilateral, moderate-to-severe, high-frequency hearing loss. Genna was unable to hear many English consonants, particularly stops and fricatives, but might have more success in the family's Lao dialect because of the additional information conveyed through pitch

changes in this tonal language. This difference may have explained the reported discrepancy in her comprehension when listening to the two languages. Genna received bilateral hearing aids soon after this evaluation.

A list of technology-based web sites is included on the accompanying CD-ROM.

Exploring New Modes to Enhance Communicative Independence

Exploring new modes, including using technology, is the second objective with emerging communicators.

Step 1: Identify Communicative Behaviors and Potential Functions for Specific Situations

Developing communicative competence for emerging communicators is an iterative process in which a variety of activities are used to broaden the modes and communicative intents. Initially, the focus should be on using any new signal for an existing familiar purpose or pragmatic function (e.g., a new way to request or accept objects or actions). Interventionists should introduce the new signal with new partners or in a new context in which the old signal is acceptable but not sufficient for communication. This approach helps avoid extinguishing an appropriate signal in the child's small repertoire. For example, a child's parents may understand that gazing toward an item is an indication that he or she wants something. Pointing to the object may be a more salient behavior at school and in the community, making it more readily understood. Thus, the new signal (pointing) would be taught in an environment other than with the learner's parents. Once the learner is reliable with this signal in the new context, then the parents may require it at home as well, and the interventionist can consider extending the new

Table 4.2.   Single-switch activities

Switch control of toys, appliances, or computer activities	Switch control of another person using single-message voice output
Robot control[1] (e.g., making a robot go forward to knock over blocks, attaching a pen and drawing circles while a switch is pressed and the robot moves, moving it to a specific place and stopping)	Requesting more action with toys (e.g., bubbles, moving cars, spinning tops)
Computer games (e.g., changing colors, sounds, or pictures when a single switch is pressed)	Requesting more action on self (e.g., massage, tickling)
Appliances[2] (e.g., building activities around a blender [making pudding], fan [blowing air on child], vibrating tube [tactile stimulation], or flashing lights)	Requesting more sensory activities (e.g., sound [singing, music], touch [feeling sand or paints])
Battery-operated toys (e.g., cars, barking dogs)	Requesting attention from others

[1]An infrared (IR)-controlled device such as Lego MindStorms; a single-switch IR control such as the Gewa Big Jack (Zygo Industries), which is available in the United States from Zygo Industries (http://www.zygo-usa.com).

[2]For example, Power Link 3 by AbleNet (http://www.ablenetinc.com).

signal to a new pragmatic purpose (e.g., pointing to comment).

The new signal may be a different vocalization, as in Genna's case, or it could involve the introduction of technology. For the latter, a **control interface** (switch) converts movement into a meaningful output. The switch might control a toy, appliance, or computer software. Alternatively, it might result in voice output that controls the action of communication partners. Interventionists should implement a straightforward approach to teach emerging communicators to use a switch in tasks with a direct, one-to-one relationship between the motor movement and the resulting output. Table 4.2 lists some of the activities in which a learner can use a single switch. None of the voice output activities involve actual symbolic communication because there is only one utterance available to the learner in each activity.

Many learners with severe sensory or motor impairments who use SGDs may request actions more readily than objects because objects are difficult to manipulate and actions bring greater social closeness (Hussey, Cook, Whinnery, Buckpitt, & Huntington, 1992). All learners require novelty and variety in order to remain engaged, regardless of these differences. Interventionists are most successful if they strive for that variety while maintaining consistency in the switch

and how it is positioned long enough for the child to become reliable with this new mode for a new purpose.

☞ *Helpful Hint*

Setting Up Single-Switch Controllers

Single-switch controllers can be set up in different ways depending on the learner's motor skills and typical behavior with a switch. Here are some suggestions that are not mutually exclusive.

- If a learner activates the switch in an apparently random manner, he or she might benefit from a **momentary switch** that is connected directly to some toy or appliance. The direct control may be more salient to the child, and the momentary nature of the switch may make it clearer that he or she is in control.

- If a learner can activate a switch but not maintain the activation, then he or she may benefit from a **latching switch** or a **switch latch and timer** so that each activation results in a consequence (e.g., music or robot control) that lasts for a period of time.

- If a learner activates and unintentionally maintains activation (e.g., resting head on the switch), then he or she may benefit from a momentary switch that activates only on release.

- If a learner tends to activate the switch repeatedly, then he or she may benefit from a **switch latch** that toggles between *on* and *off* with each activation. If the device is more interesting than the switch itself, then he or she should learn to activate it only once and enjoy the result.

All of the activities described involve using one switch to directly control an output. Although the learner is using a switch, this is essentially direct selection because there is a one-to-one association between activating the switch and the resulting effect; the learner activates one switch that results in one predetermined output.

Initially, the goal is to find any method of switch control that can work consistently for the emerging communicator, even if only in a limited context. This allows setting up opportunities in which all factors can be optimized, including the context, partners, and activity as well as the learner's positioning and the type and placement of the switch. Although these ideal circumstances may not lead directly to functional communication in everyday activities, it can maximize the likelihood of identifying the first reliable method of switch control, and that is the focus when introducing technology to emerging communicators.

Step 2: Examine Seating and Positioning in the Context of an Activity

It is important for communication to take place throughout the emerging communicator's day and, thus, to consider a variety of positions from 1) sitting in a wheelchair to 2) lying prone or supine; 3) sidelying; 4) sidesitting; 5) kneeling; 6) standing; and 7) sitting in a highchair, a corner chair, or in someone's lap (see York & Weimann, 1991). Consider these additional questions when examining seating and positioning within an activity (Cook & Polgar, 2008).

- Is the seating system comfortable for the learner and durable enough to meet the child's needs for a reasonable time?

- Does the seating system provide stability and allow for maximal performance in functional activities (e.g., transfers, weight shifts, activities of daily living)?

- Does the seating system meet the learner's goals and needs (e.g., postural control, pressure relief)?

- Is the seating system sufficiently flexible to meet the learner's changing needs (e.g., change in functional abilities, growth changes)?

- Are there resources available to ensure appropriate maintenance of the seating system?

- Can the learner's family or a third party finance the cost of the seating system?

Seating/positioning was a major obstacle for Genna. When we first met her, she was uncomfortable in her custom-built wheelchair. We attempted to set up switch exercises in a play activity with Genna positioned in her mother's lap, but the severity of her motor impairments required much more trunk support than her mother was able to provide. So, our initial focus was on finding a way to make her comfortable as she sat for brief periods. This became possible by our third session but only if her mother sat next to Genna and sang quietly to soothe her.

Step 3: Identify a Control Site and Interface for Switch Control

The interventionist can identify a **control site** once a learner is positioned comfortably. A control site is a part of the body over which the learner has the greatest volitional control. The sensory and motor screening tasks described earlier can provide important information regarding the learner's motor control, including whether it differs across activities or positions. There is a hierarchy of anatomic control sites based on the ease of interfacing and the relative degree of fine motor control typically available at each site (Cook & Polgar, 2008; Dowden & Cook, 2002). Table 4.3 shows the potential range, strength, and number of targets for different control sites for individuals with severe limitations in motor control. The interventionist should strive for an interface with the greatest number of potential targets

Table 4.3. Characteristics of switch control sites

Control site	Assuming this motor limitation	Example interface	Potential target size	Potential strength	Number of potential targets
Fingers	Poor hand/arm movement	Switch or joystick	Small	Low	Up to four
Arm	Poor finger/hand movement	Switch or joystick	Large	Large	Up to four
Head	Limited fine control	Switch or joystick	Moderate	Moderate	Up to four
Foot/leg	Limited fine control	Switch or joystick at foot	Moderate	High	Up to four
Hand	Poor finger/arm movement	Single or dual switches at hand	Moderate	Moderate	One or two
Mouth	No speech; respiration only	Sip-and-puff switch	N/A	Low	One or two
Foot	No leg movement	Single or dual switches at foot	Small	High	One or two
Leg	No foot pointing	Single or dual switches at leg or knee	Moderate	High	One or two
Eye blink	No tracking	Single switch at eye	Small	Negligible	One
Tongue	Single movement only	Tongue switch	Small	Low	One
Jaw/Chin	No head movement	Single switch at chin	Small	Low	One
Vocalization	No speech; sound only	Sound-activated switch	N/A	Low	One

From Dowden, P., & Cook, A.M. (2002). Choosing effective selection techniques for beginning communicators. In D.R. Beukelman & J. Reichle (Series Eds.) & J. Reichle, D.R. Beukelman, & J.C. Light (Vol. Eds.), *AAC series: Exemplary practices for beginning communicators: Implications for AAC* (p. 417). Baltimore: Paul H. Brookes Publishing Co.; adapted by permission.

that a learner can control at a given site (e.g., several switches with one hand). Although intervention often begins with only one switch, if the learner is able to control more switches reliably, then there are major advantages later. A thorough evaluation of all potential control sites, particularly for scanning access, can be completed using Form 4.1a on the accompanying CD-ROM. (A filled-in version of Form 4.1a [called Form 4.1b] is also found on the accompanying CD-ROM.) There are a variety of switches and other control interfaces available for most switch control sites (see Table 4.4).

Initially, the movement used to activate the control interface may be selected on the basis of the learner's existing signals (e.g., a reach toward an object is shaped into a reach to activate a switch). However, some signals are not easily converted into the high-tech equivalent. A prime example is eye gaze. Many learners rely on eye gaze for communication, and this is an easy signal for parents and teachers to interpret. Unfortunately, although technology for measuring eye gaze has improved dramatically, it is still difficult to use, especially for emerging communica-

tors. The learner must use eye movements for multiple purposes—to locate symbols, watch the cursor move, and select a location. Thus, eye gaze is a great no-tech signal but a real challenge technologically.

Finding a control site and interface for Genna was a challenge. We used the hierarchy of sites in Table 4.3 and selected a compatible switch interface from Table 4.4. It was difficult for Genna to control switches even while sitting comfortably in her wheelchair, engaged by her mother. We quickly ruled out all of the sites for control of multiple switches using the fingers, arms/hands, head, and foot. Subsequently, we ruled out a number of other sites because of Genna's strong reflexes, particularly the ATNR that frequently disrupted volitional control of her head, hand, arm, and jaw. We began to focus on control of her leg, specifically moving her right leg to activate a switch placed outside her right knee. The switch controlled a single-message voice output device that produced a recorded voice saying MORE SINGING, MOM. Although she was engaged and vocalizing, Genna was not able to control her leg well enough to activate the switch

Table 4.4. Switches and control interfaces

Category	Description	Switch name/manufacturer
Mechanical switches	Activated by applying force; generic names of switches include paddle, plate, button, lever, membrane	Pal Pads, Taction Pads (Adaptivation); Big Buddy Button, Microlight Switch, Grasp, Trigger Switch (TASH); Big Red and Jelly Bean Switches (AbleNet); Lever, Leaf, and Tread Switches (Zygo Industries); Dual-rocking, P and Wobble Switch (Prentke Romich); Access and Finger Access (Saltillo); FlexAble, Rocking Action, Plate Switch (AMDi)
Electromagnetic switches	Activated by receiving electro-magnetic energy such as light or radio waves	Fiber Optic Sensor (Adaptive Switch Laboratories); Proximity Switches (AMDi); SCATIR (Tash); Infrared/Sound/Touch Switch (Words +)
Electrical control switches	Activated by detecting electrical signals from the surface of the body	D-Box Standalone EMG Switch (Emerge Medical); Brainfingers 9 Cyberlink (Adaptivation)
Proximity switches	Activated by moving close to the detector, but without actual contact	ASL 204 and 208, Proximity Switch (Adaptive Switch Laboratories); Untouchable Buddy (Tash)
Pneumatic switches	Activated by detecting respira-tory airflow or pressure	Pneumatic Switch (Adaptivation); LifeBreath Switch, Sip and Puff Switch (Enabling Devices); ASL 308 Pneumatic Switch (Adaptive Switch Laboratories); PRC Pneumatic Switch Model PS-2 (Prentke Romich); Pneumatic Switch Model CM-3 (Zygo Industries); Wireless Integrated Sip/Puff Switch (Madentec)
Phonation switches	Activated by sound or speech	Voice Activated and Sound Activated Switches (Enabling Devices); Infrared/Sound/Touch Switch (Words +)

This table was published in Cook and Hussey's assistive technologies: Principles and practice, A.M. Cook & J.M. Polgar, p. 260, Copyright Elsevier 2008.

consistently. Her ATNRs were a signifi-cant obstacle, actually increasing through-out the trials. Her vocalizations became more persistent, and eventually, she cried from frustration.

CASE EXAMPLE

Heeding the Learner's Preference

The story of another learner, Leanne, illustrates why it is not sufficient to choose control sites based on theory alone. Leanne had a diagno-sis of cerebral palsy affecting all four limbs. Her hand movements were not well controlled, but her head control was good. In our assess-ment, we tried an enlarged keyboard with her hand, and she struggled to make selections reliably. When provided a single switch at her right hand, she was accurate and had a rela-tively fast reaction time. Leanne's best control site, however, was her head. She could control her head movements well enough to directly select with a headlight or head pointer. So, the theoretical recommendation would be to use head control for direct selection because it would be the most efficient. However, Leanne hated anything on her head. So, we opted for the second choice—good hand control for indirect selection, which she subsequently mastered.

A breakthrough in switch control did not happen for Genna until she and her team mastered a method of no-tech communica-tion. As mentioned previously, we had rec-ommended that she learn to vocalize for ac-ceptance. Once that was established and we were able to test the consistency and intelli-gibility of that signal, we introduced **Partner-Assisted Scanning (PAS)**. We taught Genna's primary partners how to do PAS, presenting items of choice sequentially, one at a time and accepting a vocalization as the signal to accept that choice. We also taught her family how to guard against partner influence using PAS.

✍ Helpful Hint

How to Teach a Learner to Engage in Partner-Assisted Scanning

Step 1: Identify a reliable response that the learner can produce on command and is readily identifiable by his or her communicative partner.

Step 2: The communicative partner menus the items of choice for the learner. This can be done verbally (slowly list the items) and/or visually (point to the items).

Step 3: When the communicative partner arrives at the desired item, the learner is prompted to produce the signal, and the item is delivered to the learner. All prompting should be eliminated quickly, and natural reinforcement should be provided upon any occurrence of the signal.

Step 4: Once PAS is established, the interventionist may consider a switch evaluation to determine if the signaling behavior can be matched to a switch.

PAS became Genna's first reliable method of symbolic communication, whether the choice set was presented in auditory form only (e.g., "Do you want . . . milk? Apple juice? Orange juice? Water?") or with the partner also pointing to pictures. Two members of the school team, along with her mother and grandmother, refined the PAS system by making consistent vocabulary displays. Upon our request, the SLP and classroom assistant were able to test Genna's reliability (operational competence) with this communication strategy, using some procedures addressed in Piché and Reichle (1991) and discussed in Chapter 3 of this text. Genna recognized symbols and made reliable selections from them in a quiet environment with one partner.

See Kovach and Kenyon (2003) and Burkhart and Porter (2006) for additional information about PAS.

Some informal measures of auditory comprehension and symbol recognition revealed that Genna recognized most simple line drawings, some words, and even some letters of the alphabet. It was only these results that began to convince some team members that Genna was communicating reliably and understood much of what was said to her.

✍ Helpful Hint

Postpone Formal Assessments in Emerging Communicators

Many emerging communicators with severe motor impairments cannot be formally evaluated for underlying language and cognitive skills. A learner who cannot reliably point to or otherwise select symbols for communication would be unable to produce reliable selections for traditional testing. Severe motor impairments also preclude a learner from being assessed through the nonverbal performance or manipulation tasks. The team must simply defer all formal questions of language or cognition until the child is able to communicate reliably and consistently via some symbolic means.

Once PAS was underway, we capitalized on Genna's vocal signal by conducting a switch evaluation with a voice-activated (sonic) switch. There were a number of challenges, however. First, Genna's switch needed to be sensitive enough to pick up intentional phonation but not other sounds (e.g., involuntary vocalization). This was a problem because Genna vocalized unintentionally when she went into an ATNR, and she had many chest colds that resulted in frequent coughing and changes to her voice quality. Mounting the switch close to Genna's mouth presented a second problem because she was small and her ATNR reflexes were substantial (involving her head, neck, and torso). We explored mounting the switch on a chest strap, picking up the sound acoustically, as well as taping the switch to her throat, picking up sound by vibration. We settled on the chest strap, and Genna began to have reliable switch control after many months of practice.

Step 4: Choose an Initial Selection Method

The control site, interfaces, and the selection technique are all functionally interrelated. Learners may be able to use direct selection at only one control site with one interface, as shown in Leanne's case example. If that site cannot be utilized for some reason, then it may be difficult to find another site-interface combination for direct selection. Yet, searching is important because of the advantages of direct selection. In general, direct selection is cognitively easier than indirect selection for any user as long as he or she has the motor control for multiple sites.

It is not easy to decide when to introduce indirect selection methods to any given child because of the difference in the cognitive aspects of direct and indirect selection. The change in access itself would only make learning discrimination more difficult. Consider the following when deciding to introduce indirect selection methods:

- When learners such as Genna have only one control site, the move to indirect selection is inevitable. Many interventionists begin with a single switch with a single function (technically still direct selection) and then move quickly to PAS or technology-assisted scanning. Discrimination can only be taught in the context of scanning, despite the challenges that presents.

- When learners have limited direct selection abilities, some interventionists teach both direct and indirect selection concurrently (e.g., Piché & Reichle, 1991). This approach requires careful consideration of the learner's skill with each selection method, however.

- Using direct selection to its utmost capacity before changing to indirect selection. For example, if a learner has the motor control to reach and activate several switches but is challenged by learning to discriminate their function, then that learner should continue to practice

with direct selection. The learner's motor control may improve with practice, allowing more switches at a later time. See the case study on Matthew about continuing to use direct selection to teach symbol association and discrimination even if indirect selection is likely to be in the learner's future.

CASE EXAMPLE

Matthew

Matthew was an emerging communicator when we met him, but his team was conducting trials during lunch with a voice output communication device with four large switches. It was set up so the voice output would request one of four snack items whenever Matthew activated any switch. He had significant motor limitations, but the greater problem was that he cried throughout much of the activity. He also activated switches repeatedly, regardless of whether he was already eating. He showed no expectation of receiving food and, in fact, often refused food given to him upon switch activation. He was referred to us to determine whether indirect selection would be more effective. It was our strong opinion that Matthew's performance would not improve if his team abandoned direct selection. He first had to learn how to use these limited direct selection targets. We did recommend, however, that he might be more successful using fewer switches, arranged differently on his lap tray, in a different activity, with different targets, and more salient symbols. Changing to indirect selection too early would only make the task more complex for Matthew.

There are two primary reasons for continuing with direct selection even if an emerging communicator can access only a few targets.

1. Activities can be designed to teach discrimination among targets when the child can use direct selection. For example, two switches can be set up with

symbols for engaging consequences (see examples of such activities in Table 4.2) and one switch (the distractor) can be left empty. Moving the distractor allows for teaching or assessing discrimination skills. These activities can assist in determining the individual's preferences once discrimination has been verified. Knowing that the child discriminates and has clear preferences will help greatly when the interventionist designs activities to teach indirect methods such as scanning.

2. Direct selection activities can improve the learner's operational competence with the switch(es). Simply being able to activate the switch is not sufficient competence for a learner to move to scanning. The learner also needs to be able to wait, activate, and release the switch appropriately in repeated attempts in a natural context. These skills can be taught with one or more switches set up for direct selection if the activity requires waiting, activating, and releasing the switch or switches in a timely manner. Table 4.5 shows how these early switch skills relate to the different types of indirect selection. The learner's skills help guide the interventionist toward different types of indirect selection. For example, if the learner cannot activate the switch easily but can hold and release well, then the interventionist should consider trials with inverse scanning. See Form 4.1a on the accompanying CD-ROM to evaluate the prerequisites skills

at all or most potential control sites. See Chapter 3 as well as Cook and Polgar (2008) and Dowden and Cook (2002) for more information on types of indirect selection.

> ### What Does the Research Say?
> #### Assessing Discrimination and Preference Via Single Switches
>
> Discrimination and preference are easy to observe when the individual can activate multiple switches (e.g., Matthew) or when the individual shows strong preferences through nonsymbolic signals (e.g., Genna). It is necessary to use some innovative procedures, however, when the individual uses only a single switch and there are no other indications of preference. A number of authors have written about establishing discrimination and preferences in individuals with severe motor impairments (Cannella, O'Reilly, & Lancioni, 2005; Lancioni, O'Reilly, Singh, Oliva, & Groeneweg, 2002; Saunders et al., 2005; Saunders, Smagner, & Saunders, 2003). They described data collection methods for examining learning, as well as procedures for identifying individual preferences for different outputs.
>
> For example, Saunders et al. (2005) described activation–deactivation activities with adults with no communication and severe motor impairments. In initial trials, switch activation turned on a consequence such as music or tactile vibration. The activity was reversed after the pattern of switch activations was clear so that the music or vibration was turned off by switch activation. This provided a means of identifying preferences that were unknown.

Once the interventionist has some idea of the most appropriate type of scanning for an individual learner, then he or she must

Table 4.5. Required tasks and relative importance for scanning

Required tasks	Automatic scanning	Step scanning	Inverse scanning	Directed scanning
Wait	High	Low	Medium	Low
Activate	High	Medium	Low	Medium
Hold	Low	Low	High	High
Release	Low	Medium	High	High
Vigilance	High	Low	High	High

From Beukelman, D.R., & Mirenda, P. (2005). *Augmentative and alternative communication: Supporting children and adults with complex communication needs* (3rd ed., p. 184). Baltimore: Paul H. Brookes Publishing Co.; adapted by permission.

Table 4.6. Sequential steps in motor training for switch use with play-based and/or functional activities

| Goals | Activity to accomplish goal | |
	Controlling environment	Controlling people
1. Time-independent switch use to develop cause and effect	Appliances (e.g., fan, blender) Battery-operated toys/radio Software that produces a result whenever the switch is pressed	Single-message device; no time constraints on use in activity (e.g., call for attention, request for singing or reading)
2. Time-dependent activities to develop switch use at the right time socially	Software that requires a response to visual or auditory stimuli to obtain a pleasant consequence	Single-message device; broad time constraints on use in activity (e.g., finish a joke, finish a song, read another page, play "more" or "again")
3. Using switch within a narrow time window to lead to multichoice scanning	Computer software requiring a response in a narrow time window	Single-message device, narrow time constraints (e.g., speak a line in a book or poem, sing refrain of a song at right moment)
4. Early symbolic communication through scanning	Simple scanning communication device with either environmental control or voice output or (more likely) both; software allowing time-dependent choice making that has a symbolic label and communicative output; use of foils to monitor accuracy.	

This table was published in Cook and Hussey's assistive technologies: Principles and practice, A.M. Cook & J.M. Polgar, p. 265, Copyright Elsevier 2008.

begin to devise activities to teach that selection method in small steps. Table 4.6 suggests a sequence for such training and the activities that might be used. None of the methods listed in Table 4.6 absolutely require technology. No-tech scanning is possible with PAS, as described previously for Genna. See Beukelman and Mirenda (2005) for more ideas on single-switch activities.

Step 5: Refine Control for Indirect Selection

The interventionist can begin to evaluate whether the learner can use indirect selection once he or she is using one switch consistently or multiple switches with some evidence of discrimination. We prefer to do this in the context of play-based activities for young children and engaging functional tasks for older individuals. Table 4.6 provides examples of tasks that can be used to identify viable control sites and gradually narrow the response time for switch activation in anticipation of trials with indirect selection. This process allows the interventionist and the learner to focus gradually on results rather than on the effort to activate

the switch. The interventionist can distinguish errors due to poor motor control from those that might be due to inattention or boredom by fully integrating task engagement into the assessment process.

Cook and Polgar (2008) recommended specific activities for each step of this motor training (see Table 4.6). Many of the same activities can be adapted to refine motor control for indirect selection. The activities must be carefully designed, however, to teach the learner finer control over the switch (Cook, Hussey, & Currier, 1996). Goals 1–3 are the focus for emerging communicators, and they lead logically to the last goal, which is the first foray into symbolic communication. The interventionist may select different activities, select different switches, or use switch latches or timers depending on the learner's skills to capitalize on the learner's strengths or compensate for his or her limitations while moving through these steps.

Positioning and switch control were successful when Genna was 8 years old. At that point, we were working at Goal 3, teaching her to use the voice-activated switch within a narrow time window. We used direct environmental control and indirect control of partners through a single voice output message. She used the switch to sing part of a song at the right moment with her mother. She used it to participate in activities at school, such as cooking, in which she mixed the cake using an appliance control connected to a blender when her classmates told her to "Go for it!" She also used the switch to play with a Lego MindStorms robot (Cook, Adams, & Harbottle, 2007; Schulmeister, Wiberg, Adams, & Cook, 2006), a robot programmed to knock over blocks or to deliver toys to her friends when a switch was activated, and a CD player with some of her favorite music. All of these gave Genna the opportunity for partial participation in an activity with her classmates, and this social opportunity greatly enhanced her engagement. We found a way to require increasingly finer timing of the switch control for each of these activities. For example, if Genna was delivering toys to a classmate, then she had to stop the robot at just the right time or the robot would not be close enough. When she delivered a repeating line in a storybook, she had to wait until just the right moment and deliver it in a timely manner.

As she increased her operational competence, we also found educational software to be particularly helpful in creating opportunities for Genna to apply her new competencies to language-based activities. Her interventionists introduced her to educational software that allowed Genna to paint and play games using on-screen scanning. Although her no-tech PAS system was known to be reliable by this time, her use of the voice-activated switch remained a challenge in this respect. By measuring her accuracy in carefully structured trials, we were able to determine a pattern to her reliability. We found that she was unreliable on days shortly before, during, or after an illness or on days when we could observe that she was congested or having many ATNR reflexes. This allowed us to establish that she was demonstrably reliable with the switch on the other days. She communicated that she greatly enjoyed the computer-based activities when she felt good. This meant it was time to conduct

trials of scanning for communication using this technology while acknowledging the limitations of a system that may be unreliable when she is ill or uncomfortable.

✍ Helpful Hint

Tips for Early Switch Control for Emerging Communicators

The following tips can be used while teaching early switch control to emerging communicators (Dowden & Cook, 2002).

- Cues to the AAC user should always be natural to the environment (e.g., silence in the middle of a song). Using explicit commands will keep the learner dependent on that prompt and impede learning (e.g., saying, "Hit the switch").

- The learner must not repeatedly or continuously activate the switch in anticipation of the right moment. This will prevent him or her from learning to wait for the cursor to be in the right position in scanning.

- It is unfair to expect communicative use of the switch/selection method before ensuring that the individual has reliable control (operational competence) over the interface itself.

Step 6: Conduct Early Scanning Trials

Mastering scanning access is challenging (Light, 1993; McCarthy et al., 2006; Mizuko et al., 1994; Petersen, Reichle, & Johnston, 2000; Piché & Reichle, 1991). Challenges may arise from the learner's intrinsic characteristics (e.g., his or her sensory or motor impairments, cognition, or language limitations). Or, challenges may be extrinsic due to poor positioning; inadequate switch choice or set up; or an inappropriate type, pattern, or speed of scanning (McCarthy et al., 2006). See the Helpful Hint about early scanning as well as Form 4.2 on the accompanying CD-ROM for ways to maximize the likelihood of success with initial scanning practice.

Although most interventionists agree that scanning evaluations should involve a small set of targets and a slow scanning speed, there is some disagreement about the optimal scanning pattern for learners with severe disabilities. Few clinicians begin with row column scanning because it is considered more cognitively challenging (Mizuko et al., 1994). Some researchers and interventionists recommend linear scanning for beginners (Mustonen, Locke, Reichle, Solbrack, & Lindgren, 1991), whereas others believe circular scanning is better (Beukelman & Mirenda, 2005). Circular scanning may be more easily understood because the cursor moves in a continuous pattern around the circle; in linear scanning, the cursor appears to jump back to the beginning when it reaches the end of a row. This discontinuity can be confusing to beginning users. Some argue that linear scanning, particularly with a small set in a single row, may be less challenging visually to some users with oculomotor impairments when compared with circular scanning (Piché & Reichle, 1991), which requires more eye movement. McCarthy et al. (2006) recommended a type of "enhanced" linear scanning in which both the presentation of options and the feedback upon selection are made exceptionally salient, both visually and auditorily to the learner.

Often, the scanning type will be changed as the skills and needs of the learner change. Initially, Genna used a linear scan with her no-tech PAS system. Later, she used her sonic switch with educational software in what was essentially a circular scan as she chose from a series of "hot spots" sequentially highlighted around the screen. Eventually, we set up communication displays on the computer using Speaking Dynamically Pro (Mayer-Johnson). This software permits the development of communication pages that are linked dynamically and can be accessed, in this case, via single-switch scanning. This set up meant that Genna could use the computer to communicate in much the same way she had been using PAS. We set it up for visual and auditory scanning because Genna's ATNR reflexes made it difficult for her to keep her head forward to watch the cursor. She learned to use the auditory cues as she had been doing with PAS. She needed to

learn the system at each stage, improving her operational competence, before she could be expected to use it for communication in a natural context.

☞ Helpful Hint

Before engaging the learner in early scanning activities, make sure there is

- At least one comfortable position for an engaging activity
- An appropriate control site and an identified switch for the learner's motor control
- A well-positioned and stable switch
- Easy movement to activate the switch
- Nearly 100% accurate switch activation upon stimulus/cue without scanning
- A scanning method that matches the learner's motor patterns (see Table 4.5)
- An initial scan speed that is 1.5 times the learner's reaction time (Lesher, Higginbotham & Moulton, 2000)
- No reward for inappropriate activations (e.g., during stimulus)
- Empty space (foil) in the scanning array in addition to targets
- A simple scanning pattern—linear or circular
- A highly salient presentation of options to the learner (McCarthy et al., 2006)
- A cue/stimulus in the same modality as the selection set items (e.g., the cue should be visual for visual scanning, the stimulus should be audible for auditory scanning)
- Use of natural cues and prompts rather than unnatural ones (e.g., "Hit the switch now")
- An ability for the learner to look at the display continuously during visual scanning
- Salient and reinforcing feedback upon selection (McCarthy et al., 2006)

Step 7: Verify the Reliability of Scanning (Operational Competence)

Interventionists know that operational competence is an essential element of technology-based scanning. Many teams forget, however, that no-tech approaches to scanning (e.g., Genna's PAS) also require operational competence. Piché and Reichle (1991) and Burkhart and Porter (2006) described practical approaches to the development of no-tech scanning.

There is a tendency to discredit the importance and difficulty of operational competency as secondary to the other three types (McCarthy et al., 2006), which can result in insufficient assessment (e.g., deciding too quickly that a switch or selection method will not work). Interventionists need to be reminded that even highly skilled typically developing individuals require many hours of practice to achieve optimal performance with controls such as head pointers and joysticks (McCarthy et al., 2006). If interventionists fail to address operational competence, then the learner's communicative acts cannot be assumed to be correctly interpreted because they might be due to motor or sensory errors. Interventionists also need to recognize that practice in operational competence can be made engaging and rewarding for the learner. If done well, the learner and interventionist can then expand their focus to include the other three areas of communicative competence.

- The time taken to achieve reliable results varies widely among children.
- Most children received parallel training from an OT using scanning games on the computer while developing scanning skills on a communication device.
- OTs were involved in all phases of scanning training, with the SLPs more involved in later stages.

Angelo (2000) reported a number of essential elements of a single-switch assessment as identified by an experienced OT. Among those reported were reliability of movement, volitional nature of movement, safety, easily performed movement, use of activities in which learners participate regularly, efficiency of movement, previous successful movements, ability to perform a timed response within a time frame, and time required between switch activations.

Cook and Polgar (2008) found that speed of response and accuracy of response are often used to compare control interfaces. Speed of response is a time-based measurement that is related to reaction time. Accuracy of response is often based on moving to the correct position, and it is, therefore, a spatial measurement. The number of correct responses out of the total number of trials is usually the standard of performance for accuracy. Speed of response and accuracy are generally inversely proportional to each other for novice users.

What Does the Research Say?

Developing Skills with Switches and Other Control Interfaces

Jagacinski and Monk (1985) evaluated the use of joysticks and head pointers by young typically developing adults. The task involved moving from a center point to one of eight lighted targets as fast as possible. The skill in using these devices for this task was acquired with some difficulty over many trials. Based on a criterion of less than 3% improvement in speed over 4 consecutive days, proficient joystick use required 6–18 days, and head pointer use required 7–29 days of practice for young typically developing participants who had good motor skills.

Jones and Stewart (2004) surveyed 56 occupational therapists (OTs) and SLPs experienced in teaching scanning to determine how they carried out this training. They indicated that *(continued)*

Watching Genna operate her computer software for entertainment or for communication was thrilling. It appeared that she had reliable control over her environment and her communication partners when she selected colors and designs for her computer artwork or requested repositioning or assistance from her mother. It was possible, however, that she was making selection errors but accepting the results. Consequently, we set up specific tasks to demonstrate that she had reliable control over this system.

We could enlist Genna's help in designing opportunities because she was now 9 years old. She agreed that she would design a picture on the computer that matched a simple picture we had already completed. We were able to determine Genna's accuracy with her new scanning system as we watched her. She was approximately 85% accurate, but she demonstrated that she could erase and correct all errors in this task, which resulted in a completely identical picture. We used picture descriptions in a barrier task in which only Genna could see the pictures, to verify her accuracy in communication. She was to describe each picture well enough for her mother to state what was depicted. Genna could not yet produce complete sentences, but she was effective at using the words she needed to describe these carefully chosen images. For example, Genna would look at a picture, select her different symbols for GIRL and RUN on her communication display, and her mother would ask, "Is it a girl running?" Genna was able to communicate 90% of all content words to her mother during these opportunities.

The preceding communication tasks verified that Genna was now actually a context-dependent communicator. She had a reliable means of symbolic communication, but it was limited to vocabulary chosen by others. This did not mean that she had finished improving her operational competence with her communication methods; indeed, many experts say that operational control never stops improving (McCarthy et al., 2006). Genna had, however, demonstrated that she had sufficient competence with this method for the focus of our intervention to change. Our next task was to expand her communication to more topics, in more contexts, with more partners, and while in positions other than just her wheelchair. This process is the focus of the next section on context-dependent communicators.

LEARNERS WHO SHOW CONTEXT-DEPENDENT COMMUNICATION

A context-dependent communicator is a learner who demonstrates intentional symbolic communication through at least one reliable means (Blackstone & Hunt Berg, 2003; Dowden & Cook, 2002). As discussed, though, communication for these individuals is highly effective only in some activities or with a limited set of partners. Victor, for

example, was not able to convey all his thoughts because it was not possible for his interventionists to anticipate and provide all the vocabulary he would ever wish to express. When Victor wanted to talk about concepts for which he had no vocabulary (e.g., talking about new friends, music, or bands) he could only hint at the missing words and hope the partner could figure it out. His communicative competence depended entirely on the context. Nonetheless, Victor demonstrated considerable competence in other ways. He had operational competence with multiple modes of communication, including his limited speech and 15 visual communication displays with 20–25 symbols each. More important, he demonstrated the social and strategic competence to use these modes with a variety of familiar and unfamiliar partners. Victor used his facial expressions and body language effectively to keep even unfamiliar partners engaged long enough to learn how to present his visual displays to him for extended conversation.

These skills were a starting point in our work with Victor. In our opinion, he needed greater independence in two respects. First, he needed a communication mode that he could operate without constant assistance. Victor's current system required the partners to position each communication display for him and to recognize and give voice to his message. Second, Victor needed vocabulary independence—he needed to be free from vocabulary selected by others and able to communicate anything on any topic in any context. In general, this second type of independence would require Victor to produce completely novel words, which is best accomplished through spelling.

Broadly speaking, serving a context-dependent communicator is quite different from serving an emerging communicator in the following ways:

- Context-dependent communicators have developed significant operational competence with their current modes, so interventionists must be cautious about changing modes or selection methods, doing so only when they are clearly inadequate.

- The context-dependent communicator has sufficient communication to participate directly in all aspects of the assessment process, although it may be necessary to provide new vocabulary to "talk about" communicating. One should begin by understanding what the AAC user likes and dislikes about his or her current communication method. Then, the interventionist must discuss each change in a manner that is appropriate to the individual's age and understanding. In most instances, the team should not proceed with changes unless the user consents.

- The learner's communication ability means that it is easier to conduct assessments in highly structured, less functional tasks. Although such tasks should not be overused, it can be faster and more informative for some initial assessments, such as spelling and literacy.

- Evaluation and intervention is different because the goal is broader. Interventionists should not look at selection methods in the context of specific tasks, as is done for emerging communicators. Solutions need to be found that can be fully integrated into all areas of the context-dependent communicator's life, with an eye toward later independence.

The following objectives will sound familiar, despite differences in the process as a whole.

- Build on current communicative competence.

- Explore new modes in order to enhance communicative independence.

Building on Current Communicative Competence

As with other communicators, our first step is to recognize and improve the individu-

al's current communicative competence. Although there may be many potential changes, this chapter focuses on those competencies that affect decision making regarding selection techniques.

Step 1: Examine Current Competencies

Vision and Hearing   Interventionists must identify any hearing or vision impairments that could confound the language testing. Screening the hearing and vision of a context-dependent communicator is not as difficult as testing emerging communicators.

We found that Victor could participate in traditional hearing screening by raising his right hand when he heard the sound in either ear. The audiologist had to provide him extra time to respond with each tone. Vision testing was a bit more complex. Victor could not speak the names of letters of the alphabet clearly enough for testing with the Snellen Chart, and we could not give him a display with all 26 letters on it for him to point to the name of letters he could see. Victor could be tested with methods that were designed for younger children, however; for example the Tumbling *E* Chart only required him to indicate whether the *E* was oriented "up" or "down" or "left" or "right." He was faster at signaling direction with his right thumb, a procedure that did not require him to take his eyes off the display. Victor's vision and hearing were found to be within normal limits.

☞ *Helpful Hint*

Tips for Assessing Vision in Context-Dependent Communicators

Consider the following testing methods when collaborating with the learner's family physician or a vision specialist (Doshi & Rodriguez, 2007):

- If the learner can name letters, then use the Snellen Chart.

- If the learner can indicate up, down, left, and right, then use the Tumbling *E* Chart.

- If the learner can recognize black line drawings on a white background and has vocabulary for *house, apple,* and *umbrella,* then use the Lea Chart.

- If the learner can recognize solid black drawings on a white background and has vocabulary for *boat, heart, circle, plus, star, flag, moon,* and *cup,* then use the Allen Chart.

See Beukelman and Mirenda (2005), Broderick (1998), DeCoste (1997), and Doshi and Rodriguez (2007) for more information on vision testing.

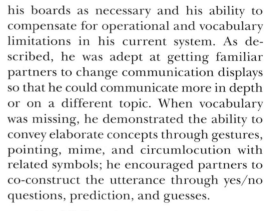

Steps for building on current communicative competence

Step 1: Examine current competencies.
Step 2: Improve current modes of communication.

Social and Strategic Competence Many interventionists turn to Social Networks (Blackstone & Hunt Berg, 2003) in the initial evaluation of context-dependent communicators. This tool examines social and strategic competence in two ways. First, an interview of the family and team (possibly including the learner) can be used to identify the "circles" of people around the learner. It is important to know something about the communication partners in the learner's life—closest family members (Circle 1), friends (Circle 2), acquaintances (Circle 3), service providers (Circle 4), and complete strangers (Circle 5). Second, interviews with many of these communication partners clarify how the learner uses his or her various modes with these partners in different contexts.

We relate the findings from Social Networks directly to competencies delineated by Light (1989) to guide intervention. For example, Victor's social competence was striking given the inherent limitations of his communication systems. He interacted with people in all circles, except complete strangers (Circle 5). He tended to rely on his speech, supplemented by his boards, when he communicated to his immediate family (Circle 1) and his closest friends (Circle 2). School personnel and others (Circle 4) could not understand much of his speech, so he relied primarily on his communication displays. Despite these strategies, there were ways in which his system limited his social competence (e.g., initiating with the displays).

Victor's strategic competence included his ability to switch between his speech and his boards as necessary and his ability to compensate for operational and vocabulary limitations in his current system. As described, he was adept at getting familiar partners to change communication displays so that he could communicate more in depth or on a different topic. When vocabulary was missing, he demonstrated the ability to convey elaborate concepts through gestures, pointing, mime, and circumlocution with related symbols; he encouraged partners to co-construct the utterance through yes/no questions, prediction, and guesses.

Linguistic Competence Victor appeared to show many more limitations in his linguistic competence than in his social or strategic competence. He had a small expressive vocabulary, and he communicated in telegraphic utterances such as PROM, MY DATE, SUSAN, TUXEDO, and FUN. Some limitations, however, might have been due to his particular communicative methods. We needed to assess his underlying linguistic competence.

Assessment of Receptive Language Receptive language can have a profound effect on AAC decision making. Information about the individual's word acquisition can guide decisions about the size of the vocabulary needed by the individual (Blockberger & Sutton, 2003). The individual's understanding of morphology (e.g., plurals, tensing) and syntax (ordered relationship between words) should guide plans for vocabulary organization and for the use of content words (e.g., nouns, verbs), functors (e.g., prepositions), and inflections (e.g., *-ing, -ed*). Perhaps most important, information on literacy skills can provide guidance about the need for the alphabet and the consideration of different **rate enhancement** methods.

Modified standard assessments may have value for some individuals when interpreted informally. Any modifications, however, may also add unforeseen challenges for the individual that dramatically affect his or her scores, invalidating even informal use of the information (Blockberger & Sutton, 2003). For example, modifications that reduce motor demands may increase cognitive demands such as memory, whereas modifications that reduce the response set may increase the odds of a correct response by chance. For this reason, interventionists should seek converging evidence whenever modifications are necessary, using the individual's performance on multiple tasks with different physical and cognitive demands.

> Chapter 3 provides additional information regarding rate enhancement.

We chose to examine Victor's lexical acquisition by giving him a modified version of the Peabody Picture Vocabulary Test–Third Edition (PPVT-III; Dunn & Dunn, 1997). Typically, the targets are organized in a field of four within a two-by-two grid. We did not need to change that format, but we had to place the pictures under a clear Plexiglass cover. Victor had to look at the pictures, find the answer, hold that in memory while he put his arm on the Plexiglass, "walk" his fingers to the right answer, and hold it there until we confirmed it. We knew this was exhausting for Victor, so we tested him in several short sessions, and we considered any result to be an underestimate of his abilities. Results suggested that Victor's receptive vocabulary was at least commensurate with a child about 2 years younger than his age of 13.

We administered the Test for Auditory Comprehension of Language–Third Edition (TACL-3; Carrow-Woolfolk, 1999) in much the same way we had administered the PPVT-III. Results suggested that Victor had skills well below his chronological age, showing difficulties in understanding inflectional morphemes such as -ed and -ing. Victor's strength was his understanding of word order.

The unique linguistic codes (Light, 2003) of AAC systems—the lexicon and the semantic-syntactic skills for combining vocabulary into complex messages—is the other aspect of linguistic competence that must be assessed in all context-dependent communicators. Of course, competence in this code depends entirely on the vocabulary that has been provided and taught. Victor had only been provided about 375 vocabulary words. It was not reasonable to assess Victor with a standardized measure of expressive language because he had been given so little vocabulary. Although we could and did observe his use of that vocabulary in context, these observations could not shed light on his potential ability to use a greatly expanded vocabulary. Thus, we postponed further assessment in this domain.

However, we did evaluate his spelling and other literacy skills required for written expression. As discussed, freedom from vocabulary chosen by others is the key to fully independent communication—the ability to spell well enough to convey meaning not available in preprogrammed vocabulary. This requires evaluation of a host of skills within the domains of phonology, morphology, and syntax, all of which contribute to the construction of novel utterances via spelling. See Beukelman and Mirenda (2005) and Sturm (2005) for an in-depth discussion.

We chose to focus on Victor's word recognition and his single-word spelling because these skills could have a major effect on his communication through spelling plus word prediction in his AAC. To assess word recognition, we used the Wechsler Individual Achievement Test–Second Edition Screener (WIAT-II; Wechsler, 2002), which required Victor to point to one of four words that described a picture. This was administered much like the PPVT-III, yielding a score that suggested skills approximately 4 years behind his chronological age of 13.

Evaluating Victor's spelling skills was more challenging because he had never had access to the entire alphabet at once. In spelling activities, he had to use two separate displays: *A* to *L* and *M* to *Z*. Therefore, we chose to begin our assessment by examining his knowledge of first letters of common words. We used the Sound Matching subtest of the Comprehensive Test of Phonological Processing (CTOPP; Wagner, Torgesen, & Rashotte, 1999). This subtest was designed for typically developing children who were 5–6 years of age; the child has to select one picture from a field of four that stands for a word with the same initial phoneme as the verbal stimulus. To our surprise, Victor quickly reached the ceiling on this task, suggesting that he had more skills in this domain than we had thought. For this reason, we went further to investigate Victor's spelling using the Peabody Individual Achievement Test (Markwardt, 1997). Typically developing children take this spelling test by writing the word spoken by the examiner. Victor had to use his existing alphabet displays and point to the letters sequentially. This method taxed his memory because he had to switch displays to complete most words, so we again considered his score to be an underestimate of his abilities. We were surprised to see that he showed at least third-grade spelling skills, even with this cumbersome assessment. Although Victor's spelling was not flawless, he demonstrated enough skills with phonology to produce invented spellings that partners could recognize, such as "lissen" for *listen*.

These assessments of linguistic competence had some important implications for current and future AAC strategies for Victor. First, it was clear from Victor's receptive vocabulary testing that he needed access to a much larger expressive vocabulary than his current set of 375 words. Second, his reading recognition suggested he could use some printed words as symbols for some vocabulary items and might benefit from word prediction software to speed communication. Third, Victor's spelling skills meant he was actually an independent communicator

because he had sufficient ability to produce novel words when given access to the complete alphabet. His invented spellings were sufficient for partners to guess the meaning, although those words might be mispronounced by a voice output device. Nonetheless, Victor needed to have the alphabet available at all times. Last, Victor's overall profile suggested he would need explicit instruction in literacy and all aspects of expressive communication.

Operational Competence It is important to examine operational competence in isolation and in the context of natural everyday communication. For context-dependent communicators such as Victor, it is easy for the interventionist to switch back and forth as needed, observing these learners during interviews or in daily activities as well as during structured tasks. Interventionists must look at the match between the individual's motor, sensory, and cognitive skills and the operational characteristics of the current communication methods. The initial goal is to make changes in motor performance and/or system configuration that might increase operational competence by improving the efficiency of motor access. Interventionists must pay attention to motor control problems that can be addressed by small changes in the way the current system is configured or used.

Victor accessed his vocabulary by slamming his arm down on the display and "walking" his fingers to point to the desired item. This was slow and required much energy. We started by examining his arm and hand control to improve his pointing ability. We used a systematic motor assessment (Cook & Polgar, 2008) to determine that the smallest size target that Victor could reliably hit was 2 inches square. We also found that he was most successful with targets close to his body (which did not require large movement) and those further away (which allowed him to keep his arm extended). This meant that the maximum number of targets for Victor was 20, arranged in four rows of 5, two rows close to his body and two at full arm exten-

Table 4.7. Control enhancers and technique modifications

Postural supports	At hands/arms	At head
Lap tray[1]	Finger splint/pointer	Mouth stick
Armrests[1]	Universal cuff with typing stick	Head pointer
Hip belt[1]	Wrist strap pointer	Head light
Chest straps[1]	Mobile arm supports[1]	Head mouse
Lateral supports[1]	Hand brace[1]	Head rest[1]
Abductor/adductor	Hand splint[1]	
Selection set design	**Interface adjustments**	**Additional aids**
Target size[1]	Acceptance time[1]	Keyguards
Spacing[1]	Delay until repeat[1]	Templates[1]
Array shape[1]	Repeat rate[1]	Shields[1]
Angle[1]	Cursor speed[1]	Hand rest[1]
Height[1]	Sensitivity[1]	
Order of items	Activation feedback[1]	

[1] These devices or equipment could also extend or enhance motor control for indirect selection.
From Dowden, P., & Cook, A.M. (2002). Choosing effective selection techniques for beginning communicators. In D.R. Beukelman & J. Reichle (Series Eds.) & J. Reichle, D.R. Beukelman, & J.C. Light (Vol. Eds.), *AAC series: Exemplary practices for beginning communicators: Implications for AAC* (p. 398). Baltimore: Paul H. Brookes Publishing Co.; adapted by permission.

sion. These findings about range and resolution did not change, even with trials with control enhancers such as armrests, pointers, keyguards, and so forth. See Table 4.7 for more ideas we considered. See also Form 4.3 on the accompanying CD-ROM, a clinical checklist for interventionists as they assess the impact of these devices and modifications.

Victor was unable to refine his motor control, despite motor training and practice. As we observed him using his communication displays, we also noted that he had great difficulty crossing midline and that the actual usable number of targets that he could reach quickly, easily, and reliably was closer to 10 than 20. Increasing the target size to 3 inches made it much easier for Victor, but the immediate selection set would be even further reduced in number. We sought to make changes in his current low-tech system before considering technology-based solutions.

Step 2: Improve Current Modes of Communication

There may be ways in which small changes in seating and positioning may be used to en-

hance access to AAC. The goal for context-dependent communicators, however, is efficient communication all day, every day, not just success in one communication activity. We had limited options with Victor's current system. We changed the size and location of the items on his communication display so that each item was 3 inches square, arranged in 4 rows of 4 items each. We moved some infrequently used, nonurgent vocabulary on the left side to improve efficiency. This made it faster and easier for Victor, but it also worked against him because it decreased the amount of vocabulary available on any one display, requiring him to have more boards. To improve his independence, we attempted to mount all of his communication displays on his lap tray with large rings and page tabs so he could turn pages and find the display he needed without his partner having to set it up. Although Victor liked the regular access to his displays, there were important disadvantages to this system. First, the mounting of the displays meant the laptray could not be used for meals or other activities in school. More important to him, once the pages were turned forward, they hung down over the front of his lap tray and he could not retrieve them. It was clear that these problems would only be solved with a technology-based system. There was one more limitation in the current system that Victor did not yet fully appreciate. His no-tech system could never provide him with rapid access to the alphabet for vocabulary independence. Victor was already capable of independent communication if he could access all of the letters plus punctuation. We needed to reevaluate access and consider indirect selection through technology to maximize his communicative independence.

Exploring New Modes to Enhance Communicative Independence

Technology may offer a number of advantages when developing independent communication. First, additional output modes are available in a high-tech device. For example, the team working with Victor wanted him to have an SGD in order to increase his independence with many partners. Voice output may also be indicated for telephone use with distant relatives or communicating with people who do not understand the symbols. In addition, infrared output could allow him to control electronic devices, including a computer.

Second, technology can result in more available vocabulary, which was the case for Victor. If he were to use a device with dynamic displays, then the amount of vocabulary would only be limited by his ability to navigate the displays. With an encoding device, he would only be limited by his ability to learn codes for retrieval. Although neither limitation is trivial, these technology-assisted strategies would clearly expand his available vocabulary beyond the current 375 words. Victor could communicate anything he could spell with access to the alphabet, allowing him to use preprogrammed vocabulary solely for rate enhancement.

Third, there is the potential to improve the rate of communication in several ways (see Table 4.7 and Form 4.4 on the accompanying CD-ROM). We had already examined the size and spacing of Victor's possible targets. We had also already considered adding

postural supports, splints, and armrests and found that they made a small difference in speed or accuracy but were exceedingly unpleasant to Victor. We had not examined the benefits of adjustments to the sensitivity, feedback, or timing of the switches or buttons on a device—a function only available with technology. We found a few settings that made a significant difference in Victor's accuracy. For example, we had to set the **acceptance time** to be very long so that the keys that he "walked" his fingers over would not activate. The keys would activate only when he held his fingers there for a set length of time before release.

Fourth, endurance can be improved through technology. Sometimes fatigue can be reduced or eliminated by changing the type or location of the switches/keys. Changes in positioning may permit the individual to use this method for more hours each day. Victor's existing direct selection system of slamming his hand down and walking his fingers to targets was exhausting.

The accessibility of the interface is another consideration. Switches and devices must be available at all times, but monopolizing a lap tray for access is not acceptable if there are other uses for that surface. Of course, any mounting system must be designed to permit easy transfer of the individual in and out of the wheelchair.

The control interface must be positioned optimally for the individual (Cook & Polgar, 2008). Typically, single switches, joysticks, and switch arrays are mounted by attachments to a table desk, or wheelchair. Commercially available mounting systems are available, although some mounting requirements are more challenging than others as shown in the following Helpful Hint. It is also possible to attach a switch or switches to a chest strap as described previously for Genna. This attachment is not as affected by changes in body position as a mount that is attached to a table or wheelchair. For example, if a switch is mounted to the arm of a wheelchair, then even a small shift in position might make it difficult or impossible for the individual to activate it.

Finally, interventionists must consider the connection between the switch interface and the communication device or computer. Most systems require a cable that can become tangled and then inconsistent due to a short circuit, which can cause frustration. Wireless interfaces solve these challenges (e.g., wireless keyboards, pointing interfaces, some switches). Separate wireless links consisting of a transmitter that is plugged into the switch and a receiver that plugs into the communication device or the computer are also available. Activating the switch transmits an infrared signal from the switch to the device, similar to the signals used with television remote controls.

☞ Helpful Hint

Advantages of Flexible and Static Mounts for Switches

Advantages for flexible mounts

- Angle can be adjusted for switch trials
- Is useful for trials with different children
- Can be moved with child from one position to another (wheelchair to highchair)

Advantages for static mounts

- Can be placed in the optimal position for the child
- Do not move when repeatedly used
- Can be an optimal mount for the particular interface
- Can be an optimal mount for the particular mounting surface

All of these steps made it clear that Victor would be better served by a carefully designed high-tech communication device. Victor would have a system that he could operate without constant assistance. If we could give him access to the alphabet, then he would be capable of independent communication, using spelling and word prediction for words or messages that were not preprogrammed. Our assessment needed to focus on two important questions—how could he access such a system and what features would be required for greatest inde-

pendence and communicative competence. Up to this point, Victor had refused to consider anything but direct selection, but we believed that some forms of indirect selection held promise for him in the long run. We wanted him to at least consider alternatives to direct selection.

Step 1: Considering a Change in Selection Method

Whether a team is considering technology-based solutions or improving a no-tech strategy, there are many reasons that a different selection method may be required (Dowden & Cook, 2002).

- A child may need a different interface and selection method for certain positions (e.g., in bed, on the floor).
- The individual might have a degenerative disease that is gradually reducing motor control.
- It may be necessary to consider another technique simply because the current method is inappropriate for achieving independent communication, as in Victor's case.

What Does the Research Say?
Different Types of Indirect Selection

Mizuko and Esser (1991) studied 12 typically developing 4-year-olds who were taught to select two- or three-symbol sequences on a circular array, either by pointing or by single-switch inverse scanning. Subsequent testing showed no significant differences in the number of correct sequences selected by the children using the two selection techniques.

Petersen et al. (2000) investigated the performance of typically developing 2- to 4-year-old children using linear and row column scanning. They found no significant differences in errors made between these two techniques, but errors increased with the number of cursor movements to the desired symbol and the number of passes the cursor made across the display.

Dropik and Reichle (2008) studied typically developing 4-year-olds using directed scanning and group item scan-

(continued)

ning. The children were more accurate with directed scanning, beginning with a good initial performance. There appeared to be no advantage for directed scanning over group item scanning, however, in terms of efficiency of response.

Venkatagiri (1999) used computer simulation tasks to compare row column and linear scanning. Results showed that row column scanning is significantly more efficient as measured by time per character.

Angelo (1992) evaluated automatic, inverse, and step scanning methods in a task involving a single target item in an array with otherwise empty boxes at slow and fast scanning speeds customized for each individual. Three individuals had been diagnosed with spastic cerebral palsy, the other three with athetoid cerebral palsy. Accuracy in this task was primarily sensorimotor in nature as there was no symbol recognition necessary. The author found that the group data showed no significant differences among the scanning methods. Angelo reported visual trends in the data, suggesting that individuals with spastic cerebral palsy were least accurate with automatic scanning, and individuals with athetoid cerebral palsy were least accurate with step scanning. Angelo cautioned, however, that individual results even within a broad diagnostic category such as cerebral palsy can vary and cannot replace trials with each method for each individual.

The findings from any of the studies with typical participants cannot be generalized to individuals who require AAC because of the unknown impact of physical or other disabilities on the performance of the task (Bedrosian, 1995).

During assessment, interventionists must consider all possible indirect selection techniques, including single- or dual-switch scanning, directed scanning, and coded access such as Morse code (Dowden & Cook, 2002). Different techniques may offer a different number of targets at a given control site (see Table 4.3). For example, if the individual has four sites, then directed scanning, with arrow keys or a joystick, would be far more efficient than single- or dual-switch scanning. Initially, use assessment tasks that minimize the cognitive and linguistic demands of all selection techniques in order to focus on sensorimotor demands. Some of the activities listed in Table 4.6 also apply to this training. For example, we are considering multi-switch directed scanning for Victor so we can use computer software that utilizes arrow keys or joystick access. It is important to compare any new mode with the context-dependent communicator's current mode. If there is not a clear advantage in terms of speed, accuracy, fatigue, vocabulary size, or independence, then the individual may choose to continue with the existing mode. This is often a difficult decision because the final (expert) skill level may be different from the initial (novice) level, and the expert level may require significant practice time for skill development (Cook & Polgar, 2008). It may be necessary to convince the individual to practice with a new mode even while relying on the old mode for communication.

Strategies to identify the most appropriate anatomical site for a learner to use in activating a switch were described earlier. The second step in the process is to select several switches that have the potential to be used successfully by the learner at that control site. Initial choices may be dictated by the available "stock" of switches and the clinician's experience. Cook and Polgar (2008) presented a set of switch characteristics that are useful in choosing interfaces that most closely match the learner's available anatomical sites. Simple tasks can be used for switch trials with emerging communicators (see Table 4.2). Many more interesting tasks can be adapted to context-dependent communicator's capabilities and interests. During these trials, it is necessary to measure the learner's speed and accuracy to objectively determine the optimal combination of switch and control site. These data can be used to compare different interfaces operated with a given site. Speed and accuracy of responses can be quantified in the controlled setting of the clinic, but they must also be examined in the classroom, home, or community at large. Accuracy of response is often based on moving to the correct position, and its measurement requires a standard of performance, which is usually the number of correct responses out of the total number of trials. Speed of response and accuracy are generally inversely proportional to each other for novice users.

Computer-assisted assessment provides several useful features (e.g., Ashlock, Koester, LoPresti, McMillan, & Simpson, 2003). First, data collection and analysis can be automated, relieving the clinician of tedious record keeping. Performance measures for each possible anatomic site/switch pair can be obtained, including the effect of different positions for the switch mounting. In this way, it is possible to compare different combinations of control sites, interfaces, and selection techniques based on measurable results. The computer can also provide a variety of contingent results (including graphics, sound, and speech) when the switch is activated, making the task more interesting and allowing for evaluation of both visual and auditory modalities.

Although initially resistant, Victor was willing to discuss the advantages and disadvantages of indirect selection methods. Once we convinced him and his team to go for a spelling-based system and demonstrated the inadequacies of his direct selection mode in that regard, we were able to use that as leverage to convince him to try indirect selection methods. We knew we could focus on directed scanning, a method that would be more efficient than any other indirect selection technique (Cook & Polgar, 2008), because Victor could easily activate four switches on his lap tray or four directions with his wheelchair joystick. We began with his existing joystick, changing it to access computer software. We found that he had some immediate difficulty moving the cursor accurately enough with the joystick. He was used to the vestibular feedback he received from moving in his wheelchair, and without it, controlling the joystick was considerably more difficult. We began to explore modifications to the joystick itself as well as the speed of the onscreen cursor, but Victor asked us to reserve the joystick for wheelchair control and explore other options for communication.

We changed the control interface to arrow keys on the computer, beginning with one switch and progressing quickly to four switches. Victor's response time was fastest with switches close to his body. He was able to reliably react to a stimulus on the screen and hit his switch quickly with this configuration. We moved to a computer game that required him to shoot down airplanes as they crossed the screen by pressing his switch when the airplane was aligned with his gun barrel. Once again, Victor was successful but only at slower speeds. He did not like the waiting and tended to tense up just as the plane appeared, which caused him to have difficulty in activating the switch, miss his target, and become frustrated. We tried an approach in which he had to hold his switch until the plane appeared and then let go to shoot it. This was only marginally easier for him.

Finally, we chose to combine all four switches into true directed scanning, using them as arrow keys to move the cursor up, down, left, or right on the screen. We set this up initially with visual targets in a structured task, teaching him that a target on the screen would be selected whenever the cursor remained over it for 3 seconds, a setting called acceptance time in Table 4.7. This was not only the easiest and fastest selection method, but it was also the method that Victor liked the best. We conducted specific trials with other fun, low-stakes activities, and his speed and accuracy continued to increase gradually over time. Later, we arranged for similar trials on an SGD. See Cook and Polgar (2008) for a detailed description of additional approaches to assessment and ways to compare different techniques in terms of speed and accuracy as well as ways to measure the effects of training over time.

Step 2: Modifying the Selection Set to Improve Efficiency

The arrangement of the elements in a scanning array can have a large effect on the rate of communication (Lesher, Moulton, & Higginbotham, 1998; Treviranus & Roberts, 2003). For example, optimization of the display for row column scanning requires the most frequently used characters to be placed where they are scanned first.

What Does the Research Say?

Increasing Efficiency with Scanning Displays for Spelling

Research by Foulds, Baletsa, and Crochetiere (1975); Lesher et al. (1998); and Reichle, York, and Sigafoos (1991) indicated that any of the following strategies can increase the efficiency of scanning:

- Arranging the matrix to minimize the number of cursor movements or pulses required to select the most frequent items

- Placing most frequently used letters at the beginning of a row column array to increase rate of communication by 35% or more

- Placing space early in the matrix because it is one of the most frequently occurring items

- Placing backspace early in the matrix so that the user can correct errors quickly

- Using prediction in which word lists are presented based on previous scanning input

- Scanning predicted words before resuming scanning of the character matrix or permitting the user to choose whether to scan the word list or the character matrix first

- Using a **dynamic matrix rearrangement** in which prediction is based on the previous four entries rather than fewer previous entries

Victor's scanning array had to match his use of the arrow keys. First, we set up the system with a fixed display so that the cursor would return to a center or "home" space after each activation. We arranged the symbols and letters so that the most frequently used vocabulary (or letters on the alphabet page) were closest to that home space. Less frequently used letters, vocabulary, and phrases were at the edges of the display.

Step 3: Trials with New Selection Methods

The interventionist is faced with the dilemma alluded to earlier whenever a new selection technique or interface is selected for a con-

text-dependent communicator. The individual's operational competence is initially limited, making the new mode less efficient and possibly less reliable than the old, familiar system. Most AAC users are justifiably frustrated if their communicative competence is decreased while they are learning the new system. Therefore, it is recommended that the individual continue to use his or her existing system in some contexts while receiving direct instruction in the new system or mode. OTs and PTs often use some of the approaches described in the following Helpful Hint when teaching scanning. The AAC user needs to develop operational skills with the new selection method in tasks that are functional but not highly demanding.

☞ Helpful Hint

Teaching Scanning to Context-Dependent Communicators

Jones and Stewart (2004) found four themes in their survey described previously.

1. The process of training scanning is progressive.

2. Training programs must be developed specifically for each individual.

3. Training scanning is inextricably linked to functional goals.

4. It is important to train both the child and the primary caregivers using a collaborative approach.

They also suggested

- Parallel training on both the AAC device and scanning computer games, particularly when a new mode or device is added to an existing mode

- Using branching arrays to teach the progression from linear to row column scanning

Goossens' and Crain (1992) recommended training the child in the skills required by the new method while using the current method for communication.

Piché and Reichle (1991) recommended training individuals in indirect selection even while refining their direct selection access if indirect access will be necessary in the future.

The communicative functions can be transferred from the old to the new mode when the operational competence with the new mode is reliable, accurate, and as efficient as possible. This new system can then be practiced and tested in natural communication exchanges in which cognitive and linguistic demands are high; in other words, in everyday communication. Blackstone (1989) recommended introducing such demands gradually to maximize success and give the individual time to learn each new component.

It is often difficult to know when to say, "It is not going to work, even with more practice" versus "keep practicing, you will get it" when moving to a new mode that requires skill acquisition. Interventionists most often quit too early rather than too late. The process of developing operational competence can be frustrating to everyone, but it is generally worth the effort to allow time to develop these skills (Treviranus & Roberts, 2003). This is not unlike any other skilled motor task such as athletics or music—all take practice to achieve high levels of skill.

Victor continued to rely on his no-tech direct selection system during the transition to indirect selection. His mocked-up voice output system using directed scanning on a computer had displays that were as similar as possible to his original no-tech communication displays. We gradually rearranged each display for maximum efficiency as Victor became accustomed to using this new access to make selections from a familiar selection set. We also introduced the alphabet and word prediction but did not remove any familiar vocabulary until he began to see that many words such as *I, he,* and *is* were so short that it was faster to spell them out than to search for preprogrammed vocabulary for rate enhancement.

We identified and acquired a voice output device for Victor once he was confident that this selection method would work for him. After we customized it with his input, our routine work with him and his team came to a conclusion. He was well on his way to communicative competence and independence with this new system added to his repertoire of communication strategies. We saw him again several years later. He was attending a local community college and advocating for computer access for students with disabilities. Victor was clearly making a place for himself as a leader among his peers, and we could only imagine where he would go in the years that follow. He had achieved the competence and independence that were the means to the goals he was pursuing with such intensity.

SUMMARY

Communicative competence and independence are the main goals whether a team is seeking the first access method for an emerging communicator or striving to improve access for a context-dependent or independent communicator. Technology should always be a means to an end, not a goal in and of itself. As we saw with Genna, technology is not the only way to improve the competence of an emerging communicator. Interventionists must consider all modes of expression and take the time to achieve that first, reliable means of symbolic communication. Serving individuals such as Victor has taught us to facilitate social, strategic, and linguistic competence while working to provide or enhance operational control for the most independent communication. Working together on all of these elements of communication gradually reveal the individual's true capabilities. Eventually, there comes a time when we have to step out of the way and allow the individual to shape his or her own communication strategies to accomplish his or her own goals.

REFERENCES

Angelo, J. (1992). Comparison of three computer scanning modes as an interface method for persons with cerebral palsy. *American Journal of Occupational Therapy, 46,* 217–222.

Angelo, J. (2000). Factors affecting the use of a single switch with assistive technology devices. *Journal of Rehabilitation Research and Development, 37*(5), 591–598.

Ashlock, G., Koester, H.H., LoPresti, E.F., Mc-Millan, W., & Simpson, R.C. (2003). *User-centered design of software for assessing computer usage skills.* Presentation at the RESNA 2003 Annual Conference, Atlanta, GA.

Bedrosian, J. (1995). Limitations in the use of nondisabled subjects in AAC research. *Augmentative and Alternative Communication, 11,* 6–10.

Beukelman, D.R., & Mirenda, P. (2005). *Augmentative and alternative communication: Supporting children and adults with complex communication needs* (3rd ed.). Baltimore: Paul H. Brookes Publishing Co.

Blackstone, S. (1989). Visual scanning: What's it all about and training approaches. *Augmentative Communication News, 2*(4), 1–5.

Blackstone, S., & Hunt Berg, M. (2003). *Social networks: A communication inventory for individuals with complex needs and their communication partners.* Monterey, CA: Augmentative Communication.

Blockberger, S., & Sutton, A. (2003). Toward linguistic competence: Language experiences and knowledge of children with extremely limited speech. In D.R. Beukelman & J. Reichle (Series Eds.) & J.C. Light, D.R. Beukelman, & J. Reichle (Vol. Eds.), *AAC series: Communicative competence for individuals who use AAC: From research to effective practice* (pp. 63–106). Baltimore: Paul H. Brookes Publishing Co.

Broderick, P. (1998). *Pediatric vision screening for the family physician.* Retrieved August 26, 2007, from http://www.aafp.org/afp/980901ap/broderic.html

Burkhart, L.J., & Porter, G. (2006). *Partner-assisted communication strategies for children who face multiple challenges.* Preconference instructional course, International Society of Augmentative and Alternative Communication, Düsseldorf, Germany.

Bush, J.S. (2003). *Practice guidelines: AAP issues screening recommendations to identify hearing loss in children.* Retrieved March 16, 2008, from http://www.aafp.org/afp/20030601/practice.html

Cannella, H.I., O'Reilly, M.F., & Lancioni, G.E. (2005). Choice and preference assessment research with people with severe to profound developmental disabilities: A review of the literature. *Research in Developmental Disabilities, 26,* 1–15.

Carrow-Woolfolk, E. (1999). *Test for Auditory Comprehension of Language–Third Edition (TACL-3).* Austin, TX: PRO-ED.

Casey, K. (1995). Play-based assessment for AAC. In G.M. VanTatenhove (Ed.), *Special interest division 12: Augmentative and alternative communication* (pp. 10–13). Rockville, MD: American Speech-Language-Hearing Association.

Cook, A.M., Adams, K., & Harbottle, N. (2007). *Lego robot use by children with severe disabilities.* Paper presented at the CSUN Conference, Northridge, CA.

Cook, A.M., Hussey, S.M., & Currier, M. (1996). *Development of a head-controlled dynamic display AAC system.* Paper presented at the ISAAC Conference, Vancouver, British Columbia, Canada.

Cook, A.M., & Polgar, J.M. (2008). *Cook and Hussey's assistive technologies: Principles and practice.* St. Louis: Mosby.

Cress, P.J., Spellman, C.R., DeBriere, T.J., Sizemore, A.C., Northam, J.K., & Johnson, J.L. (1981). Vision screening for persons with severe handicaps. *Journal of The Association for Persons with Severe Handicaps, 6,* 41–49.

DeCoste, D.C. (1997). Augmentative and alternative communication assessment strategies: Motor access and visual considerations. In S. Glennen & D.C. DeCoste (Eds.), *Handbook of augmentative and alternative communication* (pp. 243–282). San Diego: Singular Publishing.

Doshi, N.R., & Rodriguez, M.L.F. (2007). Amblyopia. *American Family Physician, 75*(3), 361–367.

Dowden, P.A. (1999). Different strokes for different folks. *Augmentative Communication News, 12*(1 and 2), 7–8.

Dowden, P., & Cook, A.M. (2002). Choosing effective selection techniques for beginning communicators. In D.R. Beukelman & J. Reichle (Series Eds.) & J. Reichle, D.R. Beukelman, & J.C. Light (Vol. Eds.), *AAC series: Exemplary practices for beginning communicators: Implications for AAC* (pp. 395–432). Baltimore: Paul H. Brookes Publishing Co.

Dropik, P.L., & Reichle, R. (2008). Comparison of accuracy and efficiency of directed scanning and group-item scanning for augmentative communication selection techniques with typically developing preschoolers. *American Journal of Speech-Language Pathology, 17,* 35–47.

Dunn, L.M., & Dunn, L.M. (1997). *Peabody Picture Vocabulary Test–Third Edition (PPVT-III).* Circle Pines, MN: American Guidance Service.

Foulds, R., Baletsa, G., & Crochetiere, W. (1975). The effectiveness of language redundancy in non-verbal communication. *Proceedings of the Conference on Systems and Devices for the Disabled,* 82–86.

Goossens', C., & Crain, M.S. (1992), *Utilizing switch interfaces with children who are severely physically challenged.* Austin, TX: PRO-ED.

Horn, E.M., & Jones, H.A. (1996). Comparison of two selection techniques used in augmentative and alternative communication. *Augmentative and Alternative Communication, 12,* 23–31.

Hussey, S.M., Cook, A.M., Whinnery, S.E., Buckpitt, L., & Huntington, M. (1992). *A conceptual model for developing augmentative communication skills in individuals with severe disabilities.* Arlington, VA: RESNA.

Iacono, T., Carter, M., & Hook, J. (1998). Identification of intentional communication in students with severe and multiple disabilities. *Augmentative and Alternative Communication, 14,* 102–114.

Jagacinski, R.J., & Monk, D.L. (1985). Fitts' Law in two dimensions with hand and head movements. *Journal of Motor Behavior, 17*(1), 77–95.

Jones, J., & Stewart, H. (2004). A description of how three occupational therapists train children in using the scanning access technique. *Australian Journal of Occupational Therapy, 51,* 155–165.

Kovach, T.M., & Kenyon, P.B. (2003). Visual issues and access to AAC. In D. Beukelman & J. Reichle (Series Eds.) & J.C. Light, D.R. Beukelman & J. Reichle (Vol. Eds.), *AAC series: Communicative competence for individuals who use AAC: From research to effective practice* (pp. 277–322). Baltimore: Paul H. Brookes Publishing Co.

Lancioni, G.E., O'Reilly, M.F., Singh, N.N., Oliva, D., & Groeneweg, J. (2002). Impact of stimulation versus microswitch-based programs on indices of happiness of people with profound multiple disabilities. *Research in Developmental Disabilities, 23,* 149–160.

Lesher, G.W., Higginbotham, J., & Moulton, B.J. (2000). *Techniques for automatically updating scanning delays.* Paper presented at the Annual Conference on Rehabilitation Technology, Orlando, FL.

Lesher, G.W., Moulton, B.J., & Higginbotham, D.J. (1998). Techniques for augmenting scanning. *Augmentative and Alternative Communication, 14*(2), 81–101.

Light, J. (1989). Toward a definition of communicative competence for individuals using augmentative and alternative communication systems. *Augmentative and Alternative Communication, 5,* 137–144.

Light, J. (1993). Teaching automatic linear scanning for computer access: A case study of a preschooler with severe physical and communication disabilities. *Journal of Special Education Technology, 12,* 125–134.

Light, J.C. (1997). Communication is the essence of human life: Reflections on communicative competence. *Augmentative and Alternative Communication, 13,* 61–70.

Light, J.C. (2003). Shattering the silence: Development of communicative competence by individuals who use AAC. In D. Beukelman & J. Reichle (Series Eds.) & J.C. Light, D.R. Beukelman, & J. Reichle (Vol. Eds.), *AAC series: Communicative competence for individuals who use AAC: From research to effective practice* (pp. 3–40). Baltimore: Paul H. Brookes Publishing Co.

Markwardt, F.C., Jr. (1997). *Peabody Individual Achievement Test.* Bloomington, MN: Pearson Assessments.

McCarthy, G.T. (1992). *Physical disability in childhood.* London: Churchill Livingstone.

McCarthy, J., Light, J., Drager, K., McNaughton, D., Grodzicki, L., Jones, J., et al. (2006). Redesigning scanning to reduce learning demands: The performance of typically developing 2-year-olds. *Augmentative and Alternative Communication, 22,* 269–283.

McLean, J.E., McLean, L.K.S., Brady, N.C., & Etter, R. (1991). Communication profiles of two types of gesture using nonverbal persons with severe to profound mental retardation. *Journal of Speech and Hearing Research, 34,* 294–308.

Mizuko, M., & Esser, J. (1991). The effect of direct selection and circular scanning on visual sequential recall. *Journal of Speech and Hearing Research, 34,* 43–48.

Mizuko, M., Reichle, J., Ratcliff, A., & Esser, J. (1994). Effects of selection techniques and array sizes on short-term visual memory. *Augmentative and Alternative Communication, 10,* 237–244.

Mustonen, T., Locke, P., Reichle, J., Solbrack, M., & Lindgren, A. (1991). An overview of augmentative and alternative communication systems. In J. Reichle, J. York, & J. Sigafoos (Eds.), *Implementing augmentative and alternative communication: Strategies for learners with severe disabilities* (pp. 1–38). Baltimore: Paul H. Brookes Publishing Co.

Olswang, L.B., & Pinder, G.L. (1995). Preverbal functional communication and the role of object play in children with cerebral palsy. *Infant-Toddler Intervention, 5*(3), 277–299.

Petersen, K., Reichle, J., & Johnston, S.S. (2000). Examining preschoolers' performance in linear and row-column scanning techniques. *Augmentative and Alternative Communication, 16,* 27–36.

Piché, L., & Reichle, J. (1991). Teaching scanning selection techniques. In J. Reichle, J. York, & J. Sigafoos (Eds.), *Implementing augmentative and alternative communication: Strategies for learners with severe disabilities* (pp. 257–274). Baltimore: Paul H. Brookes Publishing Co.

Pinder, G.L., & Olswang, L.B. (1995). Development of communicative intent in young children with cerebral palsy: A treatment efficacy study. *Infant-Toddler Intervention, 5*(1), 51–69.

Ratcliff, A. (1994). Comparison of relative demands implicated in direct selection and scanning: Considerations from normal children. *Augmentative and Alternative Communication, 10,* 67–74.

Reichle, J., York, J., & Sigafoos, J. (1991). *Implementing augmentative and alternative communica-*

tion: Strategies for learners with severe disabilities. Baltimore: Paul H. Brookes Publishing Co.

Saunders, M.D., Saunders, R.R., Mulugeta, A., Henderson, K., Kedziorski, T., Hekker, B., & Wilson, S. (2005). A novel method for testing learning and preferences in people with minimal motor movement. *Research in Developmental Disabilities, 26,* 255–266.

Saunders, M.D., Smagner, J.P., & Saunders, R.R. (2003). Improving methodological and technological analysis of adaptive switch use of individuals with profound multiple impairments. *Behavioral Intervention, 18,* 227–243.

Schulmeister, J., Wiberg, C., Adams, K., & Cook, C. (2006). *Robot assisted play for children with disabilities.* Poster presentation at the RESNA International Conference, Arlington, VA.

Sigafoos, J., Arthur-Kelly, M., & Butterfield, N. (2006). *Enhancing everyday communication for children with disabilities.* Baltimore: Paul H. Brookes Publishing Co.

Sigafoos, J., Drasgow, E., Reichle, J., O'Reilly, M., Green, V.A., & Tait, K. (2004). Tutorial: Teaching communicative rejecting to children with severe disabilities. *American Journal of Speech-Language Pathology, 13,* 31–42.

Sturm, J. (2005). Literacy development of children who use AAC. In D.R. Beukelman & P. Mirenda (Eds.), *Augmentative and alternative communication: Supporting children and adults with complex communication needs* (3rd ed., pp. 351–389). Baltimore: Paul H. Brookes Publishing Co.

Tait, K., Sigafoos, J., Woodyatt, G., O'Reilly, M.F., & Lancioni, G.E. (2004). Evaluating parent use of functional communication training to replace and enhance prelinguistic behaviors in six children with developmental and physical disabilities. *Disability and Rehabilitation, 26,* 1241–1254.

Treviranus, J., & Roberts, V. (2003). Supporting competent motor control of AAC systems. In D. Beukelman & J. Reichle (Series Eds.) & J.C. Light, D.R. Beukelman, & J. Reichle (Vol. Eds.), *AAC series: Communicative competence for individuals who use AAC: From research to effective practice* (pp. 199–240). Baltimore: Paul H. Brookes Publishing Co.

Utley, B.L. (2002). Visual assessment considerations for the design of AAC systems. In D. Beukelman & J. Reichle (Series Eds.) & J. Reichle, D.R. Beukelman, & J.C. Light (Vol. Eds.), *AAC series: Exemplary practices for beginning communicators: Implications for AAC* (pp. 353–394). Baltimore: Paul H. Brookes Publishing Co.

Venkatagiri, H.S. (1999). Efficient keyboard layouts for sequential access in augmentative and alternative communication. *Augmentative and Alternative Communication, 15,* 126–134.

Wagner, B.T., & Jackson, H.M. (2006). Developmental memory capacity resources of children retrieving picture communication symbols using direct selection and visual linear scanning with fixed communication displays. *Journal of Speech, Language, and Hearing Research, 49,* 113–126.

Wagner, R.K., Torgesen, J.K., & Rashotte, C.A. (1999). *Comprehensive Test of Phonological Processing (CTOPP).* Austin, TX: PRO-ED.

Wechsler, D. (2002). *Wechsler Individual Achievement Tests–Second Edition (WIAT-II).* San Antonio, TX: Psychological Corporation.

York, J., & Weimann, G. (1991). Accommodating severe physical disabilities. In J. Reichle, J. York, & J. Sigafoos (Eds.), *Implementing augmentative and alternative communication: Strategies for learners with severe disabilities* (pp. 239–256). Baltimore: Paul H. Brookes Publishing Co.

Instructional Strategies

Kathleen M. Feeley and Emily A. Jones

▷ CHAPTER OVERVIEW

Interventions addressing the needs of augmentative and alternative communication (AAC) users utilize **evidence-based instructional strategies** to help the learner produce desired **behaviors,** reinforce correct behaviors, and respond to learner errors. Fluency in each of these areas enables interventionists to select strategies that most effectively meet the needs of individual AAC users.

▷ CHAPTER OBJECTIVES

After studying this chapter, readers will be able to

- Plan intervention to increase the likelihood of generalization and conditional use
- Describe the foundation on which instruction is based
- Develop and implement effective prompting procedures
- Develop and implement effective reinforcement procedures
- Develop and implement procedures that address incorrect responding
- Implement instructional procedures to shape behavior
- Implement instructional procedures to teach chains of behavior
- Develop and implement procedures to enhance spontaneous use of communication skills
- Develop and implement procedures to maintain acquired skills

▷ KEY TERMS

- ▶ abolishing operations
- ▶ backward chaining
- ▶ behavior
- ▶ behavior chain interruption
- ▶ behavior interruption
- ▶ chaining
- ▶ conditional use
- ▶ consequence
- ▶ constant
- ▶ continuous schedule of reinforcement
- ▶ delay signal
- ▶ deprivation
- ▶ differential reinforcement
- ▶ discriminative stimulus (S^D)
- ▶ error correction
- ▶ establishing operations
- ▶ evidence-based instructional strategies
- ▶ fade reinforcement
- ▶ fading
- ▶ fixed ratio schedule of reinforcement
- ▶ forward chaining
- ▶ general case instruction
- ▶ generalization
- ▶ gestural prompts
- ▶ graduated guidance
- ▶ intermittent schedule of reinforcement
- ▶ interval schedule
- ▶ least-to-most prompt hierarchy
- ▶ maintenance
- ▶ modeling prompts
- ▶ most-to-least prompt hierarchy
- ▶ motivating operations
- ▶ negative reinforcement
- ▶ negative teaching examples
- ▶ physical prompts
- ▶ picture prompts

- ▶ position cues
- ▶ positive reinforcement
- ▶ positive teaching examples
- ▶ primary reinforcers
- ▶ progressive
- ▶ prompts
- ▶ ratio schedule
- ▶ reinforcement
- ▶ response generalization
- ▶ response prompts
- ▶ safety signal
- ▶ satiation

- ▶ schedule of reinforcement
- ▶ schedule thinning
- ▶ secondary reinforcers
- ▶ shaping
- ▶ spontaniety
- ▶ stimulus building
- ▶ stimulus fading
- ▶ stimulus generalization
- ▶ stimulus prompts
- ▶ stimulus shaping
- ▶ systematic preference assessment
- ▶ task analysis

- ▶ textual prompts
- ▶ three-term contingency
- ▶ time delay procedure
- ▶ token economy
- ▶ tolerance cue
- ▶ tolerance for delay of reinforcement
- ▶ total task chaining
- ▶ transferring stimulus control
- ▶ variable ratio schedule of reinforcement
- ▶ verbal prompts

PLANNING FOR GENERALIZATION AND CONDITIONAL USE

Intervention should result in a learner's acquisition of a variety of communication skills demonstrated across a range of situations (i.e., **generalization** of communication skills). Learners with severe disabilities, however, often fail to engage in generalized responding.

Stimulus generalization occurs when a learner performs a behavior under conditions different from those during intervention (Stokes & Baer, 1977). For example, a child follows a different activity schedule at home after learning to follow an activity schedule at school. Using the same communication form (e.g., raising hand) for different communicative functions (e.g., to request assistance, to request attention) is another example of stimulus generalization. Generalization across materials, partners, settings, and functions may not readily occur for learners with disabilities (Sigafoos, O'Reilly, Drasgow, & Reichle, 2002).

Response generalization occurs when a learner has multiple behaviors within his or her repertoire, and each is appropriate for a given set of stimuli. For example, a learner notices a preferred item and 1) points to the item, 2) says "want that," or 3) points to a symbol (e.g., photograph of the item). In this case, the multiple behaviors represent different communicative modes. Response generalization may also involve multiple ways of delivering the same message within a communicative mode. For example, a learner could say, "I would like coffee," "A cup of Joe," or "Coffee" in response to the question, "What do you want?" Having an array of behaviors from which to choose allows for effective communication, particularly with an unfamiliar person or when needing to repair a communication breakdown (e.g., speech is not understood by a partner, so the learner adds a gesture).

Conditional use refers to discriminating between situations that call for a communicative behavior and situations that call for the learner to refrain from using the behavior (or to use a different behavior). For example, a learner should finish an assignment that he or she can complete independently, and a learner should request assistance when he or she cannot finish a difficult assignment.

What Is General Case Instruction?

General case instruction addresses the acquisition of generalized skills and conditional use from the onset of intervention (Horner & McDonald, 1982). Carefully selected intervention opportunities sample the range of behavior forms and situations in which specific communication skills should and should not be demonstrated so that acquisition, generalization, and conditional use of skills occur concurrently.

How Do I Implement General Case Instruction?

General case instruction is relatively straight-forward to implement even though it may require additional effort on the part of the team of individuals who provide educational or in-home service for an individual. The following steps are drawn from the literature discussing general case instruction.

Step 1: Define the Instructional Universe

Specify the range of relevant stimuli (e.g., people, places, materials) likely to occasion the communicative behavior.

Step 2: Identify Teaching Examples

Identify multiple teaching examples representing the range of situations in which communication should and should not occur (e.g., across environments, in the presence of a variety of individuals and materials), and include multiple forms of communication.

- **Positive teaching examples** are opportunities when the behavior should occur.
- **Negative teaching examples** are opportunities when the behavior should not occur.

Instruction using both positive and negative examples teaches conditional use of communication from the outset (Reichle & Johnston, 1999; Reichle et al., 2005). Table 5.1 shows conditional use of communication in several situations.

Step 3: Choose Specific Teaching Examples with Which to Begin Intervention

- Sample from the range of examples within the instructional universe. For example, if communication opportunities arise at home, in the community, and at school or the workplace, then teaching opportunities should represent each environment.

Steps to implement general case instruction

Step 1: Define the instructional universe.
Step 2: Identify teaching examples.
Step 3: Choose specific teaching examples with which to begin intervention.
Step 4: Begin intervention while continuing to assess learner performance for examples not targeted for intervention.

- Initially, positive and negative teaching examples should be maximally different to enable the learner to discriminate when a response should and should not be used. The lid tightly on the container (positive) and the lid off of the container (negative) are maximally different examples to teach requesting assistance before attempting a task. Over time, make teaching opportunities less discriminable (e.g., lid partially on, loosely on the container).

- Situations in which the learner engages in challenging behavior may warrant immediate intervention.

- Consider the resources (e.g., interventionists, time) available within each situation.

Step 4: Begin Intervention While Continuing to Assess Learner Performance for Examples Not Targeted for Intervention

1. Begin with the teaching examples chosen in Step 3, and use evidence-based strategies presented throughout this chapter.

2. Conduct probes of the learner's performance in situations, including negative teaching examples, not yet targeted for intervention to examine generalization. Conduct probes more frequently if the AAC user acquires skills relatively rapidly.

3. Implement additional intervention if the communicative behavior is not demonstrated on probe opportunities. Arrange the environment or take advantage of natural opportunities when the behav-

Table 5.1.   Examples of situations requiring conditional discriminations

Type of situation	Example
Setting specific	Request a drink in a restaurant, but wait until intermission at a concert.
Person specific	Use signs with familiar partners who understand sign language, but use graphic symbols with unfamiliar people in the community.
Frequency of access	Request a second helping of cake, but reject an offer of a third piece.
Task specific	Request assistance for difficult tasks, but readily complete easy tasks.

ior should not be produced if negative teaching examples require instruction. For example, place the items within the learner's reach to establish a negative teaching example. Place the items out of the learner's reach to teach him or her to request desired items. During negative teaching opportunities, interrupt the learner's attempts to emit the communicative behavior, or consider **error correction** procedures (discussed later in this chapter) if it is difficult to interrupt the communicative behavior during negative teaching opportunities.

CASE EXAMPLE

General Case Instruction

Pablo: Requesting a Break

Pablo, an 18-year-old with autism, spent half of his day in classroom instruction and the other half in job training. He used line drawings stored in a small, multipage book to communicate but did not consistently use his book to gain access to breaks from daily activities.

Katie: Requesting Assistance

Katie was a second-grade student with severe disabilities involved in several community activities including Girl Scouts and soccer. Katie used signs to augment her speech. She tended to have tantrums, however, when she could not get her needs met.

Communicative Response

Pablo: Requesting a break using the graphic symbol for BREAK

Katie: Requesting assistance using the sign for HELP

Step 1: Define the Instructional Universe

Pablo and Katie: Range of relevant stimuli

- Activities in school with a variety of materials with different peers and staff
- Activities at home with family members
- Activities at work requiring different materials with different co-workers (Pablo only)
- Activities within the community with different community members

Pablo: Behavior variation

- Point to the graphic symbol for BREAK.
- Point to the clock to indicate time for a break.

Katie: Behavior variation

- Sign HELP.
- Bring the materials to an peer or adult.

Step 2: Identify Teaching Examples

Positive teaching examples for Pablo requesting a break

1. Learning sight words with peers
2. Playing field hockey
3. Stocking shelves at work
4. Tearing empty boxes at work
5. Playing games at home with family

Negative teaching examples for Pablo requesting a break

1. Helping to prepare a meal at home
2. Helping a customer at work
3. At home preparing to get ready for school
4. Traveling on the bus between stops

Positive teaching examples for Katie requesting assistance

1. Opening a difficult food package
2. Being asked to engage in an unfamiliar task
3. Putting on a sweater with difficult buttons

4. Trying to reach a video on a high shelf
5. Putting on shin guards at soccer

Negative teaching examples for Katie requesting assistance

1. Being provided with a package that has a history of being easily opened
2. Zipping up a jacket that she has been independently doing prior to being taught a request for assistance
3. Putting on soccer gear (other than shin guards)

Step 3: Choose Specific Teaching Examples with Which to Begin Intervention

- Pablo's intervention began during one situation at school and one at work.
- Katie's parents and teachers began intervention at home and school.

Step 4: Begin Intervention While Continuing to Assess Learner Performance for Examples Not Targeted for Intervention

Weekly positive example probes revealed Pablo generalized requesting a break to other situations at school, work, and home. Negative example probes showed he requested a break when it was not appropriate (e.g., at work while helping a customer). Pablo's interventionist prespecified a reinforcer (snack) that Pablo would receive if he did not request a break. Before going to help a customer Pablo's interventionist said, "We'll take a break and have your favorite snack as soon as you're done helping this customer" and interrupted any attempts to select the BREAK symbol by placing her hand over the symbol and saying, "You shouldn't take a break while helping a customer. You can take a break and have a snack when you're done."

Katie quickly learned to sign HELP when in need of assistance, but positive example probes in other environments

> A *probe* is a test in which one or more opportunities are presented to examine learner performance in the absence of intervention strategies (e.g., prompting, reinforcement).

revealed she did not request assistance in the community, rather she cried when in need of assistance. Katie's mother implemented intervention in the community setting.

Katie's performance during negative example probes indicated Katie readily discriminated when she did not need to use her sign for HELP and immediately attempted the task at hand.

What Does the Research Say?
General Case Instruction

Romer, Cullinan, and Schoenberg (1994) used general case instruction to teach a general sign (e.g., WANT, PLEASE) and signs for specific items (e.g., JUICE, WATER) to request within a variety of activities to four adults with severe disabilities. Probes showed all participants used the general requesting behavior (e.g., WANT) in the presence of untrained items, and three of the four also used untrained explicit requests (e.g., signs for WANT plus the novel item).

Chadsey-Rusch, Drasgow, Reinoehl, and Halle (1993) used a multiple probe design to compare general case instruction implemented in several situations (i.e., cafeteria, classroom, hallway, vocational training sites) with intervention implemented in only one situation (i.e., during mealtime) to teach requesting to three adolescent girls with severe disabilities. Compared to baseline and the single-instance condition, general case instruction resulted in fewer trials to criterion for two of three participants and marked increases in communication skills during generalization probes in different settings, with different materials, and with different partners.

WHAT HAPPENS DURING EVERY INTERVENTION OPPORTUNITY: THE THREE-TERM CONTINGENCY

Effective intervention involves well-planned teaching opportunities, not only with respect to generalization but also with respect to the components of each opportunity. The **three-term contingency,** which describes the relationship between behavior

Table 5.2. Examples of the three-term contingency for several communicative behaviors

Discriminative stimulus (S^D)	Response	Consequence
Frank's interventionist asked, "What's this?" while holding an object.	Frank produced the sign corresponding to the object.	Frank's interventionist delivered verbal praise.
John's favorite toy was on a high shelf.	John pointed to the toy.	John's mother retrieved the toy and handed it to him.
Tom's juice container was too difficult for him to open.	Tom selected the symbol HELP PLEASE on his speech-generating device.	Tom's friend opened his juice container for him.
Suzanne's teacher greeted her at the door in the morning.	Suzanne pointed to the symbols HI, HOW ARE YOU? in her communication wallet.	Suzanne's teacher said, "Fine; thank you for asking," while giving Suzanne a big smile.

and events in the environment (i.e., stimuli) that occur prior to and after that behavior, is the foundation of every intervention opportunity. The **discriminative stimulus (S^D;** the first part of the three-term contingency) cues the learner to engage in a particular behavior (the second part of the three-term contingency) because it will likely result in a certain **consequence** (the third part of the three-term contingency). The S^D may occur naturally (e.g., a sneeze) or may be contrived by an interventionist (e.g., asking "What color is this?" while holding an object). Table 5.2 provides several examples of three-term contingencies for communicative behaviors.

IMPLEMENT STRATEGIES TO PROMPT CORRECT RESPONDING

Proficient communicators readily respond to events (S^{D}s). Learners with severe disabilities may not readily respond to natural events, failing to notice some stimuli. A learner may lack the skills necessary to emit an appropriate behavior. Some learners might respond to S^{D}s related to specific skill areas in which they are more proficient, but

not respond to S^{D}s related to other skill areas. Learners with autism, for example, may be less likely to respond to an opportunity for a comment than a request; in contrast, young children with Down syndrome may be less likely to request than comment (Mundy, Kasari, & Sigman, 1995).

Interventionists often use **prompts** (i.e., some assistance to the learner to produce the correct behavior) to increase the likelihood that a learner produces a correct behavior in the presence of a naturally occurring event. Prompts can be delivered at the same time as the naturally occurring stimuli (S^D) or immediately following (see Figure 5.1).

TYPES OF PROMPTS

There are two broad types of prompts:

1. **Stimulus prompts** manipulate dimensions of a stimulus (e.g., position, size) to increase the likelihood that a learner will notice the natural cues to which he or she should respond.

2. **Response prompts** direct the learner's production of a correct behavior.

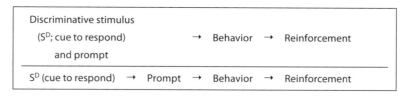

Figure 5.1. Temporal order of components of an instructional opportunity.

Stimulus Prompts

Position cues involve positioning stimuli to increase the likelihood of a correct behavior (e.g., placing the ball closer to the learner to teach receptive identification of the ball).

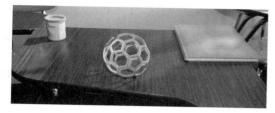

Stimuli can also be enlarged to increase the likelihood that the learner will respond correctly. For example, to teach shape identification an interventionist presented an enlarged triangle and smaller square and circle with the S^D and asked, "Where's the triangle?"

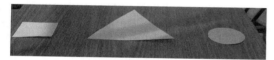

Picture prompts (or visual prompts) and **textual prompts** (or scripts) involve adding graphic symbols (e.g., photographs, line drawings) or text to materials in the environment (e.g., placed on student's placemat during snack time) to increase the likelihood that a learner performs a specific behavior.

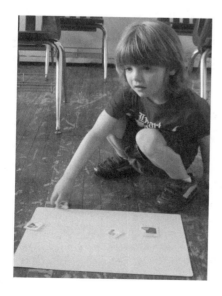

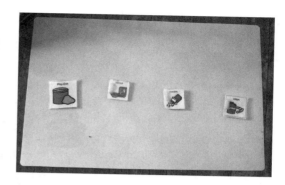

☞ Helpful Hint

Other terms are also used to describe types of prompts. *Within-stimulus prompts* focus on the inherent characteristics of the stimulus itself, emphasizing or enhancing the size, shape, color, hue, and so forth of the actual stimulus. Within-stimulus prompts direct a learner's attention to the stimulus itself. *Extra-stimulus prompts* are external to the stimulus and include physically pointing to the stimulus, focusing a light on the stimulus, or positioning a visual prompt (e.g., a photograph) next to or under the target stimulus (e.g., a sight word). Extra-stimulus prompts may distract the learner from the stimulus itself, which may be particularly problematic for some learners (e.g., those with autism; Schreibman, 1975). Generally, choose prompts that focus the learner's attention on the stimulus and its qualities instead of diverting the learner's attention to other, insignificant features presented with the stimulus (Sulzer-Azaroff & Mayer, 1991).

Picture prompts may also involve superimposing familiar stimuli (e.g., photographs) with the natural stimuli. For example, Birkan, McClannahan, and Krantz (2007) superimposed a known picture on the written word *chips* to teach sight word reading to a 6-year-old boy with autism. They then cut away the photograph to fade the stimulus prompt and replaced the remaining photograph background behind the word with plain paper (fading prompts will be discussed shortly).

Textual prompts are written words that cue behavior. Textual prompts can be single words that cue a variety of behaviors or even complete sentences (i.e., scripts) that a learner is supposed to express. For example, the interventionist created several written scripts on index cards joined on a ring for easy transport to teach appropriate spontaneous comments and requests.

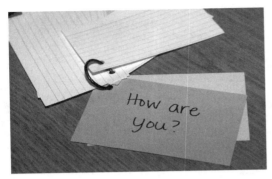

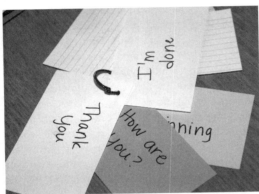

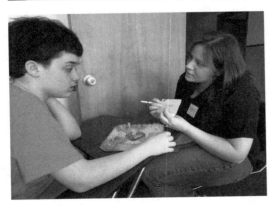

Sarokoff, Taylor, and Poulson (2001) used textual prompts in the form of multiword scripts to prompt two children with autism to engage in conversation about specific items (e.g., snack food, activities). Items were chosen that specifically contained existing naturally occurring textual cues (e.g., food item with the name on the package,

such as Skittles). The item (i.e., snack food) was mounted on a paper containing a script of several conversation statements, each starting with the text that naturally occurred on the item (e.g., "Skittles are my favorite"). Sarokoff et al. also used a gestural prompt (e.g., a gesture; discussed shortly) to direct learner attention to the textual scripts, illustrating the combined use of different prompts. Scripts were faded by gradually removing portions of the scripted words and eventually the paper, leaving just the materials (and naturally occurring textual cue on the item).

☞ Helpful Hint

Take advantage of computer technology to develop materials for picture and textual prompts. Scan symbols and manipulate the size (as well as brightness and color) of photographs, text, and drawings. Symbols can then be printed for easy use. Computer programs (e.g., Boardmaker) also provide convenient access to pictures, line drawings, and so forth.

Stimulus prompts increase the likelihood of a correct behavior by increasing the saliency (adding or exaggerating dimensions) of the stimuli cueing that behavior. More intrusive prompts are necessary for some learners to help the learner to emit the behavior. For others, it is the lack of the specific behavior in the learner's repertoire, not the saliency of the stimuli, interfering with skill acquisition. Response prompts are likely necessary in these instances.

Response Prompts

In general, the distinction between stimulus and response prompts is that stimulus prompts involve manipulation of antecedent stimuli (e.g., task materials), whereas response prompts are directed specifically at the learner's behavior.

The interventionist comments, asks questions, or provides instructions with **verbal prompts,** which assists the learner in emitting the correct behavior. For example, the presence of a favorite toy during play-

A *mand-model* procedure involves providing a verbal prompt manding for a behavior. For example, the interventionist says, "What do you want?" (mand). If the learner does not correctly respond, then the interventionist presents a model, "Say, 'I want the toy.'"

time is a natural cue for the child to request access to that toy. Interventionists might use verbal prompts including commenting, "You can ask for it if you'd like," asking a question, "What do you want?" or instructing, "Say, 'I want the toy'" to help the child request. A verbal comment prompt requires a higher level of sophistication on the part of the learner.

The interventionist performs the target skill with **modeling prompts** to demonstrate what the learner should do. For example, the interventionist could provide a verbal model of the child's request for his or her favorite toy by saying, "I want the toy." Alternatively, if the communicative behavior involved physical action (e.g., selecting a symbol on a communication board), then the interventionist's model would involve selecting the appropriate symbol on the board.

Helpful Hint

Present opportunities for the learner to imitate models of various behaviors (e.g., gestures, actions, verbalizations), with and without a verbal directive (e.g., "Do this"), while performing the model to determine if the learner imitates and if modeling prompts could be used. If the learner imitates, then modeling prompts can be used in intervention. If the learner does not readily imitate, then consider teaching imitation skills so that modeling prompts can be used in the future.

To teach imitation, begin with a gross motor movement that can be easily prompted in the presence of the model (e.g., raise hand, cover mouth [as in covering a sneeze]). Do not begin intervention with a movement requiring both hands (e.g., clapping) because the interventionist cannot provide the model while simultaneously prompting the learner to respond. Provide the instruction, "Do this," and a model. Use a physical prompt to help

the learner produce the behavior and deliver reinforcement. Teach other gross motor movements (e.g., clapping hands), followed by the more sophisticated movements that function as natural gestures (e.g., thumbs up, shrug shoulders), once the learner imitates gross motor movements that are easily prompted. See Maurice, Green, and Luce (1996) and Cooper, Heron, and Heward (2007) for additional information about teaching imitation skills.

Gestural prompts involve motions (e.g., pointing, tapping) to direct the learner's attention toward a specific behavior option (e.g., the correct item in an array, a set of symbols on a display, a learner's communication system/device).

Physical prompts involve physically assisting the learner in emitting the correct behavior. The interventionist physically guides the learner through the behavior using a small amount of pressure (e.g., light touch) in hand-over-hand and hand-under-hand guidance.

Hand-under-hand guidance can be particularly useful to help the learner see what his or her hands are doing (e.g., pointing to a symbol on a communication board).

Helpful Hint

Effectively using a prompt results in the learner engaging in the appropriate communicative behavior without any errors or errorless learning (e.g., Duffy & Wishart, 1987; Mackay, Soraci, Carlin, Dennis, & Strawbridge, 2002). Errorless learning is an important way to teach because engagement in errors increases the likelihood of repeating those errors.

TRANSFERRING STIMULUS CONTROL

Using effective prompts in the initial stages of intervention assists the learner in producing the correct behavior, but, in most instances, efforts should be made to discontinue the use of prompts so the learner responds in the presence of the natural cue/ S^D without additional assistance. This is called **transferring stimulus control** of the learner's correct behavior from the prompt to the natural cue/S^D.

Transferring Stimulus Control: Stimulus Prompts

Stimulus fading involves gradually reducing the extra or exaggerated dimensions of stimuli. For example, fade by gradually lightening color or decreasing size (e.g., making an enlarged triangle smaller over successive opportunities) depending on the dimension exaggerated.

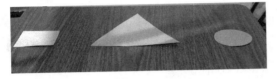

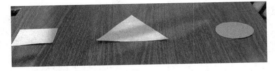

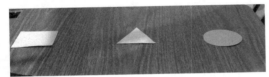

Place the correct option progressively closer to the array of choices (e.g., move the ball in line with the other items over successive opportunities) to fade position prompts.

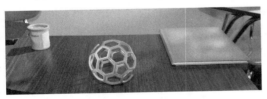

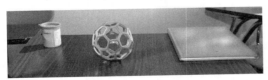

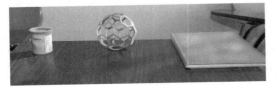

Fade additional stimuli such as picture prompts by gradually reducing the size of the picture (e.g., gradually decreasing the size of the book picture to teach sight word reading), cutting away portions, and/or even lightening the picture (see Figure 5.2).

Fading can occur on the target stimulus (e.g., making the target stimulus bigger than the distractor stimulus and gradually decreasing its size to match the distractor stimulus) or on the distractor stimulus (e.g., initially making the distractor stimulus smaller and gradually increasing its size to match the target stimulus). Evidence suggests that fading on the distractor stimulus is more effective for some learners (Schreibman & Charlop, 1981).

In addition to stimulus fading there is also **stimulus shaping** or **stimulus building**. During stimulus building, features not present in the original representation are gradually and systematically added with the expectation that the learner will continue to make correct selections. For example, a line drawing of a cat is gradually altered across opportunities to reveal the printed word *cat*. In this sequence of steps, both stimulus building and stimulus fading are occurring.

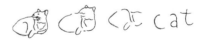

In other applications, as aspects of the target figure are faded, the features of a distractor are concurrently added to make the discriminating more challenging. For example, initially a flattened potato chip bag may be the target symbol and a tiny dot the distractor. Across successive opportunities of a learner's correct responding, the target symbol is trimmed. The potato chip bag gets smaller until only the printed word *potato chips* remains. Correspondingly, the small dot is built across successive opportunities to reveal a football. Using both stimulus building and stimulus fading simultaneously is an extremely effective strategy to teach symbol discrimination and is discussed in Chapter 8.

Stimulus prompting procedures tend to result in a more errorless approach to in-

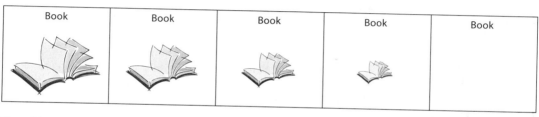

Figure 5.2. Fading stimuli such as picture prompts by gradually reducing the size of the picture.

struction with a reduced number of teaching opportunities compared with other types of instruction. Interventionists must prepare materials, plan instructional strategies, and be diligent in quickly shaping and fading, however, which is key to the successful use of stimulus prompts.

Transferring Stimulus Control: Response Prompts

A **most-to-least prompt hierarchy** begins with a prompt that reliably results in the learner performing the behavior. The prompt is faded along a hierarchy, from the current, most intrusive prompt, to lesser prompts (partial prompt to minimal prompt), to the eventual removal of the prompt altogether (i.e., independent performance), based on improvements in the learner's performance over successive opportunities. For example, the highest prompt level when teaching a learner to respond to peers' greetings might be a verbal directive, "Say 'hello' to your friend," faded to a question, "What should you say?" Alternatively, a physical prompt could consist of placing the learner's hand on the symbol on his or her speech-generating device (SGD), fading to a gesture directed to that symbol, and then fading to a gesture toward the device itself (not any particular symbol).

Graduated guidance is a strategy that is often used in a most-to-least prompt hierarchy. It refers to fading the amount of physical assistance using a most-to-least prompt hierarchy. For example, upon entering the recreation room, the interventionist prompts the learner using hand-over-hand guidance to open his or her communication book to

the correct page and select a symbol for a preferred leisure activity (e.g., checkers). The interventionist gradually decreases the physical prompts by changing the location of the prompt; for example, from hand-over-hand guidance to touching the learner at the wrist, then at the elbow, and then the shoulder. *Shadowing* refers to fading physical guidance by decreasing the amount of contact with the learner until the interventionist's hand moves simultaneously with, but does not touch, the learner's hand.

In a **least-to-most prompt hierarchy**, instead of beginning the intervention with the prompt that guarantees a correct behavior (i.e., the most intrusive prompt), the interventionist utilizes a minimal prompt level. If the learner does not respond in the presence of this minimal prompt, then the interventionist progresses through increasingly intrusive prompts until the learner performs the desired behavior. Consider teaching a learner to ask his or her teachers about their weekends by selecting the symbol on his or her SGD. If the teacher approaches and the learner does not ask the question, then the interventionist says, "Do you have something to ask Mr./Ms. ___?" (least intrusive prompt). If the learner does not respond, then the interventionist uses a more intrusive prompt, saying, "Ask Mr./Ms. ____ if he or she had a nice weekend." If the learner still does not produce a correct behavior, then the interventionist takes the learner's hand and places it on the symbol corresponding to the question, "Did you have a nice weekend?" (most intrusive prompt). Nelson, McDonnell, Johnston, Crompton, and Nelson (2007) used a least-to-most prompt hierarchy across prompt types (progressing from a verbal comment, to a model, to physical prompting) to teach preschoolers to use a symbol to initiate entry into a peer play activity.

With a **time delay procedure**, the interventionist introduces a pause between the natural cue (S^D) and the delivery of a prompt, which provides an opportunity for the learner to independently respond to the S^D prior to the prompt. The prompt is faded over time (rather than faded within or across types of prompts). For example, the teacher instructs the students, "Write the letter *a*." She waits 5 seconds before writing the letter *a* on the learner's paper (a modeling prompt). This 5-second delay provides the learner with an opportunity to emit the correct behavior without any prompt.

Constant and **progressive** (or gradual) are two types of time delay procedures (Ault, Gast, & Wolery, 1988). Intervention in both procedures begins by presenting the prompt in conjunction with or immediately following the S^D (i.e., 0-second time delay). The difference between the procedures is how the delay is increased. In a constant time delay procedure, introduce a delay of a set length of time (e.g., 10 seconds) following the S^D once the learner is correctly responding to the prompt at the 0-second delay level. If the learner produces a correct behavior before the delay ends, then the interventionist provides reinforcement. If he or she does not produce a correct behavior before the delay ends, then the interventionist provides a prompt.

In a progressive delay procedure, gradually increase the delay to some maximum once the learner correctly responds to the prompt at the 0-second delay level. That is, following a successful response in the presence of prompts delivered with a 0-second delay, introduce a small delay (e.g., 2 seconds). As the learner responds correctly, increase the delay again (e.g., total of 4 seconds). Continue until some maximum delay (e.g., 10 seconds) is reached. The result of both types of time delay procedures is that the learner eventually responds prior to the prompt (i.e., responds independently).

☞ *Helpful Hint*

Time delay can also be used when transferring stimulus control from a stimulus prompt. Consider, for example, an interventionist teaching his or her student to request missing materials. During the initial stages of intervention, the interventionist prompts by presenting a symbol corresponding to the communicative behavior (photograph of the paint set) in conjunction with or immediately following the presentation of the paper without the paint set. When the learner successfully requests in the presence of the picture prompt in conjunction with the S^D (i.e., 0-second time delay), the interventionist introduces a delay before presenting the picture prompt.

Both constant and gradual time delay procedures are effective; however, both require practice. A constant time delay may be easier to implement because there is only one change in "when" to present the prompt. A progressive time delay requires more regular increases (i.e., after correct responding at each delay interval) and also decreases in the delay following error behaviors. It may be appropriate to switch delay procedures; change to a progressive delay procedure if errors increase when using a constant time delay procedure.

How Do I Implement Prompting Procedures?

In deciding which type(s) of prompts to use, consider the skill to be taught, the materials, the situation in which the prompts will be used, and the characteristics of the learner.

Step 1: Decide on a Type(s) of Prompt(s)

Matson, Sevin, Box, Francis, and Sevin (1993) compared stimulus and response prompts when they taught three young children with autism and intellectual disabilities to initiate speech using a modeling prompt with a time delay procedure or a stimulus prompt of the target word printed on a flashcard (faded by reducing its size). Both prompting procedures were effective.

• The more closely the prompt resembles the natural cue, the less intrusive and less stigmatizing it may be and, likely, easier to fade. For example, if the natural cue is a spoken question, then a verbal prompt may blend in well. If the natural cue is a physical event (e.g., someone drops something), a gesture or physical prompt may be more appropriate (e.g., pointing to the symbol corresponding to "Uh oh").

Steps to implement prompting procedures

Step 1: Decide on a type(s) of prompt(s).
Step 2: Decide how to transfer stimulus control.
Step 3: Implement and fade prompts.

- Some prompts during natural interactions may be more intrusive and disruptive to the learner and others in the environment. For example, verbal prompts when ordering a meal at a restaurant (e.g., "Take your communication book out," "Tell the server what you want") are likely to interrupt the interaction between the AAC user and the server. If discretion is important, then picture and textual prompts (stimulus prompts) attached to the learner's possessions (e.g., key ring, binder, wallet) or held up briefly by the interventionist (at a distance if necessary) may be more appropriate.

- Physical prompts are prohibited when prompts need to be delivered at a distance from the learner (e.g., during an activity with classmates, at a job with co-workers). Verbal, gestural, and modeling prompts as well as some stimulus prompts (e.g., picture prompts) may be used more easily. "Light pointer cues" in which the interventionist shines a light on the target stimulus may be particularly useful at a distance. The learner must demonstrate good attending skills in order for prompts to be delivered at a distance.

- Response prompts and position cues do not require additional materials (either their creation or the need for transport) and, therefore, may be easier to implement than picture or textual prompts that require specific materials.

- Stimulus prompts can be particularly useful when materials can be easily manipulated.

- If the behavior is not in the learner's repertoire, then just increasing the likelihood that the learner will notice the natural stimuli through use of stimulus prompts will likely not affect the behavior. Response prompts (perhaps in conjunction with stimulus prompts) are warranted.

- Stimulus prompts may be appropriate if the learner is averse to verbal instructions (including verbal modeling) or physical interaction.

- If the learner demonstrates good imitation skills (verbal and/or physical), then a model prompt may be appropriate. Consider also using peers to provide appropriate models.

- Consider any past difficulty fading particular types of prompts for a learner. Verbal and physical prompts can create dependency in some learners. Stimulus prompts can be easier to fade than response prompts or can be maintained more naturally (e.g., graphic symbols on the refrigerator to prompt a sequence of after-school activities) because they involve manipulations of existing stimuli in the environment.

Different types of prompts can be used in isolation or combined. For example, an interventionist can combine a verbal prompt with a gesture to the correct symbol for the learner to choose in his or her communication book. Often, interventionists use response prompts in the event the learner emits an error in the presence of a stimulus prompt (Repp, Karsh, & Lenz, 1990). For example, a new symbol placed in a child's communication system might be enlarged to increase the likelihood the child selects the symbol (stimulus prompt). If the enlarged symbol does not immediately result in its use, however, then the interventionist models selection of the symbol.

After determining the type(s) of prompt(s), the interventionist must identify the form of the type of prompt that reliably results in the occurrence of the target behavior. Present a series of prompts from less to more intrusive (e.g., if a verbal modeling prompt is chosen for a verbal behavior, then present a general question, a partial model, and a complete model of the behavior). Examine the level of prompt that reliably results in the behavior.

Step 2: Decide How to Transfer Stimulus Control

Consider using stimulus fading and stimulus shaping when deciding how to transfer stimulus control (see Chapter 8 for a discussion of stimulus prompting procedures). Also, consider using a most-to-least prompt hierarchy

- When the learner has no level of proficiency with the target skill
- If the learner tends to repeat incorrect behaviors
- When intervening in the natural environment, with natural communicative partners
- When the skill is one for which an error would be dangerous (e.g., learning to ask for help with a difficult physical task) or unacceptable (e.g., remaining quiet during a presentation)

When using most-to-least prompt fading, develop a hierarchy of prompts beginning with the prompt that currently controls the communicative behavior (from Step 1)—the most intrusive or full prompt. The hierarchy progresses through gradual changes within a type of prompt (e.g., levels within physical prompting, as in graduated guidance) or across prompt types (e.g., levels move from physical to verbal) to a minimal prompt. Buzolich, King, and Baroody (1991) used a hierarchy with level changes within and across prompt type. Specifically, they faded across two levels of a verbal prompt (an indirect general question, "What could

you say?" and direct instruction, "You could say . . .") and then modeled the appropriate behavior (i.e., touching the correct symbol on the device). Be sure the prompts truly become less intrusive in a hierarchy across prompt types. For example, interventionists often consider physical prompts to be more intrusive than verbal prompts; however, verbal prompts can be extraordinarily intrusive, interrupting natural interactions and drawing undo attention to the learner, as well as being difficult to fade.

Prompt hierarchies can also be developed across response and stimulus prompts; for example, a drawing of a red heart (stimulus prompt) placed on the wall next to the bed of a child. Just before his mother left his bedside, she pointed to the red heart and modeled saying, "I love you" (response prompt), and he responded by saying, "I love you." Eventually, the model was faded and then the heart was faded in size and removed. Table 5.3 provides examples of hierarchies across and within prompt type.

The number of levels of the hierarchy depends on the complexity of the behavior and prompt, as well as the learner's existing repertoire. One rule of thumb is to fade prompts gradually but swiftly; that is, the amount of change is minimal from one level to the next (e.g., moving from physically prompting at the learner's wrist to his or her forearm and then to his or her elbow) so that the learner continues to respond to the new, less intrusive prompt level but the changes take place relatively quickly (e.g., after two consecutive opportunities for which the learner responds correctly), preventing the learner from responding to one prompt level for too many instructional opportunities. Always base changes in prompt level on the learner's success at a given prompt level.

Consider using a least-to-most prompt fading hierarchy:

- When a learner demonstrates the skill; thus, it is in his or her repertoire, but not to criteria in the desired environment/ situation.

Table 5.3. Examples of prompt hierarchies for selecting the symbol for "hello" in a communication book when a peer enters the room

Level of support	Hierarchy within one type of prompt: Physical prompt	Hierarchy within one type of prompt: Textual prompt	Hierarchy across prompt types: Physical to gestural	Hierarchy across prompt types: Stimulus and model prompts
Full	Uses physical assistance to help Michael select the symbol	Shows Michael a textual cue of the word *hello* on an index card	Provides physical assistance to Michael to select the HELLO symbol on his communication book	Shows Michael a textual cue of the word *hello* on an index card and models the use of his communication book
Partial	Presents a physical prompt at Michael's wrist to select the symbol	Shows Michael a textual cue with the first three letters of *hello*	Gestures by pointing to the HELLO symbol	Shows Michael a textual cue with the word *hello*
Minimal	Applies gentle pressure to Michael's upper arm	Shows Michael the textual cue with the first letter of *hello*	Gestures toward Michael's communication board	Shows Michael a textual cue with just the first letter of the word *hello*

- With a learner who tends to wait until a prompt is delivered rather than respond independently, the full prompt is only delivered after less intrusive prompts prove unsuccessful. Consider this choice carefully; some learners are willing to wait through each of the less intrusive prompts until the most intrusive one is presented.

- When a most-to-least prompt hierarchy was used during acquisition, it may be a good idea to switch to a least-to-most hierarchy so that more intrusive prompts are only presented if the learner responds incorrectly. For example, a picture prompt representing "hello" was faded using a most-to-least prompt hierarchy in which the picture representing "hello" was made smaller to teach a learner to greet his peers. If the learner did not appropriately greet his peers following mastery, then interventionists used least-to-most prompting, introducing the most recently used small-sized picture as a prompt and then increasing the prompt level (moving to progressively larger pictures until the learner responds correctly).

Consider using a time-delay procedure:

- When the skill is not yet in the learner's repertoire. This procedure begins with immediate prompting (10-second delay) of the behavior that will result in reinforcement.

- When the goal is to increase spontaneous use. The use of a time delay provides an opportunity to spontaneously engage in communicative behavior.

Helpful Hint

Fading procedures can be used in isolation or combined. For example, combine a time delay procedure with a most-to-least prompt hierarchy (e.g., Gee, Graham, Goetz, Oshima, & Yoshioka, 1991; Jones, Carr, & Feeley, 2006) so that fading occurs from a higher prompt level to a lower prompt level delivered immediately following the S^D. Introduce a delay once the learner responds in the presence of the less intrusive prompt. Gee et al. (1991) taught switch activation to three learners with profound intellectual, physical, and sensory disabilities using physical prompts faded through a combination of a time delay and most-to-least prompt hierarchy.

Step 3: Implement and Fade Prompts

- Make sure the materials for prompting (e.g., picture cards) are readily accessible.

- Clearly indicate the current prompt level (e.g., on a performance monitoring form).

- Include the S^D, a behavior, and a consequence, with prompts added as necessary, in every teaching opportunity.

- Provide prompts in conjunction with or immediately following the S^D when addressing a new skill to ensure the learner emits a correct behavior (i.e., errorless learning).

- Initially, prompted opportunities should result in reinforcement; however, once the learner begins to produce independent behaviors, reserve a more potent reinforcer for independent behaviors or reserve reinforcement altogether only for independent behaviors (i.e., reinforcement would not be delivered following a prompted behavior). Moving from reinforcing every behavior (regardless of prompting) to reinforcing only independent behaviors involves a change in schedule of reinforcement.

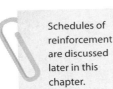

Schedules of reinforcement are discussed later in this chapter.

However, ensure reinforcement continues to be delivered frequently enough to increase responding. If the learner stops responding independently, then consider delivering reinforcement for some of the prompted behaviors.

- If an error occurs (even in the presence of a prompt), then follow through with error correction procedures and deliver the S^D for a new opportunity. Delivering prompts immediately following an error (without first delivering consequences and then the S^D for a new opportunity)

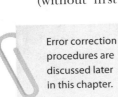

Error correction procedures are discussed later in this chapter.

increases the likelihood that the learner will respond only in the presence of the prompt and not the S^D. He or she might also learn an undesirable chain of behaviors involving the S^D, error behavior, prompt, and the correct behavior followed by reinforcement.

When using a most-to-least prompt fading procedure,

- Present the natural cue and provide the most intrusive prompt (i.e., full prompt) at the beginning of instruction. Reinforce correct behaviors in the presence of this prompt.

- Decide when to fade to the next prompt level:

   Fade to the next level in the hierarchy when the learner meets preidentified criterion (e.g., 90% correct performance across two consecutive sessions).

   Present probes to examine learner behaviors in the presence of less intrusive prompts and fade to just below the level at which the learner responds.

- If the learner makes an error at a given prompt level,

   Use error correction procedures

   Increase the prompt level (i.e., using a more intrusive level) on subsequent opportunities

- If errors persist, then return to a previous level of the prompt (a level at which the learner successfully responded) and identify and implement finer levels of the prompt hierarchy.

- Continue until all prompts are faded and the learner responds independently to the natural cue.

When using a least-to-most prompt fading procedure,

- Present the natural cue and provide the least intrusive prompt (i.e., minimal prompt, no prompt at all) at the beginning of instruction.

- If the learner emits a correct behavior, then proceed with reinforcement procedures.

- If the learner emits an incorrect behavior, then introduce a more intrusive prompt.

   If the learner emits a correct behavior, then deliver reinforcement.

If the learner emits another incorrect behavior, then introduce the next more intrusive prompt in the hierarchy. Continue providing more intrusive prompts until the learner emits a correct behavior and then deliver reinforcement.

- Start with the least intrusive prompt on the next instructional opportunity.

When using a time delay,

- Present the natural cue and immediately (0-second time delay) deliver the prompt at the beginning of instruction. Deliver reinforcement once the learner responds.

- Begin to delay the prompt when the learner responds to criterion or after a set number of instructional opportunities/ sessions. Wait the identified delay interval after presenting the natural cue. If the learner does not respond by the end of the interval, then prompt a correct behavior. If the learner makes an error, then use error correction.

- If using a progressive time delay, then gradually increase the delay up to the maximum delay.

CONSEQUENCES FOR LEARNER RESPONSES

Consequences should be designed to specifically increase correct responding in the future (i.e., **reinforcement**). Consequences must also be designed to specifically correct errors (i.e., error correction procedures).

Reinforcement

Reinforcement strategies enhance the learner's communicative performance because their delivery following the behavior maintains or increases the future likelihood of the behavior. There are two types of reinforcers. **Primary reinforcers** are stimuli that have biological importance and include food, liquid, sleep, shelter, and sex. These stimuli are likely to be highly motivating to most learners because they are unlearned and necessary for the continuation of the spe-

cies. **Secondary reinforcers** do not have biological importance; rather, the individual has learned the value of these items/events. Verbal praise, tokens, and toys may function as secondary reinforcers because of their history of association with other reinforcers.

There are two ways reinforcement occurs. **Positive reinforcement** is the contingent presentation of a stimulus (i.e., something in the environment) following a behavior that maintains or increases the future rate of the behavior. Consider a young child who selects the symbol for COOKIE on her board and immediately receives a cookie, increasing her selection of the COOKIE symbol in the future. Similarly, a young adult enjoyed interacting with his roommates. His roommates chatted with him each time he used his SGD, increasing his use of the SGD in their presence. Both are examples of positive reinforcement.

Negative reinforcement is the contingent removal of a nonpreferred stimulus following a behavior that results in the maintenance or increase in the future rate of that behavior. A stimulus is presented in positive reinforcement. The "negative" in negative reinforcement refers to the removal of a stimulus contingent on the target behavior. The future rate of responding maintains or increases in both cases. For example, a young child was presented with a food he does not like, he selected the symbol NO, THANK YOU on his communication board, and the item was removed. The removal of the nonpreferred food item resulted in an increase in his use of the NO, THANK YOU symbol. Removing the nonpreferred item was negative reinforcement.

⌖ Helpful Hint

The terms *negative* and *positive* reinforcement are often confusing. Reinforcement results in an increase or maintenance of a behavior in all cases. The term *positive* means something is presented to the learner as a consequence for the behavior. The term *negative* means something (nonpreferred or aversive) is removed as a consequence for the behavior.

Interventionists must consider the extent to which a specific reinforcer will enhance learner performance at a given point in time when using reinforcement strategies. For example, if video games were identified as a reinforcer, then there might be times when they are more or less reinforcing than others. Playing a brand new video game is likely very reinforcing, but playing that video game may be less reinforcing when a learner is stuck at a certain level of a video game. **Motivating operations** (MOs) are conditions that affect the quality of a reinforcer (i.e., the extent to which that reinforcer will enhance a learner's performance; Cooper et al., 2007; Laraway, Snycerski, Michael, & Poling, 2003). There are two types of MOs:

1. **Establishing operations** (EOs) are in effect when there is an increase in the value of a reinforcer and frequency of behavior associated with that reinforcer. If a learner is in a state of **deprivation** (i.e., he or she has not had access to the reinforcer), then it is likely the reinforcer will be more valuable to the learner at that point in time. For example, if a learner is being taught to request food, and it has been 2 or 3 hours since his last meal, then acquiring food should be extremely reinforcing, and its use should be quite effective in teaching communicative requests.

2. **Abolishing operations** (AOs) are in effect when there is a decrease in the value of a reinforcer and the frequency of behavior associated with that reinforcer. For example, the learner is not likely to be hungry shortly after a meal; rather, he is in a state of **satiation** with respect to food as a reinforcer. That is, the delivery of the food item will likely have little or no reinforcing value. Similarly, when a learner has free access to a particular toy, the reinforcing value of that toy during instruction is likely less than if the toy was only available during instruction. Therefore, free access to a toy can be an AO that decreases the effectiveness of the toy as a reinforcer.

Implementing Reinforcement Procedures

Failure to implement effective reinforcement procedures is a primary culprit in the failure of instructional procedures. It is extremely important to make sure that powerful reinforcers are available contingent on correct responding. The steps described next represent ones that have been associated with effective intervention strategies.

Steps to implementing reinforcement procedures

Step 1: Identify a pool of potential reinforcers.
Step 2: Choose a potential reinforcer.
Step 3: Choose a schedule of reinforcement.
Step 4: Deliver reinforcement.
Step 5: Fade reinforcement.

Step 1: Identify a Pool of Potential Reinforcers

It is important for interventionists to identify items/activities that potentially function as reinforcers. The term *potentially* is used because something is not technically considered a reinforcer until it has been demonstrated to increase or maintain behavior. It is uncertain at this point if identified items truly have reinforcing value.

Begin communication intervention with situations in which the natural consequences are likely to function as reinforcers for a learner. For example, begin with highly preferred activities when teaching requesting access to activities; use nonpreferred items when teaching rejecting so that their removal is reinforcing (i.e., negative reinforcement). A highly preferred or highly disliked item will often evoke a comment (e.g., "That tastes awful!") when teaching commenting.

Sometimes the natural consequences for communicative behaviors are not reinforcing to a learner. For example, the natural consequence for commenting to a peer is interaction with that peer. Interaction with a peer, however, may not function as a reinforcer for some learners. Present other reinforcers in this situation to increase communicative behaviors.

Use interviews and **systematic preference assessments** to identify potential reinforcers. During an interview, interventionists ask about a variety of activities and items in an interview to determine what the learner enjoys (and might function as reinforcers). Create a list of potential reinforcers, sampling a range of types of materials and activities (e.g., foods, sports, arts and crafts). It is likely the learner will not be able to respond to these questions unless he or she already has some means of communicating. In this case, interview people who are familiar with the learner, including parents, siblings, peers, teachers, and significant others. The interview can be in person, in the form of a checklist, or in the form of a rating scale. An example of a rating scale is provided in Form 5.1 on the accompanying CD-ROM. Both blank (Form 5.1a) and filled-in (Form 5.1b) versions of Form 5.1 are on the accompanying CD-ROM.

Asking the learner and/or individuals who know the learner is a good way to begin identifying potential reinforcers. It is not the most reliable method for identifying reinforcers, however (Green et al., 1988). Although an item may be one the learner prefers, it might not consistently result in an increase in performance (i.e., not function as a reinforcer). Reinforcers also change over time (Carr, Nicholson, & Higbee, 2000). Therefore, use interviews and checklists in conjunction with observational methods.

Systematic preference assessment involves observing the learner when he or she is given either free access to or a choice of potentially reinforcing items. The free access condition includes the following (e.g., Ortiz & Carr, 2000).

- Identify several potentially preferred items (e.g., through interview or checklist).

- Position items so that the learner has access to all the items (e.g., spread them around the room in the learner's view and reach).

- Observe the learner on several occasions.

- Document the first item (and next item) the learner approaches and the total duration of time the learner engages with each item (see Chapter 7 for information about measurement systems). The first

items and those with which the learner engages the longest are presumably more preferred.

Figure 5.3 is an example of a free access preference assessment used with Dana. Form 5.2 is a blank version of this assessment and is included on the accompanying CD-ROM.

The forced choice condition includes the following steps (e.g., Piazza, Fisher, Hagopian, Bowman, & Toole, 1996).

- Identify several potentially preferred items (e.g., through interview or checklist).

- Present items in pairs. Randomize the presentation of the items in pairs and order of pairs. This will prevent the same item from being presented several times in a row. In addition, be sure to randomize the position of the items during presentation (e.g., each of the items should be presented on both the right and left side of the learner). This will show if the learner has a "position" bias—he or she only chooses items placed to one side. If this is the case, then it is not possible to determine the learner's true preference.

- Document the item in each pair the learner selects.

Figure 5.4 is an example of a forced choice preference assessment used with Sam (Light Shriner & Johnston, 1992). Form 5.3 is a blank version of this assessment and is included on the accompanying CD-ROM.

Free choice and forced choice preference assessments often effectively identify potential reinforcers, even though they are lengthy to complete (Ortiz & Carr, 2000). Research shows, however, that similar, but brief assessments, conducted on a regular basis (e.g., just before instruction, at the beginning of the school day) can be just as effective (e.g., DeLeon et al., 2001; Graff & Libby, 1999). For example, an interventionist presented two potential reinforcers and asked the learner, "Which one?" before beginning a job task. Conducting more frequent, but shorter, preference assessments accounts for learner's changing preferences (which can sometimes change daily or even hourly).

Learner's name: _Dana_   Length of sessions: _20 minutes_

Instructions: Fill in the items or activities across the top row. Fill in the date in the far left column. Fill in the time span (e.g., 11:15–11:20) that the learner engaged with each item/activity. Indicate the first item approached each day with an asterisk (*). Add the total amount of time spent with each item/activity over all days.

Date	Items/activities			
	Listening to music	Reading magazine	Video game	Playing cards
8/11	11:15–11:20		11:00–11:15*	
8/12	12:10–12:15	12:08–12:10	12:00–12:08* 12:15–12:20	
8/13	11:09–11:11		11:00–11:09* 11:11–11:20	
8/14	1:47–1:50	1:42–1:47	1:30–1:42*	
Total duration	15 minutes	7 minutes	58 minutes	0 minutes

Figure 5.3. Free access preference assessment used with Dana. (*Note:* This is a filled-in version of Form 5.2, Free Access Preference Assessment. A blank, printable version appears on the accompanying CD-ROM.)

Learner's name: _Sam_

Instructions: Write the name of each item next to each of the letters below. Present the two corresponding items to the learner during each opportunity, being sure to attend to the right and left position of the item. Circle the letter that corresponds to the chosen item.

A: _Bubbles_   B: _Playdough_

C: _Book_   D: _Toy cars_

E: _Action figures_   F: _Riding toy_

1.	D	(F)	11.	(E)	B	21.	(C)	D
2.	(B)	A	12.	(D)	E	22.	(F)	A
3.	A	(B)	13.	F	(C)	23.	(B)	E
4.	E	(D)	14.	(D)	A	24.	B	(F)
5.	(C)	E	15.	(C)	B	25.	(F)	B
6.	(F)	D	16.	E	(C)	26.	A	(E)
7.	D	(C)	17.	C	(F)	27.	(B)	D
8.	A	(C)	18.	(C)	A	28.	(E)	F
9.	D	(B)	19.	(B)	C	29.	(E)	A
10.	(F)	E	20.	A	(D)	30.	A	(F)

Item A was chosen _0_/10 times   Item B was chosen _6_/10 times

Item C was chosen _8_/10 times   Item D was chosen _4_/10 times

Item E was chosen _4_/10 times   Item F was chosen _8_/10 times

Figure 5.4. Forced choice preference assessment used with Sam. (From Light Shriner, C., & Johnston, S.S. [1992]. *Conducting forced choice preference assessments.* Unpublished manuscript; adapted by permission.) (*Note:* This is a filled-in version of Form 5.3, Forced Choice Preference Assessment. A blank, printable version appears on the accompanying CD-ROM.)

Step 2: Choose a Potential Reinforcer   Natural consequences will function as reinforcers to maintain and increase communication skills for many learners. For example, signing MORE to request food items at the dinner table resulted in the natural consequence of receiving food items. The rate of signing MORE should increase in the future as long as the food at the dinner table functions as a reinforcer. Selecting the symbol for NO, THANK YOU resulted in the natural consequence of removal of the nonpreferred food item. The removal of a nonpreferred food item may also function as a natural reinforcer increasing the use of NO, THANK YOU (in this case, negative reinforcement).

Natural consequences may not always function as reinforcers. Consider a learner who is not motivated to interact with peers. Interventionists may pair other known reinforcers with the natural (but not reinforcing) consequence. For example, each time the learner interacted with a peer, his interventionist provided an edible reinforcer (i.e., a piece of pretzel) and a high five (another known reinforcer), and the peers provided natural consequences of continuing to interact with the learner. The peers' reactions began to function as reinforcers because of this pairing. The interventionist gradually faded the edible reinforcer and high fives. Pairing additional reinforcers should be viewed as a temporary situation.

Choose potential reinforcers to use during instruction

- That are readily available and easily accessible for the interventionist's use
- That are as natural/social as possible
- That are age appropriate
- That can be paired with neutral items to expand the range of items that function as reinforcers for a learner
- For which the learner will not quickly satiate:

    If possible, choose items to which the learner does not have frequent access

    Choose items for which the learner's access can be controlled

Choose several potential reinforcers to vary across instructional opportunities to help decrease the likelihood the learner will satiate on one particular reinforcer

Choose a potential reinforcer that can be delivered in small amounts (e.g., eating one cookie rather than the entire bag, reading one short story rather than an entire book)

Step 3: Choose a Schedule of Reinforcement
The **schedule of reinforcement** refers to how often reinforcement will be delivered. A **continuous schedule of reinforcement** involves delivery of a reinforcer every time the learner engages in a particular behavior. For example, to teach Jason to use his communication book to comment to his peers (e.g., "This is fun"), every time Jason approached a peer and selected a comment symbol in his communication book, the peer responded (e.g., saying, "Thank you," and adding her own comment) with natural consequences. Jason's interventionist also presented a sticker—a known reinforcer.

During instruction, natural consequences may not naturally occur on a continuous schedule. Interventionists can artificially increase their frequency, however, resulting in a continuous schedule of reinforcement. For example, each time a learner signed to request a break during the initial stages of intervention, he received a break from the activity.

Use continuous reinforcement when

- The skill is new to the learner
- The skill is being taught to specifically replace challenging behavior
- A new intervention is being introduced to the learner
- A new interventionist provides instruction to a learner. The new interventionist should initially deliver reinforcers more often, but thin reinforcement over time.

Reinforcers are provided following some, but not all, occurrences of the behavior on an **intermittent schedule of reinforcement.** For example, after Jason learned to comment to his peers, his interventionist moved from a continuous schedule of reinforcement (in which every comment resulted in additional reinforcers [e.g., food item]) to an intermittent schedule (in which every three comments resulted in additional reinforcers) to maintain commenting during peer interactions. Use an intermittent schedule of reinforcement when

- The goal is maintenance of the communicative behavior

- Moving from a continuous to a more natural schedule of reinforcement in which reinforcement is delivered less frequently

- There is a need to control for satiation (e.g., when a primary reinforcer is being used)

Ratio and interval are two types of intermittent schedules. A **ratio schedule** of reinforcement involves delivery of reinforcers after a specific number of occurrences of the behavior. The learner's rate of responding determines when and how often reinforcement is delivered. A ratio schedule can, therefore, be used to increase the rate of behavior to higher levels. For example, to increase the number of times a learner spontaneously used his device, the interventionist provided reinforcement after the learner emitted a specified number of spontaneous behaviors. There are two types of ratio schedules:

1. A **fixed ratio schedule of reinforcement** identifies a specific number of behaviors and delivers reinforcement following the last occasion of the behavior. This schedule is termed *fixed* because the number of behaviors required for reinforcement does not vary across opportunities. For example, reinforcement was delivered with a fixed ratio 4 (FR4) schedule of reinforcement after the fourth occurrence of the response.

   A fixed schedule provides predictable reinforcement.

   A fixed schedule of reinforcement is effective in establishing new communicative behaviors.

Placing a behavior on a FR2, FR3, FR4, and so forth is an effective way to make a transition from a continuous to an intermittent schedule of reinforcement.

2. A **variable ratio schedule of reinforcement** varies the number of behaviors required prior to the delivery of reinforcement. This schedule is termed *variable* because the number of behaviors required for reinforcement varies across opportunities around an average number of behaviors the learner must emit. For example, the interventionist delivered reinforcement on a variable ratio 4 (VR4) schedule following the third correct behavior, then following another six correct behaviors, and then another three correct behaviors, so the average number of behaviors was four (VR4).

   A variable ratio schedule is not recommended for instruction on new skills due to the unpredictable schedule of reinforcement.

   Behaviors associated with a variable schedule of reinforcement may be better maintained.

Reinforcement is delivered after the passage of a specified amount of time with an **interval schedule** of reinforcement. The rate of responding does not determine the delivery of reinforcement, rather the passage of time dictates the availability of reinforcement. For example, an interventionist delivered reinforcement every minute the learner was on task to increase his or her engagement with the task. There are fixed and variable interval schedules. The first occurrence of the target behavior following the interval results in reinforcement with a fixed interval schedule. The intervals vary with a variable interval schedule of reinforcement, averaging to the identified time interval.

Step 4: Deliver Reinforcement

- Provide reinforcers (both natural consequences and additional reinforcers identified in Steps 1 and 2) immediately following a correct behavior.

- Reinforcement must be contingent on the target behavior (i.e., the learner cannot gain access to the reinforcer unless he or she engages in the target behavior).

☞ *Helpful Hint*

A **token economy** or token reinforcement system is one application of reinforcement. Tokens (e.g., poker chips, pennies, stickers, checkmarks) are provided and then exchanged for a back-up reinforcer (i.e., identified in Step 1). For example, a learner earned a checkmark each time he initiated interaction with a peer using his SGD. When the learner received a predetermined number of checks, he exchanged them for the back-up reinforcer (e.g., computer time).

Interventionists teach self-regulatory skills by increasing the number of tokens required because the learner waits longer periods before receiving access to the back-up reinforcer. For example, a learner whose behaviors resulted in receipt of food as a reinforcer may at first need to earn one token before gaining access to the reinforcer, then two tokens, and so forth.

Step 5: Fade Reinforcement There is no need to **fade reinforcement** when using natural reinforcers. Fading reinforcement is important, however, so that natural consequences maintain communication in situations where it is necessary to increase the frequency of naturally available reinforcers or utilize additional reinforcers. The decreased use of additional reinforcers may also allow communicative interactions to proceed more naturally (e.g., in the absence of disruption or interference by the delivery of edibles or tokens).

The frequency of reinforcement delivery in **schedule thinning** can be used to fade reinforcement, which is gradually decreased from a dense schedule of reinforcement (e.g., continuous) to a sparse schedule of reinforcement (e.g., intermittent). Increase the number of required behaviors or interval in small increments. *Ratio strain* occurs when the ratio of behaviors to time to reinforcement increases too much and learner performance declines. Base changes in the schedule of reinforcement on successful performance at the current schedule.

CASE EXAMPLE

Reinforcement and Schedule Thinning

Marina's interventionists used continuous reinforcement during the initial stages of intervention to teach her to request attention by selecting symbols such as READ A BOOK WITH ME, or PLAY CARDS WITH ME. Reinforcement involved both natural consequences (i.e., engaging Marina in the activity she indicated) and additional reinforcers (i.e., a sticker). Marina's interventionists thinned the schedule of delivery of the additional reinforcers (i.e., stickers) once she consistently used symbols to request attention. They began with a FR2 schedule, in which stickers were delivered every second time Marina requested attention (while the naturally occurring reinforcer remained on a continuous schedule; e.g., her interventionist read to her each time she requested). The schedule behavior requirements increased by one after every 2 days of successful use of the communicative behavior (i.e., FR3, FR4).

Delaying the delivery of the reinforcer is another way to fade reinforcement. Reinforcement should be delivered immediately after the communicative behavior is emitted, especially at the beginning of intervention. There are many instances, however, in which it is appropriate for the learner to wait before a reinforcer is delivered. For example, a child may request access to a preferred activity that is not available at the time of the request. To teach **tolerance for delay of reinforcement,** which is the ability to wait for a reinforcer (Carr et al., 1994):

1. Deliver the **tolerance cue** to indicate to the learner that he or she will receive the reinforcer soon. Tolerance cues can be time-based (e.g., "One more minute") or task-based (e.g., "Do one more problem") delays. Deliver a tolerance cue following the learner's request for a reinforcer.

2. Deliver a release cue or **safety signal** (or **delay signal**) to inform the learner that he or she is about to receive reinforcement (e.g., "Here it is"; "Sure, take a break"). Deliver the tolerance cue and immediately deliver the release cue/safety signal when first teaching tolerance for delay.

3. Gradually increase the amount of time or number of tasks expected before the learner receives the reinforcer by specifically stating the tolerance cue (e.g., increase from "Do one more problem" to "Do two more problems"). If the learner emits a communicative behavior before the delay elapses, then alternate between reinforcing communication and delivering the tolerance cue. In this way, the learner's independent communication continues to result in reinforcement.

CASE EXAMPLE

Tolerance for Delay of Reinforcement

Adam's interventionists taught him to select photographs of magazines from his communication wallet to request them instead of screaming to gain access to them. Then, Adam began requesting magazines throughout classroom activities, however. His interventionists decided to teach tolerance for delay of reinforcement to increase the length of time Adam engaged in classroom activities prior to gaining access to the magazines. When Adam requested magazines, his interventionist said, "Sure, you can have your magazines, but first, let's pay attention for 1 minute" (tolerance cue) and then immediately delivered the release cue, "Okay, Adam, you paid attention; let's get your magazines," resulting in Adam obtaining the magazines. A 1-minute delay was inserted between the tolerance and release cues when Adam successfully (i.e., no screaming on three occasions) responded to the introduction of the tolerance and release cues. As Adam continued to be successful, the interventionist increased the amount of the delay by 2 minutes until Adam waited 30 minutes (the approximate duration of a class activity).

CONSEQUENCES FOR ERROR RESPONSES

Despite use of prompting procedures and reinforcement following correct behaviors, learners may still make errors in which they emit an incorrect behavior (e.g., when the learner was asked, "Where did you go yesterday?" he or she selected the symbols corresponding to something he or she did last week) or no behavior (e.g., refraining from answering the question). It is important to keep error behaviors to a minimum because the more often a learner engages in incorrect behaviors, the more likely he or she is to continue that behavior. The interventionist may devise an errorless learning procedure during the early stages of acquisition to prevent any errors. An occasional error behavior may occur once prompts are faded. It is important for interventionists to decide how to respond to errors to enhance skill acquisition (Rodgers & Iwata, 1991; Worsdell et al., 2005).

How Do I Consequate Error Behaviors?

Step 1: Decide What to Do When an Error Occurs

Implement **behavior interruption** before the learner produces an incorrect behavior (e.g., physically block the learner from gaining access to the incorrect materials, touch the learner's hand to stop him or her from pointing to the incorrect symbol in his or her communication book). After interrupting, bring the learner's hand back to a starting point. Next, impose a brief pause. Subsequently, deliver the least intrusive prompt that will ensure that the learner selects the correct target symbol. The delay imposed is to ensure that the learner does not acquire a chain of behavior in which he or she learns to respond randomly to obtain a response prompt to the correct response. If prompted responses are reinforced, the undesirable

Steps for consequating errors

Step 1: Decide what to do when an error occurs.

Step 2: Decide what to do on the next opportunity.

response chain may result in the quickest path to reinforcement for the learner.

Behavior interruption may be difficult to implement in situations in which the interventionist cannot maintain close proximity to the learner. Behavior interruption may not be socially valid in some situations (e.g., during peer interactions). Many motor movements are easily interrupted, whereas verbal behaviors are less easily interrupted. Behaviors that occur rapidly may occur too quickly to interrupt. In this case, manipulating materials can make the use of behavior interruption easier. For example, symbols were placed far apart and at a distance from the learner when teaching discrimination between two graphic symbols. This resulted in the learner making broader motor movements and/or taking more time to respond, providing the interventionist with time to interrupt an incorrect behavior.

Implement **error correction** procedures once an error has been made.

- If the learner attempts the behavior or an approximation, then the interventionist provides verbal praise and feedback acknowledging the attempt. For example, a learner missed the timing for selecting a symbol on her scanning device, so the interventionist said, "Nice try; you almost got to the symbol" and then began a new opportunity.

- The interventionist provides corrective non–behavior-specific feedback (e.g., "Try again") before presenting a new opportunity.

- The interventionist provides corrective behavior-specific feedback (e.g., "That's not the sign for MORE") before presenting a new opportunity.

- The interventionist provides corrective feedback and then prompts the correct behavior before presenting a new opportunity. For example, the interventionist said, "That's not the sign for MORE. This is the sign for MORE" and prompted the learner to correctly sign MORE.

The interventionist should deliver feedback in a different tone of voice than what he or she uses for verbal praise. This is particularly important for learners who may not discriminate spoken content but can discriminate intonations.

Implement procedures to decrease the likelihood of future errors.

- Bring the reinforcer forward to give to the learner when he or she emits a correct behavior. Move the reinforcer away from the learner or out of the learner's sight when he or she emits an incorrect behavior.

- Turn away from the learner following an incorrect behavior. This can be particularly effective for learners whose behaviors are reinforced by social interaction.

- There may be natural consequences that should decrease the likelihood of future errors. For example, a server provided a food item after a learner chose its symbol on his SGD. The learner had incorrectly chosen ketchup instead of mustard, however, and the server presented ketchup. These natural consequences may not be sufficient to decrease future errors, but could be paired with other strategies.

Step 2: Decide What to Do on the Next Opportunity

Determine how to implement the next opportunity following an error and consequence.

- Increase the prompt level on the next opportunity to ensure the learner will make a correct behavior. This may be more appropriate during the beginning of skill acquisition.

- Deliver another opportunity just like the previous one (using the same prompt level or no prompt). This may be more appropriate for behaviors the learner has already acquired.

  Deliver reinforcement if the learner makes a correct behavior on this second opportunity.

  Present another opportunity if the learner makes another error, increasing the prompt level to ensure the learner makes a correct behavior.

Multiple opportunities in which the learner makes an error behavior can increase the likelihood the learner continues to make that error. Therefore, in general, it is not recommended that multiple opportunities be provided in the absence of prompting procedures to help the learner produce a correct response.

📭 Helpful Hint

In some instances, interventionists may choose not to provide any direct consequence following incorrect behavior (e.g., no feedback or error correction implemented; no prompts delivered on the following opportunity). Instead, the interventionist continues to provide many opportunities until the learner performs the correct behavior and then delivers high-quality reinforcement. For example, if a learner engages in high rates of challenging behavior in response to feedback or prompts, then reinforcement following correct behaviors might be the only consequences used.

APPLICATIONS

Shaping and chaining are two common applications that combine various strategies described in this chapter.

Shaping

Shaping is used to establish skills that are not currently part of a learner's repertoire by reinforcing successive approximations of a specified behavior. For example, when teaching a learner to activate a symbol on his SGD, the target (desired) behavior was the learner pressing a specific symbol, and the initial behavior was approaching the device, with several approximations in between. As the learner demonstrates that initial behavior, interventionists use **differen-**

> Differential reinforcement is used to reinforce one approximation of the target behavior, whereas previously produced behaviors are no longer reinforced.

tial reinforcement in which the next approximation of the desired behavior results in reinforcement, but the previous one does not.

Response shaping involves reinforcing successively better approximations of a behavior. It is useful when a behavior is not occurring at all and/or is difficult to prompt. Behavior can be shaped with respect to

- Form
- Duration of the behavior (e.g., increasing duration of sitting)
- Latency (e.g., decreasing time to open communication book to respond to a question)
- Rate (e.g., increasing the number of behaviors during playtime)
- Force (e.g., increasing the amount of pressure the learner exerts to activate a keypad)

Shaping can be a lengthy process if there are many approximations to the final behavior. During shaping, interventionists need to wait for the next approximation to occur before proceeding. It requires careful observation of subtle changes in behavior closer to the next approximation; thus adequate training of interventionists is imperative. Shaping may take considerably longer than using prompting procedures. Learners may not respond at all, however, in the presence of a relevant prompt for a particular behavior (e.g., learner who does not respond to an imitative model to say, "Mom") or learners may react negatively to the only effective (for that learner) prompt for a particular behavior (e.g., learner engages in challenging behavior when physically prompted to produce signs and does not imitate models). Shaping may be much more effective in these cases.

📭 Helpful Hint

Combine shaping with prompting to help the learner produce specific approximations to the desired behavior, which then increases the effectiveness of shaping. Prompts increase the learner's practice of the behavior and access to reinforcement, while also likely decreasing the overall time taken to acquire the skill.

What Does the Research Say?

Shaping

Mirenda and Santogrossi (1985) taught an 8-year-old girl to touch a picture to request an item using shaping. The shaping procedure progressed from reinforcing, with a small amount of the corresponding item, any accidental touch of the picture to reinforcing deliberate touching of the picture. Both the item and the symbol were gradually moved farther away and eventually out of site of the participant. Finally, more picture symbols (a total of four) were added. The participant spontaneously touched picture symbols to request items and generalized from the clinic setting to her home and school.

How Do I Implement Shaping?

Steps to implement shaping

Step 1: Identify the desired final behavior.
Step 2: Identify the first behavior to reinforce.
Step 3: Develop a list of potential approximations to the desired final behavior.
Step 4: Decide on criterion for establishing each approximation.
Step 5: Implement intervention and monitor performance.

Step 1: Identify the desired final behavior. Define the communicative behavior (the desired final behavior).

Step 2: Identify the first behavior to reinforce. The learner should already demonstrate this first behavior at some minimum frequency.

Step 3: Develop a list of potential approximations to the desired final behavior. Identifying potential approximations increases the likelihood that interventionists will notice and reinforce those approximations. Identify approximations by consulting others (e.g., a teacher), examining normative data, and/or observing one-

self and/or others performing the behavior. Approximations should reflect small enough changes that the learner can move through them easily, but not be so small that the entire shaping process becomes unnecessarily lengthy.

Step 4: Decide on criterion for establishing each approximation. Criterion should be sufficient so the learner clearly demonstrates the approximation, but allow the learner to move quickly through successive approximations. Limit the number of opportunities at each approximation so that one approximation does not result in reinforcement for such an extended period of time that it becomes firmly established.

Step 5: Implement intervention and monitor performance.

- Deliver reinforcement following the first approximation.

- Only deliver reinforcement for the next approximation once the learner reaches criterion for performance of one approximation, and do not reinforce previously reinforced approximations (those farther from the desired final behavior).

- Continue until the desired final behavior is achieved.

- If the learner fails to perform the behavior following a criterion, then increase to the next approximation, drop back to the previously successful approximation and increase in smaller increments, or add prompts to increase the likelihood the learner emits the new target approximation.

- Continue to deliver reinforcement following desired final behavior.

CASE EXAMPLE

Shaping

Jocelyn, a 6-year-old girl, was learning to use the sign ALL DONE during naturally occurring opportunities throughout the day (e.g., when finished with a meal, when finished with a workbook page). Jocelyn's interventionists initially delivered reinforcement (by terminating the activity) using shaping when Jocelyn brought her hands together in front of her body. After 2 days of Jocelyn successfully bringing her hands together, her interventionists changed the criterion approximation to Jocelyn bringing her hands together and then dropping them.

Chaining

Chaining involves linking individual behaviors into a specific sequence or chain in which each behavior is associated with a particular stimulus condition. For example, requesting can consist of chaining together a general request (e.g., expressed through using a symbol for WANT) with an explicit request for a specific object (e.g., choosing the symbol for COOKIE). Gaining access to a communication book can consist of a series of smaller steps proceeding from locating the book to selecting the target symbol. Identify the specific sequence of learner behaviors in a chain through a **task analysis** in which the chain is broken down into a series of smaller teachable units (see Figure 5.5, which is a filled-in version for Form 5.4 on the accompanying CD-ROM).

There are three procedures to teach behavior chains.

1. **Total task chaining** teaches each step in the task analysis, during each instructional session, until performance meets criterion.

2. **Forward chaining** teaches the sequence of behaviors in the task analysis in temporal order. That is, teach the first behavior in the sequence first, with the interventionist completing the rest of the steps in the chain. Instruction continues once the first step of the chain is mastered, adding one additional behavior within the chain at a time.

3. The interventionist begins **backward chaining** by completing all the behaviors in the task analysis, except for the last behavior in the chain, and teaches the last behavior first. Once the learner masters the last behavior in the chain, the interventionist completes all the behaviors in the task analysis, except for the last two behaviors, and teaches the second to last behavior. Teaching proceeds to the third behavior and so forth until the behavior chain is mastered.

What Does the Research Say?
Chaining
Hinderscheit and Reichle (1987) taught an adult with severe developmental delays a chained behavior involving touching both the color and object symbols on an SGD.

How Do I Implement Chaining Procedures?

Chaining represents an instructional procedure that is frequently used during the implementation of multistep task analyses. The following steps are designed to help the interventionist organize the implementation of a chaining procedure.

Step 1: Construct a Task Analysis   Construct a task analysis by observing oneself and/or others perform the desired behaviors and/or consulting with experts (see Form 5.4 on the accompanying CD-ROM). Test a draft task analysis by following the steps to complete the task. Modify the task analysis, as necessary, if steps were omitted. Determine whether the task analysis should be broken down into multiple smaller steps or whether steps that may be too small can be combined. The task analysis for Matt's use of his communication book with peers is shown in Figure 5.5.

Steps to implement chaining

Step 1: Construct a task analysis.
Step 2: Assess the learner's existing proficiency with the chain.
Step 3: Choose a chaining procedure.
Step 4: Implement intervention and monitor performance.

Learner's name: ___Matt_____   Task: ___Use of communication book with peers__

Instructions: Fill in the steps of the task analysis. Fill in the date in the first row, and record the learner's performance for each step of the task in the column corresponding to that date. Record a plus (+) if the learner completed the step and a minus (–) if he or she did not complete the step. Additional information about learner performance may include whether the interventionist presented a prompt (i.e., record a *P* for that step) or the learner did not respond for that step (i.e., record an *NR* for no response).

Step	Pretest					Intervention										
Date	4/2	4/4	4/4			4/5	4/5	4/6	4/6	4/9	4/10					
1. Locate communication book	+	+	+			+	+	+	+	+	+					
2. Find page with needed symbols	–	–	–			P	P	+	+	+	+					
3. Select symbols	–	–	–			P	P	P	P	+	+					
4. Place on sentence strip	+	+	+			+	+	+	+	+	+					
5. Hand to peer	+	+	+			+	+	+	+	+	+					

Figure 5.5. Behavior chain for communication book use. (*Note:* This is a filled-in version of Form 5.4, Task Analysis Development and Performance Monitoring Form. A blank, printable version appears on the accompanying CD-ROM.)

Step 2: Assess the Learner's Existing Proficiency with the Chain Assess the learner's competence with each of the component behaviors by observing the learner engaging in the task and noting his or her ability to perform each step. Error behaviors include behaviors performed incorrectly, not performed at all, or performed out of order.

Step 3: Choose a Chaining Procedure Snell and Brown (2000) noted that total task chaining may be a more natural approach to intervention than forward or backward chaining procedures.

- Can the learner perform many of the steps in the task analysis? Total task presentation may be appropriate if the learner can perform many steps in the task analysis.

- Consider switching to total task chaining if a number of the steps of the task analysis have been learned (e.g., through forward and backward chaining).

- Are there many opportunities to practice the chain? If not, total task presentation may be better. Alternatively, plan to create additional instructional opportunities.

- Does the final step in the chain result in a naturally occurring reinforcing end? If so, backward chaining may be the procedure of choice.

- Total task chaining may be a more natural approach to intervention than forward or backward chaining procedures.

- Forward or backward chaining may be better than total task presentation if the chain is long.

- How much time is available to master the skill? Initial acquisition of individual components of the task may be faster with forward and backward chaining. Acquisition of the entire chain, however, may be slower than with total task presentation. Therefore, total task presentation may be best to increase overall acquisition rate.

- How much time is available to devote to each instructional session? An advantage of forward and backward chaining is that the entire chain is completed relatively quickly (as the interventionist is completing steps that have not yet been taught).

- The interventionist must complete the unlearned portion of the task with forward and backward chaining.

Step 4: Implement Intervention and Monitor Performance   Identify prompting and reinforcement procedures. Teach each step in the task analysis during each instructional session when using total task chaining. Provide prompting as needed for any step the learner does not complete independently. Reinforce criterion performance for each step.

Initially, teach and deliver reinforcement following performance when using forward chaining, meeting criterion for only the first step in the task analysis. Once the learner masters the first behavior in the chain, teach the second behavior by presenting the opportunity, allowing the learner to complete the first behavior (already mastered), teaching the second behavior, and delivering reinforcement for meeting criterion for performance of both the first and second behaviors. Continue with subsequent behaviors in the chain, delivering reinforcement for criterion performance on the target step and any preceding steps, until mastery of all behaviors.

Complete the entire chain except for the last step when using backward chaining. Provide instruction on the last step, and deliver reinforcement only when the learner meets criterion for performance of the last step. Once the learner's performance meets criterion, complete the entire chain except for the last two steps, provide instruction on the second to last step, and deliver reinforcement when the second to last and last steps are performed to criterion, and so forth. Record performance on a form such as the task analysis form in Figure 5.5 or Form 5.4 on the accompanying CD-ROM.

CASE EXAMPLE

Chaining

Matt is a 15-year-old boy learning to use his communication book. Figure 5.5 shows the steps of this chain. Pretest performance indicated that Matt readily performed the first and final two steps in the chain. His interventionist used total task chaining for intervention because Matt had some proficiency with the steps in this relatively short chain.

ADDITIONAL CONSIDERATIONS

Consider spontaneity and maintenance of communication skills once acquired when planning intervention.

Spontaneity

Many learners with developmental disabilities show a lack of spontaneous use of communication skills (Carr, 1982; Carter, 2002, 2003; Carter & Hotchkis, 2002; Kaczmarek, 1990; Reichle & Sigafoos, 1991). Communication is described as prompt dependent, only occurring following specific questions, directions, or physical/gestural prompts (Carter, 2003; Reichle, York, & Eynon, 1989). Although such prompts may be effective during initial instruction, they limit the options for communication and independence. **Spontaneity** has been defined as communication that occurs in the absence of explicit vocal directives (Charlop, Schreibman, & Thibodeau, 1985) or in response to unobtrusive or not readily observable cues (Halle, 1987). Spontaneity can be thought of on a continuum with regard to the cues that occasion behaviors (Carter, 2003; Halle, 1987). The more obvious or intrusive the cue, the less spontaneous the behavior. Behaviors that occur in the presence of specific objects and those that occur in reaction to internal stimuli (e.g., hunger pains, headache) are more spontaneous. Two strategies are often used to develop spontaneous communication.

1. Time delay is the prompt fading procedure in which interventionists insert a delay between the natural cue (i.e., S^D) and the delivery of prompts to provide the learner with the opportunity to emit the behavior independently (i.e., spontaneously) in the presence of naturally available stimuli (e.g., a preferred game that is out of reach).

2. **Behavior chain interruption** involves creating an instructional opportunity in the midst of an activity. For example, the teacher withholds the required cards for a player's turn to create an opportunity for spontaneous requesting while playing a board game. Behavior chain interruptions might involve withholding the presentation of needed items, blocking access to needed items (or placing them out of reach), or delaying assistance.

---

al., 1994; Romer & Schoenberg, 1991), and use of graphic symbols to make requests (e.g., Goetz, Gee, & Sailor, 1985; Grunsell & Carter, 2002; Hunt, Goetz, Alwell, & Sailor, 1986; Roberts-Pennell & Sigafoos, 1999). Studies demonstrate generalization to novel routines (e.g., Gee et al., 1991; Grunsell & Carter, 2002; Hunt et al., 1986; Roberts-Pennell & Sigafoos, 1999), different interruptions within the same routine (e.g., initiation of an activity rather than continuation; Alwell, Hunt, Goetz, & Sailor, 1989; Roberts-Pennell & Sigafoos, 1999), and routines with different interruptions (e.g., Grunsell & Carter, 2002). Gee et al. used both the behavior chain interruption and time delay procedures along with physical prompting to teach three students with developmental disabilities to activate a switch to request continuation of activities.

What Does the Research Say?

Spontaneity

Time Delay

Charlop et al. (1985) taught seven children with autism to spontaneously request food using a verbal model prompt and time delay procedure. Intervention began with a 2-second delay. The delay was increased in 2-second increments to a total of 10 seconds when the child either correctly imitated the prompt or spontaneously requested food on 3 consecutive opportunities. Participants spontaneously requested food and generalized to unfamiliar people, places, and items. Charlop and Trasowech (1991) and Charlop and Walsh (1986) used a time delay to teach spontaneous expressions of affection, commenting, question asking, and greetings. Charlop-Christy, Carpenter, Le, LeBlanc, and Kellet (2002) and Tincani, Crozier, and Alazetta (2006) used a time delay to teach the Picture Exchange Communication System (PECS).

Behavior Chain Interruption

Behavior chain interruption has been used most often to teach requesting skills (Carter & Grunsell, 2001), including spoken requests (e.g., Duker, Kraaykamp, & Visser, 1994; Sigafoos & Littlewood, 1999), signed requests (e.g., Duker et al., 1994; Roberts-Pennell & Sigafoos, 1999; Romer et

---

How Do I Implement a Behavior Chain Interruption Procedure?

After designing an intervention procedure that involves chaining, it is implemented. There are well-established evidence-based strategies for implementing behavior chain interruption procedures. What follows are steps that a number of investigations have used in implementing procedures that include chaining.

• *Step 1:* Identify an activity.

Identify a regularly occurring activity in which the learner can practice the target communicative behavior. Although new rou-

Steps to implement a behavior chain interruption procedure

Step 1: Identify an activity.
Step 2: Identify the communicative behavior to be taught.
Step 3: List the steps in the behavior chain (task analysis).
Step 4: Identify potential strategies for interruption.
Step 5: Conduct pretest observations.
Step 6: Develop instructional strategies.
Step 7: Implement intervention and monitor performance.

tines can be used, an activity with which the learner has some level of independence provides opportunities so that he or she can independently complete the next step of the activity once the interruption occurs. Choose a routine with each step initiated by the learner (even if the learner cannot complete the behavior independently) and at least three steps in the chain (Hunt & Goetz, 1988). This allows the opportunity to be inserted mid-activity rather than at the beginning of an activity in an effort to increase the learner's motivation to continue the activity.

☞ Helpful Hint

Consider choosing several activities in which the same target behaviors can be taught to increase the number of opportunities and the likelihood of generalization. For example, use the behavior chain interruption strategy to teach a learner to use his or her communication system to request assistance during food preparation, dressing, and a leisure activity (e.g., making crafts).

- *Step 2*: Identify the communicative behavior to be taught.
- *Step 3*: List the steps in the behavior chain (task analysis).
- *Step 4*: Identify potential strategies for interruption.

  Minimize using verbal questions such as "What do you want?" because the goal is spontaneity.

  Block the learner from proceeding to the next step.

  Delay presentation of a needed item.

  Place a needed item out of the learner's reach.

  Remove an item needed for the routine.

  Present natural obstacles (e.g., containers the learner cannot open independently).

  Present only part/some of needed items/materials.

- *Step 5*: Conduct pretest observations.

Observe the learner during interruptions in the activity. Interruptions should result in the learner attempting to continue the activity, by using behaviors already in his or her repertoire such as facial expressions or other body movements. Each interruption can be scored for attempts to continue the activity (e.g., on a 3-point scale ranging from "no attempt" to "very clear indication of desire to continue the activity;" Hunt & Goetz, 1988). Pretests reveal

Routines in which the learner attempts to continue with moderate distress (rather than high or low levels of distress).

The specific interruptions associated with moderate distress. Interruptions associated with significant distress are not the best for intervention because prompting communication may be difficult due to interfering challenging behavior.

- *Step 6*: Develop instructional strategies.
- *Step 7*: Implement intervention and monitor performance.

Hunt and Goetz (1988) recommended terminating the routine and reevaluating the routine and planned interruptions if interruptions repeatedly result in incorrect behaviors. Identify new routines and/or interruptions if the learner shows low motivation for participation in the routine.

CASE EXAMPLE

Behavior Chain Interruption

Leila, a 17-year-old girl with developmental disabilities and no speech, was being taught to use her SGD to request access to materials during self-care routines (e.g., brushing her teeth, fixing her hair, polishing her nails). While engaged in the activity, her interventionist implemented a behavior chain interruption procedure by placing her hand in front of the item at the points within each activity when Leila reached for each item (e.g., hairbrush, mirror, clips).

Maintenance

Maintenance of skills refers to the extent to which a learner continues to perform the target behavior after terminating a portion or all of the intervention strategies. For example, Sam continued to sign HELLO in the absence of the prompts and token reinforcement that had been used to teach the sign. Natural opportunities may be available to practice skills. Additional continued practice may be needed, however, for many learners with developmental disabilities. The frequency of practice necessary to ensure skill maintenance varies by learner and task. If performance decreases with a given schedule of maintenance practice, then consider increasing the frequency of maintenance sessions and/or the number of opportunities during each maintenance session.

🖝 Helpful Hint

To monitor maintenance performance:

- Simultaneously assess previously acquired target skills when teaching new skills.

- Set up a maintenance book, folder, or chart with performance monitoring forms (e.g., a master list) listing all the skills the learner has acquired. Decide on the frequency these skills need to be reviewed with the learner (e.g., biweekly, one to two times per week).

SUMMARY

These instructional strategies are an integral part of the interventions described throughout this book. Interventionists addressing the needs of learners using AAC should consider the selection of teaching opportunities and components of those opportunities, including stimuli that occasion the behavior, types of prompts, and reinforcement and correction strategies. Proficient use of these instructional strategies enables interventionists to design interventions that meet the diverse and individualized needs of AAC users.

🖝 Helpful Hint

See Alberto and Troutman (2006), Cooper et al. (2007), and Snell and Brown (2000) for additional information about instructional strategies.

REFERENCES

Alberto, P.A., & Troutman, A.C. (2006). *Applied behavior analysis for teachers* (7th ed.). Upper Saddle River, NJ: Merrill Prentice Hall.

Alwell, M., Hunt, P., Goetz, L., & Sailor, W. (1989). Teaching generalized communicative behaviors within interrupted behavior chain contexts. *Journal of The Association for Persons with Severe Handicaps, 14,* 91–100.

Ault, M.J., Gast, D.L., & Wolery, M. (1988). Comparison of progressive and constant time-delay procedures in teaching community-sign word reading. *American Journal of Mental Retardation, 93,* 44–56.

Birkan, B., McClannahan, L.E., & Krantz, P.J. (2007). Effects of superimposition and background fading on the sight-word reading of a boy with autism. *Research in Autism Spectrum Disorders, 1,* 117–125.

Buzolich, M.J., King, J.S., & Baroody, S.M. (1991). Acquisition of the commenting function among system users. *Augmentative and Alternative Communication, 7,* 88–99.

Carr, E.G. (1982). Sign language. In R. Koegel, A. Rincover, & A. Egel (Eds.), *Educating and understanding autistic children* (pp. 142–157). San Diego: College-Hill.

Carr, E.G., Levin, L., McConnachie, G., Carlson, J.I., Kemp, D.C., & Smith, C.E. (1994). *Communication based intervention for problem behavior: A user's guide for producing positive change.* Baltimore: Paul H. Brookes Publishing Co.

Carr, J.E., Nicholson, A.C., & Higbee, T.S. (2000). Evaluation of a brief multiple-stimulus preference assessment in a naturalistic context. *Journal of Applied Behavior Analysis, 33,* 353–357.

Carter, M. (2002). Communicative spontaneity in individuals with high support needs: An exploratory consideration of causation. *International Journal of Disability, Development, and Education, 19,* 225–242.

Carter, M. (2003). Communicative spontaneity of children with high support needs who use augmentative and alternative communication systems I: Classroom spontaneity, mode, and function. *Augmentative and Alternative Communication, 19,* 141–154.

Carter, M., & Grunsell, J. (2001). The behavior chain interruption strategy: A review of research and discussion of future directions. *Journal of The Association for Persons with Severe Handicaps, 26*, 37–49.

Carter, M., & Hotchkis, G.D. (2002). A conceptual analysis of communicative spontaneity. *Journal of Intellectual and Developmental Disability, 27*, 168–190.

Chadsey-Rusch, J., Drasgow, E., Reinoehl, B., & Halle, J. (1993). Using general-case instruction to teach spontaneous and generalized requests for assistance to learners with severe disabilities. *Journal of The Association for Persons with Severe Handicaps, 18*, 177–187.

Charlop, M.H., Schreibman, L., & Thibodeau, M.G. (1985). Increasing spontaneous verbal responding in autistic children using a time delay procedure. *Journal of Applied Behavior Analysis, 18*, 155–166.

Charlop, M.H., & Trasowech, J.E. (1991). Increasing autistic children's daily spontaneous speech. *Journal of Applied Behavior Analysis, 24*, 747–761.

Charlop, M.H., & Walsh, M.E. (1986). Increasing autistic children's spontaneous verbalizations of affection: On assessment of time delay and peer modeling procedures. *Journal of Applied Behavior Analysis, 19*, 307–314.

Charlop-Christy, M.H., Carpenter, M., Le, L., LeBlanc, L.A., & Kellet, K. (2002). Using the Picture Exchange Communication System (PECS) with children with autism: Assessment of PECS acquisition, speech, social-communicative behavior, and problem behavior. *Journal of Applied Behavior Analysis, 35*, 213–231.

Cooper, J.O., Heron, T.E., & Heward, W.L. (2007). *Applied behavior analysis* (2nd ed.). Upper Saddle River, NJ: Pearson.

DeLeon, I.G., Fisher, W.W., Rodriguez-Cater, V., Maglieri, K., Herman, K., & Marhefka, J.M. (2001). Examination of relative reinforcement effects of stimuli identified through pretreatment and daily brief assessments. *Journal of Applied Behavior Analysis, 34*, 463–473.

Duffy, L., & Wishart, J.G. (1987). A comparison of two procedures or teaching discrimination skills to Down's Syndrome and non-handicapped children. *British Journal of Educational Psychology, 57*, 265–278.

Duker, P., Kraaykamp, M., & Visser, E. (1994). A stimulus control procedure to increase requesting with individuals who are severely/profoundly intellectually disabled. *Journal of Intellectual Disability Research, 38*, 177–186.

Gee, K., Graham, N., Goetz, L., Oshima, G., & Yoshioka, K. (1991). Teaching students to request the continuation of routine activities by using time delay and decreasing physical assistance in the context of chain interruption.

Journal of The Association for Persons with Severe Handicaps, 16, 154–167.

Goetz, L., Gee, K., & Sailor, W. (1985). Using a behavior chain interruption strategy to teach communication skills to students with severe disabilities. *Journal of The Association for Persons with Severe Handicaps, 10*, 21–30.

Graff, R.B., & Libby, M.E. (1999). A comparison of presession and within-session reinforcement choice. *Journal of Applied Behavior Analysis, 32*, 161–173.

Green, C.W., Reid, D.H., White, L.K., Halford, R.C., Brittain, D.P., & Gardner, S.M. (1988). Identifying reinforcers for person with profound handicaps: Staff opinion versus systematic assessment of preferences. *Journal of Applied Behavior Analysis, 21*, 31–43.

Grunsell, J., & Carter, M. (2002). The behavior chain interruption strategy: Generalization to out-of-routine contexts. *Education and Training in Mental Retardation and Developmental Disabilities, 37*, 378–390.

Halle, J.W. (1987). Teaching language in the natural environment: An analysis of spontaneity. *Journal of The Association for Persons with Severe Handicaps, 12*, 28–37.

Hinderscheit, L.R., & Reichle, J. (1987). Teaching direct select color encoding to an adolescent with multiple handicaps. *Augmentative and Alternative Communication, 3*, 137–142.

Horner, R.H., & McDonald, R.S. (1982). Comparison of single instance and general case instruction in teaching a generalized vocational skills. *Journal of the Association for the Severely Handicapped, 7*, 7–20.

Hunt, P., Goetz, L., Alwell, M., & Sailor, W. (1986). Using an interrupted behavior chain strategy to teach generalized communication behaviors. *Journal of The Association for Persons with Severe Handicaps, 11*, 196–204.

Jones, E.A., Carr, E.G., & Feeley, K.M. (2006). Multiple effects of joint attention intervention for children with autism. *Behavior Modification, 30*, 782–834.

Kaczmarek, L.A. (1990). Teaching spontaneous language to individuals with severe handicaps: A matrix model. *Journal of The Association for Persons with Severe Handicaps, 15*, 160–169.

Laraway, S., Snycerski, S., Michael, J., & Poling, A. (2003). Motivating operations and terms to describe them: Some further refinements. *Journal of Applied Behavior Analysis, 36*, 407–414.

Light-Shriner, C., & Johnston, S.S. (1992). *Conducting forced choice preference assessments.* Unpublished manuscript.

Mackay, H.A., Soraci, S.A., Carlin, M.T., Dennis, N.A., & Strawbridge, C.P. (2002). Guiding visual attention during acquisition of match-to-sample. *American Journal on Mental Retardation, 107,* 445–454.

Matson, J.L., Sevin, J.A., Box, M.L., Francis, K.L., & Sevin, B.M. (1993). An evaluation of two methods for increasing self-initiated verbalizations in autistic children. *Journal of Applied Behavior Analysis, 26,* 389–398.

Maurice, C., Green, G., & Luce, S.C. (Eds.). (1996). *Behavioral intervention for young children with autism: A manual for parents and professionals.* Austin, TX: PRO-ED.

Mirenda, P., & Santogrossi, J. (1985). A prompt-free strategy to teach pictorial communication system use. *Augmentative and Alternative Communication, 1,* 143–150.

Mundy, P., Kasari, C., & Sigman, M. (1995). Nonverbal communication and early language acquisition in children with Down syndrome and in normally developing children. *Journal of Speech and Hearing Research, 38,* 157–167.

Nelson, C., McDonnell, A.P., Johnston, S.S., Crompton, A., & Nelson, A.R. (2007). Keys to play: A strategy to increase the social interactions of young children with autism and their typically developing peers. *Education and Training in Developmental Disabilities, 42,* 165–181.

Ortiz, K.R., & Carr, J.E. (2000). Multiple-stimulus preference assessments: A comparison of free-operant and restricted-operant formats. *Behavioral Interventions, 15,* 345–353.

Piazza, C.C., Fisher, W.W., Hagopian, L.P., Bowman, L.G., & Toole, L. (1996). Using choice assessment to predict reinforce effectiveness. *Journal of Applied Behavior Analysis, 29,* 1–9.

Reichle, J., & Johnston, S. (1999). Teaching the conditional use of communicative requests to two school-age children with severe developmental disabilities. *Language, Speech, and Hearing Services in School, 30,* 324–334.

Reichle, J., McComas, J., Dahl, N., Solberg, G., Pierce, S., & Smith, D. (2005). Teaching an individual with severe intellectual delay to request assistance conditionally. *Educational Psychology, 25,* 275–286.

Reichle, J., & Sigafoos, J. (1991). Establishing spontaneity and generalization. In J. Reichle, J. York, & J. Sigafoos (Eds.), *Implementing augmentative and alternative communication: Strategies for learners with severe disabilities.* (pp. 157–171). Baltimore: Paul H. Brookes Publishing Co.

Reichle, J., York, J., & Eynon, D. (1989). Influence of indicating preferences for initiating, maintaining, and terminating interactions. In F. Brown & D.H. Lehr (Eds.), *Persons with profound disabilities: Issues and practices* (pp. 191–211). Baltimore: Paul H. Brookes Publishing Co.

Repp, A.C., Karsh, K.G., & Lenz, M. (1990). A comparison of two teaching procedures on ac-

quisition and generalization of severely handicapped persons. *Journal of Applied Behavior Analysis, 23,* 43–52.

Roberts-Pennell, D., & Sigafoos, J. (1999). Teaching young children with developmental disabilities to request more pay using the behavior chain interruption strategy. *Journal of Applied Research in Intellectual Disabilities, 12,* 100–112.

Rodgers, T.A., & Iwata, B.A. (1991). An analysis of error-correction procedures during discrimination training. *Journal of Applied Behavior Analysis, 24,* 775–781.

Romer, L.T., Cullinan, T., & Schoenberg, B. (1994). General case training of requesting: A demonstration and analysis. *Education and Training in Mental Retardation and Developmental Disabilities, 29,* 57–68.

Romer, L.T., & Schoenberg, B. (1991). Increasing requests made by people with developmental disabilities and deaf-blindness through the use of behavior interruption strategies. *Education and Training in Mental Retardation, 26,* 70–78.

Sarokoff, R.A., Taylor, B.A., & Poulson, C.L. (2001). Teaching children with autism to engage in conversational exchanges: Script fading with embedded textual stimuli. *Journal of Applied Behavior Analysis, 34,* 81–84.

Schreibman, L. (1975). Effects of within-stimulus and extra-stimulus prompting on discrimination learning in autistic children. *Journal of Applied Behavior Analysis, 8,* 91–112.

Schreibman, L., & Charlop, M.H. (1981). S+ versus S- fading in prompting procedures with autistic children. *Journal of Experimental Child Psychology, 31,* 508–520.

Sigafoos, J., & Littlewood, R. (1999). Communication intervention on the playground: A case study on teaching requesting to a young child with autism. *International Journal of Disability, Development, and Education, 46,* 421–429.

Sigafoos, J., O'Reilly, M.F., Drasgow, E., & Reichle, J. (2002). Strategies to achieve socially acceptable escape and avoidance. In D. Beukelman & J. Reichle (Series Eds.) & J. Reichle, D.R. Beukelman, & J.C. Light (Vol. Eds.), *AAC series: Exemplary practices for beginning communicators: Implications for AAC* (pp. 157–186). Baltimore: Paul H. Brookes Publishing Co.

Snell, M.E., & Brown, F. (2000). *Instruction of students with severe disabilities* (5th ed.). Upper Saddle River, NJ: Merrill.

Stokes, T., & Baer, D. (1977). An implicit technology of generalization. *Journal of Applied Behavior Analysis, 10,* 349–367.

Sulzer-Azaroff, B., & Mayer, G.R. (1991). *Behavior analysis for lasting change.* Fort Worth, TX: Harcourt Brace.

Tincani, M., Crozier, S., & Alazetta, L. (2006). The Picture Exchange Communication System: Effects on manding and speech development for school-aged children with autism. *Education and Training in Developmental Disabilities, 41,* 177–184.

Worsdell, A.S., Iwata, B.A., Dozier, C.L., Johnson, A.D., Neidert, P.L., & Thomason, J.L. (2005). Analysis of behavior repetition as an error-correction strategy during sight-word reading. *Journal of Applied Behavior Analysis, 38,* 511–527.

Intervention Intensity

Developing a Context for Instruction

Emily A. Jones and Kathleen M. Feeley

6

▷ CHAPTER OVERVIEW

Interventionists identify specific skills that need to be addressed and corresponding evidence-based intervention strategies (see Chapter 5). In addition, they must address the intensity with which intervention will be delivered. In the past, intervention intensity has been gauged largely by the number of hours of intervention across a time period (e.g., day, week, month) (Warren, Fey, & Yoder, 2007). Numbers of hours per time period is not the only measure of intervention intensity, however, and is not reflective of all of the active ingredients of an intervention. Interventions may differ greatly but still consist of a similar number of hours, weeks, or months of intervention (Eldevik, Eikeseth, Jahr, & Smith, 2006). Warren et al. described intervention intensity as the number of teaching opportunities, how those opportunities are presented, the frequency with which intervention sessions are implemented, and the time period over which intervention is implemented (e.g., for several weeks, months, years). Few researchers have empirically examined these aspects of intervention, and often, interventions are not described with the level of detail to allow for firm conclusions or direct comparisons (LeChago & Carr, 2008).

This chapter poses a series of questions related to intervention intensity. The answers to these questions determine the way instructional opportunities will be presented—referred to collectively as the **context for instruction.** A continuum of intervention intensities with three general anchor points of empirically based contexts for instruction are described to help tailor augmentative and alternative communication (AAC) intervention to each learner's needs.

▷ CHAPTER OBJECTIVES

After studying this chapter, readers will be able to

- Define intervention intensity and context for instruction
- Answer key questions to determine intervention intensity and develop a context for instruction
- Consider learner strengths and weaknesses to determine intervention intensity and develop a context for instruction
- Provide examples of three general contexts for instruction (i.e., naturalistic instruction, instruction embedded within an activity, and discrete trial instruction)
- Summarize empirical evidence supporting three general instructional contexts

---

- activity-based intervention
- context for instruction
- continuum of instruction
- discrete trial instruction
- embedded instruction
- incidental teaching
- instruction embedded within an activity
- joint action routines
- milieu teaching
- modified incidental teaching
- naturalistic instruction
- pivotal response treatment
- prelinguistic milieu teaching
- verbal behavior

DETERMINING INTERVENTION INTENSITY: KEY QUESTIONS

Some questions about intervention intensity relate to how instructional opportunities will occur (e.g., the environment, consequences), referred to as the "form" of intervention by Warren et al. (2007), whereas other questions concern the amount of intervention (e.g., number of opportunities). The range of answers to these questions reflects a continuum of the extent to which intervention mirrors how the communicative response would occur within natural interactions. Opportunities reflect natural interactions and, likely, less intensive intervention at one end of the continuum, and opportunities are more structured/prescribed and, likely, reflect more intensive intervention at the other end of the continuum.

In Which Environments Will Instruction Occur?

Instruction can occur in the natural environment where the communication skill will be used when mastered (e.g., during play, lunch at school, leisure activities) (e.g., Hart & Risley, 1974; Johnston, Nelson, Evans, & Palazolo, 2003) or (at the other end of the continuum) in a separate location (e.g., Buffington, Krantz, McClannahan, & Poulson, 1998). Instruction in natural environments may increase the likelihood of generalization because the skill is acquired (and demonstrated) in relevant settings. Alternatively, a separate location may provide fewer distractions and/or support a larger number of instructional opportunities that improve acquisition for some learners. Intervention could also involve a combination of natural and more structured environments. For example, educators can implement structured opportunities at school, whereas family members can capitalize on naturally occurring opportunities in the home. The **continuum of instructional** environments is illustrated in Figure 6.1.

Who Will Be the Communicative Partner?

Instruction can occur with natural communicative partners (e.g., Hart & Risley, 1974; Johnston et al., 2003) or specially trained professionals (e.g., Charlop, Schreibman, & Thibodeau, 1985; Whalen & Schreibman, 2003). When natural communication partners are used, external validity is enhanced. An interventionist (e.g., teaching assistant, speech-language pathologist) as the communicative partner may allow for more opportunities and the delivery of highly salient instructional cues and powerful reinforcers. Natural communication partners can be trained to act as interventionists (e.g., parents teaching joint attention [Jones & Feeley, 2007]; peers teaching communicative/interaction skills [McGee, Almeida, Sulzer-Azaroff, & Feldman, 1992]), or a combination of natural partners and interventionists (e.g., teachers teaching joint attention skills and then parents [Jones, Carr, & Feeley, 2006]) can be used. The continuum of those with whom instruction might occur is shown in Figure 6.2.

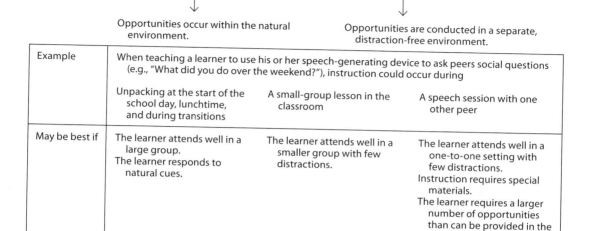

Figure 6.1. Continuum of environments in which instruction will occur.

Will the Learner or Interventionist Initiate Instructional Opportunities?

Learner-initiated opportunities occur when the learner starts communicating (e.g., Hancock & Kaiser, 2002; McGee et al., 1992) by expressing an interest in something or someone (e.g., looking, reaching, manipulating something, vocalizing). For example, a learner reaching for a book on a shelf cre-

ated a learner-initiated opportunity to teach more sophisticated requesting skills (e.g., pressing the BOOK symbol on a speech-generating device [SGD]). Learner initiations may also express that something is undesirable, such as turning his or her head away from a nonpreferred food or pushing a nonpreferred activity onto the floor, creating opportunities to practice more sophisticated rejecting skills (e.g., signing NO).

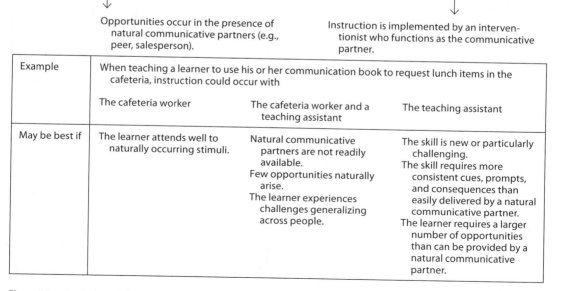

Figure 6.2. Continuum of who the communicative partner will be during instruction.

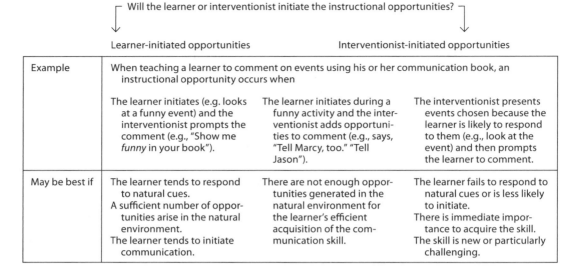

Figure 6.3. Continuum of learner-initiated or interventionist instructional opportunities.

Interventionist-initiated opportunities occur when the interventionist sets up relevant materials and delivers a cue (i.e., a specific question ["What's this?"] or instruction ["Give me____"]) to which the learner should respond. Interventionists also initiate opportunities using nonverbal stimuli (e.g., Charlop et al., 1985), such as holding an item out of reach for the learner to request access (Jones, Feeley, & Blackburn, 2010) or presenting a novel item about which the learner should request information (e.g., Koegel, Camarata, Valdez-Menchaca, & Koegel, 1998). The learner is already attending to and motivated by the relevant stimuli during learner-initiated opportunities, and the natural consequences are likely to function as reinforcers. The interventionist ensures instructional opportunities occur, controls the number of opportunities, and controls access to the materials during interventionist-initiated activities—important aspects of effective intervention. The continuum of learner- or interventionist-initiated instructional opportunities is illustrated in Figure 6.3.

What Consequences Will Follow a Learner's Communicative Act?

Consequences following communication range from those that naturally occur as a result of a response (e.g., receipt of requested object [Hart & Risley, 1974; Sigafoos, Laurie, & Pennell, 1996]; answer to a question [Koegel et al., 1998]) to highly individualized consequences chosen because of their effectiveness (e.g., token [Buffington et al., 1998]; piece of food [Chiara, Schuster, Bell, & Wolery, 1995]; verbal praise [Buffington et al., 1998; Chiara et al., 1995; Sigafoos et al., 1996]). If more natural consequences (e.g., praise) are effective, then more intense and complex strategies are not necessary (Fabiano et al., 2007). Natural consequences may not function as reinforcers for some learners and/or communication skills, requiring intensive and individualized reinforcement systems (e.g., pairing natural consequences with a powerful reinforcer).

Corrective feedback for incorrect communicative acts also includes natural consequences, such as delivering a nonpreferred food item after the learner incorrectly selects the corresponding symbol. Natural consequences, however, may not always result in a subsequent decrease in the learner's incorrect responses, warranting additional error

Chapter 5 discusses consequence strategies.

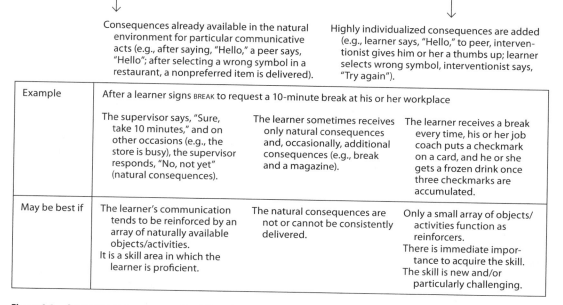

Figure 6.4. Continuum of consequences that follow a learner's communicative act.

correction strategies (e.g., interventionist says, "No, Charles, that was the wrong symbol"). The continuum of consequences that follow a learner's communicative act are presented in Figure 6.4.

How Many Instructional Opportunities Will Be Implemented During What Time Frame?

The number of instructional opportunities implemented within a specified time frame, or *dose*, ranges from few to many, with either very short or relatively longer periods of time between opportunities (Warren et al., 2007). Relatively few opportunities can be distributed throughout a day (e.g., Wolery, Anthony, & Heckathorn, 1998), or a few opportunities can be clustered at various times each day (e.g., during art, snack [Daugherty, Grisham-Brown, & Hemmeter, 2001; Venn et al., 1993], transitions [Wolery, Anthony, Caldwell, Snyder, & Morgante, 2002]). A greater number of opportunities could be presented within brief sessions providing rapid repeated practice. Factors that affect

the number of teaching opportunities include the rate of opportunities per unit of time (e.g., per minute/hour); the length of the instructional session (e.g., 10 minutes, 60 minutes); the spacing or distribution of opportunities (e.g., 1 per minute, 1 every 5 minutes); and the frequency with which intervention sessions are implemented (e.g., 1 time per day, 4 times per day), a factor discussed next.

Some learners may benefit from multiple and closely spaced instructional opportunities within a specific time frame (Smith, 2001); others may not require as many opportunities to acquire a skill or may lose interest in the task and fail to attend to multiple opportunities. Increased opportunities improve acquisition of some skills for learners with specific language impairments (Gray, 2003; Rice, Oetting, Marquis, Bode, & Pae, 1994; Riches, Tomasello, & Conti-Ramsden, 2005). Response form, target skills, and diagnosis influence the benefits of number and spacing of opportunities. The continuum of the number of instructional opportunities is presented in Figure 6.5.

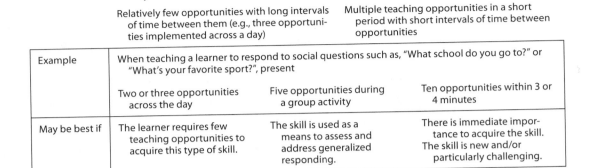

Figure 6.5. Continuum of number of instructional opportunities.

How Often Will Intervention Sessions Be Implemented?

How often intervention sessions are implemented, or *dose frequency*, is typically reported as hours per week of intervention or sessions per day or week (Warren et al., 2007). This aspect of intensity is more often reported and examined than others. Lovaas's (1987) initial study of early intensive behavioral intervention for children with autism compared 40 hours per week versus 10 hours per week of intervention, with the group receiving 40 hours per week showing significant improvement. Research continues to support the conclusion that more total hours per week of early intensive behavioral intervention is associated with better outcomes (Granpeesheh, Dixon, Tarbox, Kaplan, & Wilke, 2009; Reichow & Wolery, 2009); however, there are reports of similar outcomes for 12–27 hours versus 28–43 hours of intervention per week (Sheinkopf & Siegel, 1998).

An increase in hours or sessions often results in increases in the number of opportunities and the number and range of environments in which intervention is implemented (Hunt, Alwell, & Goetz, 1991)—two other aspects of intervention intensity. Empirical study of the number of opportunities per some time period and number of sessions is also confounded with the duration of the evaluation period of the study. There

are few direct comparisons of one of these aspects of intensity with the other aspects held constant. Warren et al. (2007) used the term *cumulative intervention intensity* to indicate the interaction of these variables. The continuum of how often intervention sessions will be implemented is presented in Figure 6.6.

What Will Be the Duration of the Intervention?

Duration refers to how long an intervention is implemented (e.g., only a few weeks [low intensity] or a full year [high intensity]). Luiselli, O'Malley, Cannon, Ellis, and Sisson (2000) found that the overall duration of participation in home-based early intervention predicted improvements in communication, cognition, and social-emotional functioning (but not gross or fine motor or self-care skills) for children with autism. In contrast, hours of intervention per week did not predict outcomes. Smith (2001) noted the best evidence regarding duration of early intensive behavioral intervention suggests several years of intervention result in positive improvements in IQ, other standardized tests, and educational placement.

Although likely an important variable, there are few direct comparisons of duration of intervention. Reed, Osborne, and

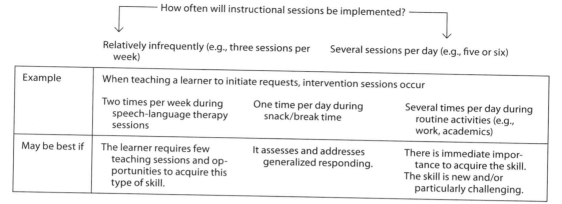

Figure 6.6. Continuum of how often instructional sessions will be implemented.

Corness (2007) compared 12 hours per week with 30 hours per week of behavioral intervention for children with autism for a duration of 9–10 months. The group of children with autism who received 30 hours per week made greater gains, but, in contrast to findings by Lovaas (1987), there was no change in the autism severity rating for any of the participants. The authors attributed this to the much shorter duration of the study (9–10 months versus 2 or more years in Lovaas's study). Warren et al. (2008) evaluated responsive education (parent training focusing on recognizing and reinforcing children's communication attempts) and **prelinguistic milieu teaching** (intervention focused on children's use of gaze, gestures, and vocalizations to comment and request) and suggested the relatively brief duration (6 months) of intervention may relate to the lack of effects they found at 6- and 12-month follow-ups, although this remains to be empirically examined.

Consider the learner's general rate of skill acquisition to help identify a priori how long (i.e., the duration) an intervention should be implemented and the time frame in which to expect acquisition of a particular skill. For example, if history suggests a learner requires 100 teaching opportunities to acquire specific skills (e.g., receptively identifying graphic symbols, spontaneously using signs) but only 10 opportunities are presented each week, then it is likely acquisition will require several weeks. A more in-

tensive spacing of teaching opportunities may yield 25 teaching opportunities in a day, with acquisition within only 4 days, significantly decreasing the overall duration of intervention. Thus, the duration of an intervention will be tailored to individual learners, recognizing that variations may occur across skills (i.e., some skills may warrant longer implementation of intervention than others). Carefully monitoring learner performance (as described in Chapter 7) will allow for ongoing evaluation of the intervention and provide useful information for future decision making about the expected duration of an intervention. Estimate an expected duration that allows sufficient time for evidence of learner acquisition, but limited time to ensure changes can be made quickly to an ineffective intervention. The continuum of the duration of intervention is presented in Figure 6.7.

DECIDING THE INTENSITY WITH WHICH AAC INTERVENTION SHOULD BE IMPLEMENTED

When developing intervention strategies for any given learner, there are a number of considerations (Smith, 2001; Turnell & Carter, 1994; Warren et al., 2007). General strengths and weaknesses exhibited by a learner may affect choices regarding intervention intensity. Cognitive and communication profiles may be directly related to the etiology of a learner's disability (e.g., Down

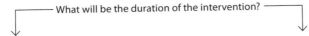

	What will be the duration of the intervention?		
	Intervention will be implemented within a relatively short period of time (e.g., 3 months).		Intervention will be implemented continuously with no specific time line identified.
Example	When teaching a learner to identify symbols representing new vocabulary, the duration of intervention may be		
	Two months during the summer to prepare the learner for vocabulary needed for that school year	Over the course of the entire school year to expand vocabulary	Continuous, as the need for new symbols/vocabulary will not come to an end
May be best if	The learner acquires well-generalized skills in a timely fashion. It is a foundational skill (e.g., verbal imitation) that is likely to remain in the learner's repertoire once it is acquired. The skill prepares the learner for an upcoming event (e.g., new school).	There is a finite set of skills that needs to be acquired.	There is an ongoing need to address an expanding or changing skill repertoire (e.g., expanding vocabulary, changing social/communicative demands).

Figure 6.7. Continuum of the duration of intervention.

syndrome, Williams syndrome). For example, based on Fidler and colleagues' (Fidler, Philofsky, Hepburn, & Rogers, 2005) findings of impaired requesting skills in children with Down syndrome, Jones et al. (2010) and Feeley, Jones, Blackburn, and Bauer (2010) used a high-intensity intervention (adult-directed, multiple, and closely spaced instructional opportunities implemented with carefully chosen materials and consequences) to teach requesting.

In contrast, the relative strengths in social development in children with Down syndrome suggest that social skills may be addressed through less intensive intervention opportunities. Other characteristics of children with Down syndrome (e.g., lower task persistence [Warren et al., 2007]) could influence the intensity of intervention.

Autism spectrum disorders have received perhaps the most attention with respect to the intensity of intervention. Lovaas (1987) and a number of replications (Eikeseth, Smith, Jahr, & Eldevik, 2002, 2007; Eldevik et al., 2006) demonstrated the effects of intensive intervention involving individualized instruction with multiple repeated opportunities for intervention conducted 40 hours per week across multiple years (e.g., 2 or more).

Also consider individual learner interests to determine the intensity of intervention. A learner with strong interest in sports may readily acquire skills related to sports (e.g., expansive vocabulary, range of communicative functions) with only a few learner-initiated opportunities. Also consider the learner's existing skill repertoire. If a learner is highly attentive and often engages with relevant stimuli, then intervention can likely be conducted in the natural environment with a range of communicative partners. If a learner demonstrates poor persistence and/or lack of engagement with stimuli relevant for instruction, however, then teacher-directed opportunities with individualized reinforcers may be more effective.

The urgency of skill acquisition may lead to the choice of a highly intensive intervention in some situations because of the likelihood of faster acquisition. For example, Sam's parents taught school-related vocabulary through many opportunities over the summer to prepare him for preschool in September. If a learner engages in challenging behavior, then consider a more intense intervention approach to quickly and efficiently replace those behaviors with more appropriate communicative responses.

These factors should result in consideration of multiple contexts of instruction to most efficiently and effectively meet the variety of needs of a specific learner. Although differences across learners may influence intervention intensity, differences within learners may suggest intervention can be best implemented in a certain way/with a certain level of intensity for some skills and in a different way/with a different level of intensity for other skills for the same learner. The case example of Marcel illustrates the process of choosing instructional context for three skills for an individual learner.

CASE EXAMPLE

Developing Contexts for Instruction for Marcel

Marcel was a 13-year-old boy in eighth grade. He used a multipage communication book with line-drawn symbols that he directly selected using his index finger. Marcel readily engaged in relevant requesting opportunities in his classroom, such as seeking out his teacher (e.g., walked to her) to obtain materials for tasks (e.g., markers, globe). As a result, there were a sufficient number of learner-directed opportunities for Marcel to acquire additional requesting skills within the natural environment. Natural consequences were also likely to function as reinforcers for these requests. Intervention mirroring natural interactions was likely to be an effective context for instruction.

In contrast, Marcel showed difficulty indicating his turn appropriately in the presence of his peers, and he often grabbed items. His interventionists decided to intervene in the presence of peers within a highly motivating activity (i.e., cooking) in which several teaching opportunities could be easily embedded (within each cooking class) with salient and valuable natural consequences in place that functioned as reinforcers (e.g., a turn to use the cooking appliance). Thus, a more intense intervention was used for requesting a turn than for requesting materials.

Marcel often needed new symbols in his communication book because of his busy schedule. Marcel required numerous teaching opportunities to acquire new graphic symbols in the past, so his interventionists chose to use a very intense intervention implemented as often as possible with numerous opportunities presented in a short period of time within a distraction-free environment. This approach was thought to increase the likelihood Marcel would acquire new vocabulary items in a timely manner. Marcel's day, therefore, involved addressing different skills within different contexts, with different levels of intensity, enabling him to receive instruction that effectively and efficiently addressed his various communication needs.

EXAMPLES OF CONTEXTS FOR INSTRUCTION

The remainder of this chapter is dedicated to three general contexts for instruction that address each of the previous questions in different ways, reflecting a continuum from less to more intense intervention. Each context is described with examples of empirically based intervention approaches and step-by-step procedures for developing interventions consistent with each context.

Naturalistic Instruction

Naturalistic instruction capitalizes on ongoing interactions about materials/activities within the learner's environment to prompt more sophisticated communicative acts with an intensity that mirrors naturally occurring opportunities to practice a given skill. For example, when a learner reaches for a doll, the interventionist prompts the learner to form the sign for DOLL before providing the doll.

- Instruction occurs within interactions in the environments in which the communication skills should be used.

- Interactions involve communication partners with whom the skills are meant to be directed.

- Opportunities are learner initiated or follow the learner's lead (e.g., instruction occurs when the learner approaches a desired toy) or generated as a result of ongoing interactions/activities (e.g., the learner finishes his or her dinner, generating a natural opportunity to practice asking to be excused).

- Natural consequences are used (e.g., when a learner signs HELLO, his or her friend responds in kind; when a learner requests, "May I have a drink?" his or her parent delivers a drink).

- Naturally occurring events embedded throughout a learner's day dictate opportunities, which results in relatively few opportunities spread across longer periods of time (e.g., a child learns to sign EXCUSE ME to pass someone during the few naturally occurring opportunities each day).

- The duration of intervention varies with relatively longer duration if naturalistic instruction involves training communicative partners and skills relevant across environments and time.

Schepis, Reid, Behrmann, and Sutton (1998) used a naturalistic instruction context to teach the use of an SGD to 4 children (3–5 years of age) with autism. Children initiated opportunities during snack and play activities that lasted an average of 11 and 9 minutes, respectively, for a total duration of 1–13 months across children. Johnston et al. (2003) used a naturalistic intervention to teach three preschoolers with autism to use a graphic symbol CAN I PLAY? to join peers in play. Interventionists used modeling, least-to-most prompt hierarchy, time delay, and natural consequences when the child initiated interest in interaction (evidenced by gazing toward the activity) during free play-time each day. Children used the graphic symbol and/or vocalizations and showed generalization to a novel activity.

Hamilton and Snell (1993) taught spontaneous use of a communication book to an adolescent with autism using a **milieu teaching** approach. Intervention occurred across settings during learner-initiated opportunities (e.g., the adolescent looked at a particular object) or interventionist-created opportunities (e.g., interventionist placed needed items out of reach). Approximately 20 opportunities occurred in each environment (in the classroom 5 days per week, home every day, community 1–2 days per week, and cafeteria 3 days per week). Prompting (expectant look and mand model) and reinforcement (praise and natural consequences, e.g., providing the item requested) increased the learner's spontaneous use of his communication book that maintained at 2–3 months and 1 year follow-up.

What Does the Research Say?

Naturalistic Instructional Approaches

Incidental Teaching

The interventionist requests more sophisticated communication (e.g., by delaying the provision of the item or prompting, "Tell me what you want" or "Say, 'book'") following a learner's initiation of an interaction about materials/activities in his or her environment (e.g., reaching for a book). Both praise and natural consequences (e.g., access to the book) following communication.

Hart and Risley (1974, 1975) first described using **incidental teaching** procedures with disadvantaged preschool children to teach more sophisticated speech. Children learned nouns, adjective–noun combinations, and compound sentences with incidental teaching during 2 half-hour free play sessions each day, spanning a total of 113 days (Hart & Risley, 1974).

Requesting (e.g., Cavallaro & Poulson, 1985) and using prepositions (e.g., McGee, Krantz, & McClannahan, 1985) and verbs (e.g., Cavallaro & Poulson, 1985) are other communication skills addressed with incidental teaching. Incidental teaching has been implemented by peers and teachers (Haring, Neetz, Lovinger, Peck, & Semmel, 1987; MacDuff, Krantz, MacDuff, & McClannahan, 1988; McGee et al., 1992).

Modified Incidental Teaching Sessions

Instruction occurs within the natural environment, with natural materials and partners, using natural consequences, during learner-initiated opportunities. The interventionist provides additional opportunities, however, following the learner's initiation and the interventionist's first request for more sophisticated communication.

(continued)

Charlop-Christy and Carpenter (2000) compared traditional incidental teaching involving 2 opportunities a day, discrete trial teaching involving a session of 10 opportunities a day, and **modified incidental teaching.** Three opportunities followed every learner initiation during modified incidental teaching (for a total of six opportunities a day). Intervention lasted 5 weeks. Modified incidental teaching resulted in acquisition and generalization of spontaneous speech for the three children with autism. Two participants acquired spontaneous speech during discrete trial instruction and one acquired it during incidental teaching.

Pivotal Response Treatment

Interventionists use specific motivational strategies, such as following the learner's lead, varying tasks to maintain interest, and interspersing maintenance tasks between novel tasks, reinforcing attempts and correct responses using natural reinforcers (Koegel & Koegel, 2006), during naturally occurring and learner-initiated opportunities across environments and partners. Use of **pivotal response treatment** with children with autism shows that addressing pivotal skill areas (e.g., motivation, self-initiations) results in collateral changes in other important skills.

Demonstrations of the effectiveness of pivotal response treatment to address communication skills are numerous (e.g., Koegel, Carter, & Koegel, 2003; Koegel, Koegel, & Surratt, 1992; Schreibman, Stahmer, & Pierce, 1996). Pierce and Schreibman (1995) taught peers to implement pivotal response treatment during 10-minute play sessions with two 10-year-old boys with autism. Children showed immediate improvements in maintaining interactions and, after several weeks, some increases in initiations. Koegel, Bruinsma, and Koegel (2006) examined parent-implemented pivotal response treatment for five children with autism less than 3 years of age. All five (four of whom demonstrated no spoken words prior to intervention) showed improvements in expressive language.

Milieu Teaching and Prelinguistic Milieu Teaching

Intervention occurs in the natural environment during ongoing interactions with a specific focus on using the learner's interests and initiations for teaching opportunities. Typically, a less intrusive prompt (e.g., time delay; see Chapter 5) is used before more intrusive prompts (e.g., specific questions and models). Prompting may include using a mand-model procedure (Rogers-Warren & Warren, 1980; see Chapter 5). Responses result in natural consequences (e.g., continuation of interaction) and specific praise (e.g., "Yes, that's *read*").

Kaiser and colleagues used milieu teaching and prelinguistic milieu teaching to address a variety of communication skills (Hancock & Kaiser, 2002; Warren & Kaiser, 1988) and taught parents to use milieu strategies (Kaiser, Hancock, & Nietfeld, 2000; Kaiser, Hancock, & Trent, 2007). Yoder and Stone (2006b) found 6 months of prelinguistic milieu teaching (with a parent education component) implemented 3 times per week in 20-minute sessions improved requesting and joint attention for children who began intervention with some level of initiating joint attention. The comparison intervention, the Picture Exchange Communication System (PECS), resulted in greater increases in requests, however, for children who began with low levels of initiating joint attention. Children with autism with relatively high object exploration showed faster growth rates in novel words with 6 months of the PECS, but children showing lower object exploration showed faster growth rates with prelinguistic milieu teaching (Yoder & Stone, 2006a).

Yoder and Warren (2002) found prelinguistic milieu teaching resulted in declines in development in children with Down syndrome. Fey et al. (2006) found no such differences for children with Down syndrome with prelinguistic milieu teaching implemented on average 3.32 times per week for 20-minute sessions over 6 months. Effects did not maintain 6 and 12 months later, however. In addition to diagnosis and preintervention abilities, parental responsivity to child communication also influences outcomes of prelinguistic milieu teaching (Yoder & Warren, 1998, 2001).

How Do I Implement Naturalistic Instruction?

Step 1: Identify the Communication Skills   Identify skills (e.g., specific graphic symbols) to teach for each goal (e.g., language comprehension). Specific materials for Marcel to request were a pencil, laptop, and tape recorder.

Step 2: Identify Instructional Opportunities

- Opportunities are learner initiated (vocalizing, gesturing, crying, looking, smiling) and/or generated by an activity (e.g., put toothpaste on the toothbrush).

- Identify the environments in which naturalistic opportunities will take place

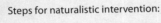

Steps for naturalistic intervention:

Step 1: Identify the communication skills
Step 2: Identify the instructional opportunities
Step 3: Identify instructional strategies
Step 4: Implement intervention procedures
and monitor performance

(e.g., traveling to work, at work, during breaks).

- Base the number of opportunities on individual learner characteristics.

- Identify how often naturalistic instruction will be implemented within each environment (e.g., one time during break, two to three times during a work shift).

- Identify the duration of intervention. Consider the number of opportunities available to the learner and his or her usual rate of acquisition. Make sure to evaluate the intervention at appropriate intervals to prevent implementing ineffective intervention strategies and allow for adjustments or changes to enhance performance.

Marcel's interventionists identified opportunities when he initiated a need for instructional materials (e.g., by looking or reaching) and at natural points within the activity (e.g., the teacher saying, "Make sure you have your globe"). They planned for at least three opportunities every day during every academic period.

Step 3: Identify Instructional Strategies

Use information in Chapter 5 to choose prompting, reinforcement, and correction procedures. Identify natural consequences (e.g., providing the item about which the learner communicated). Consider combining these with praise or a more powerful reinforcer during the early stages of instruction. Use the intervention

Form 6.1, Intervention Planning Form, is useful across instructional contexts to document specific procedures and help ensure consistent implementation.

planning form to document instructional strategies (see Figure 6.8 for Marcel; Form 6.1 is a blank version and is included on the accompanying CD-ROM).

Step 4: Implement Intervention Procedures and Monitor Performance

Attend to learner initiations within the natural environment and other opportunities from Step 2 and use instructional strategies from Step 3, including natural consequences following the learner's communication. Record learner performance on a form like the one Marcel's interventionists used (see Figure 6.9; Form 6.2 is a blank version and is included on the accompanying CD-ROM). Regularly convert performance data into a visual display (see Figure 6.10 for Marcel; Form 6.3 is a blank version and is included on the accompanying CD-ROM). Data show that Marcel mastered requesting his pencil, laptop, and tape recorder and intervention can begin for several new items (e.g., calculator, globe, and microscope in Marcel's science class).

A naturalistic instructional context reflects an intensity similar to naturally occurring interactions. There may be skills for which acquisition is not likely within a natural context (e.g., a sufficient number of teaching opportunities cannot be generated), however. A more intense intervention context may be more appropriate (e.g., instruction embedded within an activity).

See Chapter 7 for information about displaying performance.

Instruction Embedded within an Activity

Instruction embedded within an activity represents a midpoint on the continuum of instructional contexts and intervention intensity. It refers to the planned implementation of several instructional opportunities during a specific activity (e.g., a learner was taught to label household items, complete specific cleaning tasks, request materials, and so forth while doing household chores). Opportunities can be implemented in a va-

Learner's name: _Marcel_____   Start date: _3/27_____

Setting (circle one):   HOME   (SCHOOL)   COMMUNITY   WORK

Communication skill/function: ___Use of communication (book) to request materials_____

Opportunities

When: _Throughout the day_____

Where: _In classrooms during instructional periods_____

Minimum opportunities per day/session: _At least three opportunities across skill/academic period/day_

Context for instruction: _Naturalistic instruction_____

Set up: ___Instructional material is not available and/or teacher indicates to students that
they need to use that item (e.g., teacher says, "Write this down." or "Take out your pencils.")

Materials: _Communication book, pencil, laptop, and tape recorder_____

Target Behavior

Mode: _Graphic_____

Augmentative and alternative communication system features: _Direct selection of line-drawn symbols___

Vocabulary: _Pencil, laptop, and tape recorder_____

Instructional Strategies

Skill sequence/steps: _1) Observe Marcel during classroom instruction for times he needs materials;
_2) prompt by pointing to the communication book and relevant symbol; and 3) provide the
_item and verbal praise if Marcel uses his book to request._____

Prompts: _Gesture to the correct symbol._____

Consequences

    Correct response: _Provide access to the instructional material, and give verbal praise.____

    Incorrect response (no response or error response): _Model use of Marcel's communication book.__

Prompt fading: _Begin immediately prompting the correct response; fade using time delay of
_10 seconds (when Marcel requests for 1 session at 80% correct)._____

Generalization: _Family members will implement procedures at home._____

Maintenance: _Following mastery, check and record performance one time per week._____

Criterion for Mastery

_Marcel will show 80% independent correct requesting across 2 days._____

Performance Monitoring

_Record performance on each opportunity._____

Figure 6.8. Intervention planning form for naturalistic instruction of requesting for Marcel. (*Note:* This is a filled-in version of Form 6.1, Intervention Planning Form. A blank, printable version appears on the accompanying CD-ROM.)

Instructions: Fill in the goal and specific skills or responses at the top of each column. Fill in the date, and circle the symbol corresponding to the learner's performance for each observation. Circle a plus (+) if the learner independently demonstrated the correct response, a *P* if the learner demonstrated the correct response following a prompt, or a minus (–) if the learner did not demonstrate the correct response or demonstrated an incorrect response.

Learner's name: __Marcel__

Goal: Requesting
Response: Pencil

Date	Performance		
3/27	+	(P)	–
3/27	+	(P)	–
3/27	+	(P)	–
3/27	+	(P)	–
3/27	+	(P)	–
3/28	+	(P)	–
3/28	(+)	P	–
3/28	+	(P)	–
3/28	(+)	P	–
3/28	(+)	P	–

Goal: Requesting
Response: Laptop

Date	Performance		
3/27	+	(P)	–
3/27	+	(P)	–
3/27	+	(P)	–
3/27	+	(P)	–
3/27	+	(P)	–
3/28	+	(P)	–
3/28	+	(P)	–
3/28	(+)	P	–
3/28	(+)	P	–
3/28	(+)	P	–

Goal: Requesting
Response: Tape recorder

Date	Performance		
3/27	+	(P)	–
3/27	+	(P)	–
3/27	+	(P)	–
3/27	+	(P)	–
3/27	+	(P)	–
3/28	+	(P)	–
3/28	(+)	P	–
3/28	(+)	P	–
3/28	(+)	P	–
3/28	(+)	P	–

Goal: Requesting
Response: Pencil

Date	Performance		
3/29	(+)	P	–
3/29	+	(P)	–
3/29	(+)	P	–
3/29	(+)	P	–
3/29	(+)	P	–
3/30	(+)	P	–
3/30	(+)	P	–
3/30	(+)	P	–
3/30	(+)	P	–
3/30	(+)	P	–

Goal: Requesting
Response: Laptop

Date	Performance		
3/29	(+)	P	–
3/29	(+)	P	–
3/29	+	(P)	–
3/29	(+)	P	–
3/29	(+)	P	–
3/30	(+)	P	–
3/30	(+)	P	–
3/30	(+)	P	–
3/30	(+)	P	–
3/30	(+)	P	–

Goal: Requesting
Response: Tape recorder

Date	Performance		
3/29	(+)	P	–
3/29	+	(P)	–
3/29	(+)	P	–
3/29	(+)	P	–
3/29	(+)	P	–
3/30	(+)	P	–
3/30	(+)	P	–
3/30	(+)	P	–
3/30	(+)	P	–
3/30	(+)	P	–

Figure 6.9. Performance monitoring form for naturalistic instruction for requesting for Marcel. (*Note:* This is a filled-in version of Form 6.2, Performance Monitoring Form for Naturalistic Instruction. A blank, printable version appears on the accompanying CD-ROM.)

Instructions: Label the *x* axis (e.g., days, sessions). Label the *y* axis to indicate the behavior being graphed (e.g., percent correct). Place a mark (e.g., a dot) for each observation on the *x* axis at the value corresponding to the learner's performance on the *y* axis.

Figure 6.10. Marcel's performance data converted into a visual display. (*Note:* This is a filled-in version of Form 6.3, Graph for Displaying Performance Monitoring Information. A blank, printable version appears on the accompanying CD-ROM.)

riety of ways but reflect changes in intensity from naturalistic instruction.

- Instruction occurs within the natural environment or a more distraction-free setting.

- Interactions involve partners from the natural environment (e.g., peers) or interventionists.

- Opportunities are learner initiated, interventionist directed, or both.

- Available natural consequences within the activity are used, and, if necessary, individualized reinforcers not related to the activity (e.g., token system) are used.

- The activity dictates the number of opportunities and session/times the activity occurs per day or week (e.g., having snack time every day, playing a game only two or three times per week). Often, several goals (e.g., requesting, commenting, counting, identifying colors) are addressed within one activity, interspersing opportunities for different skills.

- Duration can be ongoing and relatively long or short (McConnell et al., 2002).

Instruction embedded within an activity differs from naturalistic instruction in that the activities are specifically designed to generate a number of teaching opportunities. Johnson, McDonnell, Holzwarth, and Hunter (2004) used **embedded instruction** with three students with developmental disabilities. An average of 6–8 opportunities

were presented each day to an 8-year-old child with autism to teach requests using her SGD (for break, help, and food items). Mastery occurred after 131 opportunities to request help, 177 opportunities to request a break, and 229 opportunities to request a food item during snack. Johnson and McDonnell (2004) used embedded instruction to teach the sign for HELP to one of three participants with developmental disabilities. Acquisition occurred within 20 sessions with 2 opportunities for each of 5 difficult tasks within specific activities. The SCERTS® Model (Prizant, Wetherby, Rubin, Laurent, & Rydell, 2006) incorporates instruction embedded within an activity (e.g., **activity-based intervention** applications; Bricker, Pretti-Frontczak, & McComas, 1998) as well as other naturalistic approaches (e.g., pivotal response training; Koegel & Koegel, 2006). An evidence base for SCERTS has yet to emerge because of its relatively recent development.

What Does the Research Say?

Instruction Embedded within an Activity

Activity-Based Intervention

Several teaching opportunities related to the activity are embedded within specific activities (Bricker et al., 1998). Teaching opportunities are often initiated by the learner. Materials are varied and inherent to the activity (e.g., identifying colors while playing with a toy garage using the toy

(continued)

cars and the clothing on the toy people). Natural consequences involve continuation of the activity (e.g., providing materials requested).

Bricker and colleagues reported positive outcomes (e.g., in cognitive and language development) for participants with disabilities in **activity-based intervention** programs (Bailey & Bricker, 1985; Bricker, Bruder, & Bailey, 1982; Bricker & Gumerlock, 1988; Bricker & Sheehan, 1981). Losardo and Bricker (1994) examined activity-based intervention delivered in 15-minute intervention sessions 3 times each week for 6 weeks with 6 preschoolers with or at risk for developmental delays. Both activity-based intervention and a comparison intervention involving repeated interventionist-directed opportunities (discrete trial instruction, discussed shortly) were effective in teaching identification of target objects. Acquisition was faster for skills taught with discrete trial instruction, however, whereas generalization was greater with skills taught in activity-based intervention.

Joint Action Routines

Bruner and colleagues (Bruner & Sherwood, 1976) discussed the role of **joint action routines** in child language acquisition. Joint action routines refer to turntaking interactions during which caregivers present language. Routines are interactive with clearly defined roles and a predictable, logical sequence of events that repeat each time the routine occurs.

Snyder-McLean, Solomonson, McLean, and Sack (1984) demonstrated the use of joint action routines with both preschoolers and adolescents with disabilities to improve communication skills. Holdgrafer, Kysela, and McCarthy (1989) taught mothers of four young children (approximately 2 years old) with developmental delays to use joint action routines to extend the length of interactions and model words associated with their child's actions during the routine (e.g., saying "balloon" as the child pulled on the balloon string). Children increased their use of object words during joint action routines over 10 weeks.

Embedded Instruction

Opportunities are presented during ongoing activities in **embedded instruction**; however, the skills may not be related to the activity (e.g., opportunities to practice sight words presented during transitions between classes). Specific materials (e.g., flashcards) may be created to allow for repeated practice. The interventionist directs opportunities by presenting materials and delivering specific instructions. Responses result in natural consequences and/or contrived reinforcers.

McDonnell, Johnson, Polychronis, and Risen (2002) examined embedded instruction during classroom management activities (e.g., attendance, lunch count, transitions) to teach vocabulary to four high school students with moderate intellectual disabilities. Paraprofessionals provided at least three opportunities for each word during activities (e.g., by presenting flashcards with one vocabulary word printed on each and the instruction, "Read these words"). Opportunities consisted of the delivery of an instruction, followed by a time delay, error correction (e.g., interventionist said, "No," repeated instruction, and prompted correct response) if needed, and social reinforcement. All four students learned all vocabulary words. Studies of embedded instruction have involved as few as 2 (McDonnell et al., 2002) to 6 opportunities per day (Wolery et al., 1998) to 10 opportunities within an hour (Johnson & McDonnell, 2004).

How Do I Implement Instruction Embedded within an Activity?

Embedding instruction within an activity provides the learner an opportunity to acquire new behavior in the context in which it is apt to be used. The steps of the activity that occur immediately prior to the skill being taught may come to serve as a natural prompt for the learner to engage in the target behavior. This is particularly apt to happen when, initially, a prompt that ensures the production of the target behavior is paired with the natural prompt. Subsequently, as the more intrusive prompt is gradually removed, the natural cue is a sufficient reminder for the learner to engage in the target behavior. Below are some steps that help to ensure the successfulness of embedded instruction.

Steps for instruction embedded within an activity

Step 1: Identify the communication skills.
Step 2: Identify an appropriate activity in which to embed opportunities to teach the specific communication skills.
Step 3: Identify instructional opportunities.
Step 4: Identify instructional strategies.
Step 5: Implement intervention and monitor performance.

Step 1: Identify the Communication Skills Identify several different skill areas to embed within one activity (Bricker et al., 1998). Interventionists identified communication goals for Marcel (indicating his turn, commenting, and using adjectives).

Step 2: Identify an Appropriate Activity in Which to Embed Opportunities to Teach the Specific Communication Skills Doll corner, block play, or water table might be appropriate for young children; board games, academic tasks, and sports for school-age children; games, meal preparation, and chores for adults. Marcel's team embedded opportunities during cooking in home economics class. Consider activities that

- Are implemented often enough to enhance skill acquisition

- Provide several opportunities for each skill

- Are motivating to the learner and his or her peers

- Are age appropriate

- Successfully engage the learner, allowing the interventionist to concentrate on teaching skills rather than facilitating the activity

- Involve predictable opportunities for interactions

Identify how often (e.g., three times per day) and the duration for which intervention will be implemented. Consider the number of opportunities available to the learner and his or her usual rate of acquisition. Evaluate the intervention at appropriate intervals to prevent the implementation of ineffective intervention strategies and allow for adjustments or changes to enhance performance.

Step 3: Identify Instructional Opportunities Prior to starting the intervention, carefully plan at which point to address each skill within the activity. Opportunities can be created by learner initiations and/or generated by the interventionist (e.g., the interventionist withholds a needed game piece until the learner requests using his or her

graphic communication system). Increase the number of teaching opportunities if individual learner characteristics suggest this is necessary.

Step 4: Identify Instructional Strategies See Chapter 5 to choose instructional strategies. Marcel's interventionists used a gestural point to his communication book to prompt him to request a turn and gestured "thumbs up" from across the room as a consequence. They used verbal directives (e.g., "Tell us how that tastes") to prompt Marcel to comment on the food. Commenting was a particularly challenging skill for Marcel, so reinforcers included praise and the delivery of tokens exchanged for computer time.

Step 5: Implement Intervention and Monitor Performance Attend to instructional opportunities as they arise (Step 3) and follow instructional strategies (Step 4). Record learner performance. Figure 6.11 (Form 6.4 is a blank version and is included on the accompanying CD-ROM) shows the form used by Marcel's team, which provides space for monitoring performance of several skills. Regularly convert performance to a visual display. Figure 6.12 shows Marcel mastered the communication skills embedded within cooking activities.

Instruction embedded within an activity reflects a midpoint of intervention intensity. Still, there are skills for which a learner may benefit from an even more intensive and individualized approach to intervention; in this case, discrete trial instruction may be more appropriate.

Discrete Trial Instruction

Discrete trial instruction is a different level of intensity from the other two contexts—skills are broken down into small clearly defined discrete units of instruction.

- Intervention is conducted in a relatively quiet, distraction-free setting within a highly structured, often one-to-one (i.e., interventionist and learner) situation. There are examples of group (e.g., two

Learner's name: _Marcel_ _____ Activity: _Cooking during home economics class_

Instructions: Fill in each goal for the activity indicated above. In the Set up column, describe what the interventionist should do within the activity to provide the learner with an opportunity to practice that goal. Fill in the date of an observation, and record the learner's performance on that goal. For example, record a plus (+) if the learner demonstrated the correct response for that goal and a minus (–) if he or she did not demonstrate a correct response or demonstrated no response. Additional information about learner performance may include whether the interventionist presented a prompt (e.g., record a *P*) or the learner did not respond at all (e.g., record an *NR* for no response).

Goal	Set up	Performance
Marcel will indicate his turn by selecting the corresponding symbol in his communication book during 90% of the opportunities.	Prompt Marcel to indicate his turn when a peer is using an appliance (e.g., blender, microwave oven) and it appears he or she is close to finishing.	Date: _3/27_ Interventionist's initials: _LB_ `P	P	P	+` Date: _3/28_  Interventionist's initials: _MC_ `P	P	+	+	+` Date: _3/29_  Interventionist's initials: _LB_ `+	+	P	+	+	+`

Goal	Set up	Performance
Marcel will comment on his food or a peer's food by selecting the corresponding symbol from his communication book during 80% of the opportunities.	When Marcel tastes a food item (either his or his peer's), prompt him to comment on the taste of the item (good, bad, great).	Date: _3/27_ Interventionist's initials: _LB_ `P	+	P	+	+	+` Date: _3/28_  Interventionist's initials: _MC_ `P	P	+	+` Date: _3/29_  Interventionist's initials: _LB_ `+	+	P	+	+	+`

Goal	Set up	Performance
Marcel will use adjectives to describe materials related to the cooking lesson.	Prompt Marcel to respond with the appropriate adjective (e.g., crunchy, chocolate) when asked a question such as, "How do you like your cookies?" or "What flavor do you want to put in the mix?"	Date: _3/27_ Interventionist's initials: _LB_ `P	P	P	+	+	+	+	+` Date: _3/28_  Interventionist's initials: _MC_ `P	P	+	+	P	+	+	+` Date: _3/29_  Interventionist's initials: _LB_ `+	+	+	+	+	+	+`

Figure 6.11. Performance Monitoring Form for Instruction Embedded within an Activity for Marcel. (*Note:* This is a filled-in version of Form 6.4, Performance Monitoring Form for Instruction Embedded within an Activity. A blank, printable version appears on the accompanying CD-ROM.)

to three students) discrete trial instruction (e.g., Chiara et al., 1995).

- Intervention is implemented with partners who may or may not be the eventual recipients of the communication skills

(e.g., adult interventionists practice skills for use with peers).

- The interventionist directs opportunities by presenting the cue/stimulus to which the learner should respond.

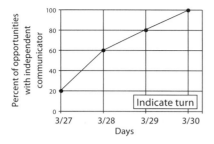 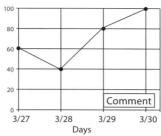 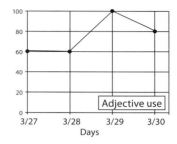

Figure 6.12. Marcel's performance data converted into a visual display. (*Note:* This is a filled-in version of Form 6.3, Graph for Displaying Performance Monitoring Information. A blank, printable version appears on the accompanying CD-ROM.)

- Consequences are individually tailored to the learner using items/activities with a history of functioning as reinforcers. Nonrelated reinforcers may be used alone (e.g., the interventionist presents a food item to the student as a reinforcer for correct responses when he or she is learning to identify a pail and shovel) or combined with natural consequences (e.g., learner selects symbol for JACK IN THE BOX, gaining access to the toy and a food item as a reinforcer).

- Multiple intervention sessions for the same skill(s) are conducted over the course of a day or a week. Sessions involve the rapid delivery of numerous opportunities, with only a brief interval between, within a fixed, predictable time interval. Opportunities could be for the same skill (e.g., repeated opportunities to select the symbol for CUP) or for several skills (e.g., opportunities to select the symbol for CUP, then FORK, then SPOON).

- Duration varies. Discrete trial instruction may result in the acquisition of basic skills that prepare some learners for more naturalistic learning situations (Smith, 2001). Other learners may require discrete trial instruction on an ongoing basis (e.g., a few hours per week) in order to continue to acquire new skills. Use of discrete trial instruction may be intermittent, with implementation in short durations on an as needed basis for select skill areas.

Smith (2001) suggested that discrete trial instruction may be particularly useful for teaching new behaviors, including communication, and discriminations. Discrete trial instruc-

tion may be a powerful teaching approach because of the presentation of many opportunities with a beginning and end that clearly segments instruction. Discrete trial instruction is often implemented in a one-to-one setting; thus, it can be easily tailored to the unique needs of the individual learner.

Discrete trial instruction has been used to teach sign language (e.g., Carr, Binkoff, Kologinsky, & Eddy, 1978; Roark, Collins, Hemmeter, & Kleinert, 2002; Romski, Sevcik, & Pate, 1988) as well as graphic symbol use. Sigafoos et al. (1996) taught two participants with Rett syndrome (12 and 17 years old) to request using a WANT symbol on a communication board. After presenting preferred items and the communication board, the interventionist delivered the instructional cue (discriminative stimulus [S^D]), "Let me know if you want something," along with verbal and gestural prompts if the learner did not respond. If the child touched the symbol, then the interventionist provided praise and access to the item. Twelve and thirty-five sessions of ten opportunities three times per week resulted in acquisition for the two participants. Using similar procedures, two other participants (7 and 15 years old) learned to select a picture of a preferred item and activate a switch to make requests.

What Does the Research Say?
Discrete Trial Instruction

Discrete trial instruction has been the primary context for instruction in several studies demonstrating improvements

(continued)

for young children with developmental disabilities; most notably, children with autism (e.g., Lovaas, 1987; McEachin, Smith, & Lovaas, 1993; Smith, Groen, & Wynn, 2000). Outcomes reveal gains in IQ, adaptive functioning, language, and communication skills, as well as increased access to general education classroom placements, outcomes that are significantly better than those observed for comparison groups receiving fewer hours (10–12 hours per week) of discrete trial instruction (Eldevik et al., 2006; Lovaas, 1987) or a more eclectic intervention approach (Eikeseth et al., 2002, 2007). Most of these studies evaluated intervention over the early childhood years, a duration of approximately 2 years.

Examples of discrete trial instruction with learners with diagnoses other than autism and for specific skills also support the effectiveness of this instructional context. Feeley and Jones (2008) addressed specific communication skills in young children with Down syndrome by teaching one child with Down syndrome spontaneous communication skills during 1–2 instructional sessions per day that consisted of 10 closely spaced teaching opportunities. Intervention lasted until the child mastered the target response, in this case between 3 and 14 sessions. Jones et al. (2010) taught two infants with Down syndrome to use their eye gaze and vocalizations to request interaction with a toy during intervention sessions of 10 opportunities, with each session lasting 7–10 minutes. Intervention sessions oc-

curred 2–4 times per day, 2 days per week for one participant. Intervention sessions occurred 1 time per day, 2–4 days per week for the other participant.

See de Boer (2007); Leaf and McEachin (1999); Lovaas (1981); Maurice, Green, and Foxx (2001); and Maurice, Green, and Luce (1996) for additional information about discrete trial instruction.

Steps to develop discrete trial instruction intervention

Step 1: Identify the communication skills.
Step 2: Identify instructional opportunities.
Step 3: Identify instructional strategies.
Step 4: Implement intervention and monitor performance.

How Do I Implement Discrete Trial Instruction?

Step 1: Identify the Communication Skills Marcel's interventionists identified several graphic symbols (i.e., SNORKEL, WET SUIT, SURFBOARD) for an upcoming vacation (see the master list in Figure 6.13; Form 6.5 is a blank version and is included on the accompanying CD-ROM).

Learner's name: __Marcel__ Program: __Receptive vocabulary__

Instructions: Fill in the specific response to teach for this goal. Record the start date when intervention begins for a specific response. Record the mastery date when a response is mastered. Record the date under Maintenance as performance is monitored after mastery, and record the learner's performance (e.g., record a plus [+] if the learner demonstrates the correct response, a minus [–] if he or she does not demonstrate the correct response, or an *NR* if the learner does not respond at all).

Response	Start date	Mastery date	Maintenance Date						
			3/17	3/20	3/21	3/23	3/24	3/30	3/17
Snorkel	3/10	3/16	+	+	+	+	+	+	+
Wet suit	3/17	3/21				+	+	+	
Surfboard	3/22	3/30							

Figure 6.13. Master List for Marcel's discrete trial instruction program. (*Note:* This is a filled-in version of Form 6.5, Master List. A blank, printable version appears on the accompanying CD-ROM.)

Form 6.5, Master List, is used to document skills targeted for intervention, providing interventionists with a means to record maintenance of mastered skills and a guide for progressing to new skills when previous ones are mastered.

Step 2: Identify Instructional Opportunities

- Identify a relatively distraction-free space (e.g., a separate room [resource room or study] or partitioned space within a room) containing age- and size-appropriate furniture and intervention materials, reinforcers, and easily accessible performance monitoring forms.

- Use a cue or directive as close to the natural one as possible. For example, use a ringing telephone as the natural cue to teach a learner to answer the telephone (rather than saying, "Answer the telephone"). Be careful not to use additional cues that might be difficult to fade.

- Base the number of opportunities within a relatively short time frame (e.g., 5–10 minutes) on individual learner characteristics. Some learners may require the consecutive presentation of many opportunities (e.g., 10) within a 5-minute session, whereas others may require only 3–5 opportunities within the same time frame to acquire a skill.

- Identify how often discrete trial instruction sessions will be implemented within each environment depending on learner and skill characteristics as well as the total number of skills targeted for discrete trial instruction.

- Identify the duration for which intervention will be implemented based on the number of opportunities available to the learner and his or her usual rate of acquisition. Evaluate the intervention at appropriate intervals to prevent the implementation of ineffective intervention strategies and allow for adjustments or changes to enhance performance.

Step 3: Identify Instructional Strategies

Choose prompting, reinforcement, and error correction procedures as described in Chapter 5. Document intervention procedures on the intervention planning form as they were for Marcel (see Figure 6.14; Form 6.1 is a blank version and is included on the accompanying CD-ROM).

Step 4: Implement Intervention and Monitor Performance

- Obtain the learner's attention by saying his or her name, moving into his or her line of vision, or touching his or her arm.

- Present the instruction (S^D) and, if the learner responds correctly (independently or following the presentation of a prompt), provide reinforcement. If the learner fails to respond or responds incorrectly, implement error correction procedures.

- After delivering reinforcement or error correction, the learner consumes or interacts with the reinforcer during the intertrial interval (e.g., 3–5 seconds), and the interventionist records the performance and prepares the next opportunity.

- Address another skill(s) within the discrete trial context, engage the learner in a different instructional context (e.g., instruction embedded within an activity), or provide "free time" for the learner once the designated number of opportunities is completed.

- Record performance on a form similar to the one in Figure 6.15 (Form 6.6 is a blank version and is included on the accompanying CD-ROM). Typically, record performance for every teaching opportunity. Less frequent recording, however, can still provide an illustration of performance (e.g., record twice a week or on the first opportunity per day/session only).

- Indicate the date of mastery in the corresponding column on the master list (Form 6.5 on the accompanying CD-ROM) when the learner achieves mastery

Learner's name: _Marcel_   Start date: _3/10_

Setting (circle one):   HOME   (SCHOOL)   COMMUNITY   WORK

Communication skill/function: _Identify (i.e., touch, point to) new vocabulary items._

Opportunities

When: _Individualized instruction period_   Where: _Resource room_

Minimum opportunities per day/session: _10 opportunities per instructional session_

Context for instruction: _Discrete trial instruction_

Set up: _"Show me the [item]." "Where is the [item]?" "Touch the [item]."_

Materials: _Communication book_

Target Behavior

Mode: _Graphic_

Augmentative and alternative communication system features: _Direct selection of line-drawn symbols_

Vocabulary: _Snorkel, wet suit, surfboard_

Instructional Strategies

Skill sequence/steps: _1) Sit across from Marcel and present three line drawings (the new vocabu-lary item and two distractor symbols; e.g., line drawing of a box of tissues); 2) deliver the discriminative stimulus (S^D) (e.g., "Show me [item]"); 3) immediately prompt Marcel to select the correct symbol; 4) deliver reinforcement (e.g., praise, high five) when Marcel points to the correct symbol; 5) as Marcel is successful, present opportunities for him to identify previously acquired symbols._

Prompts: _Gestural prompts_

Consequences

     Correct response: _Give verbal praise and a high five or thumbs up._

     Incorrect response (no response or error response): _If no response, then repeat the S^D and physi-cally prompt the response by tapping the top of Marcel's arm. If Marcel makes an error, then provide verbal feedback ("That's not the right one"), repeat the set up, and immediately prompt Marcel by touching the correct symbol._

Prompt fading: _Begin immediately prompting the correct response; fade using time delay of 10 seconds (when Marcel requests for 1 session at 80% correct)._

Generalization: _Following mastery with a vocabulary item, determine if Marcel identifies it in his communication book and teach productive use of symbols._

Maintenance: _Following mastery, check and record performance one time per week._

Criterion for Mastery

Marcel will demonstrate 80% independent correct responding across two sessions and 2 days.

Performance Monitoring

Record performance on every opportunity.

Figure 6.14.   Intervention Planning Form for Marcel's discrete trial instruction program. (*Note:* This is a filled-in version of Form 6.1, Intervention Planning Form. A blank, printable version appears on the accompanying CD-ROM.)

Learner's name: _Marcel_

Program: _Receptive vocabulary_ Set up: _"Show me [item]."_

Instructions: Fill in the learner's name, the program, and the set up identified on the Intervention Planning Form for this program. Fill in the date on which intervention occurs and the target response. Record the learner's performance on each opportunity (e.g., record a plus [+] if the learner demonstrates the correct response, a minus [−] if he or she does not demonstrate the correct response, an *NR* if the learner does not respond at all, or a *P* if the learner only responds following a prompt). Calculate percentage correct by dividing the number of opportunities during which the learner made a correct response by the total number of opportunities presented, multiplied by 100. Fill in the percentage and the initials of the interventionist.

Date	Response	Performance										%	Interventionist
3/10	Snorkel	P	P	P	P	−	P	P	−	−	P	0%	LB
3/13	Snorkel	P	P	P	P	P	P	P	P	+	+	20%	LB
3/14	Snorkel	P	P	P	P	P	P	+	+	+	+	40%	MC
3/15	Snorkel	+	+	+	+	−	+	+	+	+	+	90%	MC
3/16	Snorkel	+	+	+	−	+	+	+	+	+	+	90%	LB
3/17	Wet suit	P	P	P	P	P	P	P	P	P	P	0%	MC
3/20	Wet suit	P	P	+	+	+	+	+	+	+	+	80%	LB
3/21	Wet suit	P	P	+	+	+	+	+	+	+	+	80%	MC

Figure 6.15. Performance Monitoring Form for discrete trial instruction for Marcel. (*Note:* This is a filled-in version of Form 6.6, Performance Monitoring Form for Discrete Trial Instruction. A blank, printable version appears on the accompanying CD-ROM.)

criterion, and begin intervention with the next identified skill. After mastering each new vocabulary item, Marcel's interventionists recorded the date on the master list and then periodically recorded maintenance performance (see Figure 6.13). Performance data should be regularly converted into a visual display, regardless of the frequency with which they are collected (see Figure 6.16).

Discrete trial instruction can be an effective and efficient instructional context in situations in which an intense level of intervention is warranted, due to the characteristics of the learner or individual skills, or based on the need to acquire the skill in a relatively short period of time.

CONCLUSION

In choosing the intensity of intervention, it is likely that instruction will occur across multiple contexts for instruction for a given learner with intervention for some skills oc-

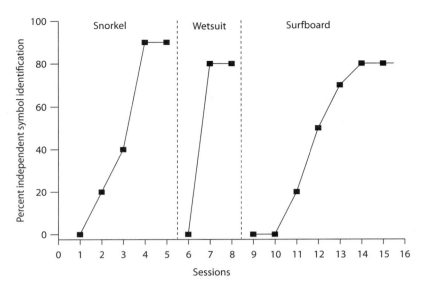

Figure 6.16.   Visual display of Marcel's progress independently identifying symbols.

curring in only one context, intervention for other skills occurring in multiple contexts simultaneously, and intervention for other skills beginning in a more intensive context with plans to progress to less intense contexts as the learner acquires skills. Many package interventions and programs specifically incorporate multiple contexts for instruction to best meet learners' needs. **Verbal behavior** intervention involves both discrete trial instruction and natural environment training, which is similar to naturalistic instruction (Sundberg & Michael, 2001; Sundberg & Partington, 1999). Sundberg and Partington (1998) suggested exhausting efforts toward developing vocal communication before considering an AAC system, despite contrary evidence that supports the potential benefits of AAC on speech development.

The PECS also capitalizes on more than one context during instruction. Teaching occurs within a one-to-one setting early in intervention to exchange one symbol for the corresponding reinforcer (Bondy & Frost, 1994). Symbols are placed around the room for exchange throughout the day as the learner acquires this skill. Carr and Felce (2007) implemented the PECS in 15 hours of intervention over 4–5 weeks, sampling a

range of situations during classroom activities (e.g., group activities, snack) and one-to-one teaching sessions.

SUMMARY

The range of contexts for instruction described in this chapter all rely on the same fundamental principles of behavior change, but differ with respect to key questions regarding the intensity of intervention. A context for instruction is created by considering the characteristics of the learner and the individual skill(s). As a result, a variety of communication skills can be addressed through a range of instructional contexts, or intensities of intervention, allowing for AAC needs to be addressed in a systematic and effective manner for individual learners.

REFERENCES

Bailey, E.J., & Bricker, D. (1985). Evaluation of a three-year early intervention demonstration project. *Topics in Early Childhood Special Education, 5,* 52–65.

Bondy, A., & Frost, L. (1994). The Picture Exchange Communication System. *Focus on Autistic Behavior, 9,* 1–19.

Bricker, D., Bruder, B., & Bailey, E. (1982). Developmental integration of preschool children. *Analysis and Intervention in Developmental Disabilities, 2,* 207–222.

Bricker, D., & Gumerlock, S. (1988). Application of a three-level evaluation plan for monitoring child progress and program effects. *Journal of Special Education, 22,* 66–81.

Bricker, D., Pretti-Frontczak, K., & McComas, N. (1998). *An activity-based approach to early intervention* (2nd ed.). Baltimore: Paul H. Brookes Publishing Co.

Bricker, D., & Sheehan, R. (1981). Effectiveness of an early intervention program as indexed by measures of child change. *Journal of the Division for Early Childhood, 4,* 11–27.

Bruner, J.S., & Sherwood, V. (1976). Early rule structure: The case of peek-a-boo. In J.S. Bruner, A. Jolly, & K. Sylva (Eds.), *Play: Its role in development and evolution* (pp. 277–286). Harmondwoth, England: Penguin.

Buffington, D.M., Krantz, P.J., McClannahan, L.E., & Poulson, C.L. (1998). Procedures for teaching appropriate gestural communication skills to children with autism. *Journal of Autism and Developmental Disorders, 28,* 535–545.

Carr, D., & Felce, J. (2007). The effects of PECS teaching to phase III on the communicative interactions between children with autism and their teachers. *Journal of Autism Developmental Disorders, 37,* 724–737.

Carr, E.G., Binkoff, J.A., Kologinsky, E., & Eddy, M. (1978). Acquisition of sign language by autistic children: I. Expressive labeling. *Journal of Applied Behavior Analysis, 11,* 489–501.

Cavallaro, C.C., & Poulson, C.L. (1985). Teaching language to handicapped children in natural settings. *Education and Treatment of Children, 8,* 1–24.

Charlop, M.H., Schreibman, L., & Thibodeau, M.G. (1985). Increasing spontaneous verbal responding in autistic children using a time delay procedure. *Journal of Applied Behavior Analysis, 18,* 155–166.

Charlop-Christy, M.H., & Carpenter, M.H. (2000). Modified incidental teaching sessions: A procedure for parents to increase spontaneous speech in their children with autism. *Journal of Positive Behavior Interventions, 2,* 98–112.

Chiara, L., Schuster, J.W., Bell, J.K., & Wolery, M. (1995). Small-group massed-trial and individually-distributed-trial instruction with preschoolers. *Journal of Early Intervention, 19,* 203–217.

Daugherty, S., Grisham-Brown, J., & Hemmeter, M.L. (2001). The effects of embedded skill instruction on the acquisition of target and nontarget skills in preschoolers with developmental delays. *Topics in Early Childhood Special Education, 21,* 213–221.

de Boer, S.R. (2007). How to do discrete trial instruction. In R.L. Simpson (Ed.), *PRO-ED series on autism spectrum disorders.* Austin, TX: PRO-ED.

Eikeseth, S., Smith, T., Jahr, E., & Eldevik, S. (2002). Intensive behavioral treatment at school for 4- to 7-year-old children with autism: A 1-year comparison controlled study. *Behavior Modification, 26,* 49–68.

Eikeseth, S., Smith, T., Jahr, E., & Eldevik, S. (2007). Outcome for children with autism who began intensive behavioral treatment between ages 4 and 7. *Behavior Modification, 31,* 264–278.

Eldevik, S., Eikeseth, S., Jahr, E., & Smith, T. (2006). Effects of low-intensity behavioral treatment for children with autism and mental retardation. *Journal of Autism and Developmental Disabilities, 36,* 211–224.

Fabiano, G.A., Pelham, W.E., Gnagy, E.M., Burrows-MacLean, L., Coles, E.K., Chacko, A., et al. (2007). The single and combined effects of multiple intensities of behavior modification and multiple intensities of methylphenidate in a classroom setting. *School Psychology Review, 36,* 195–216.

Feeley, K.M., & Jones, E.A. (2008). Teaching spontaneous responses to a young child with Down syndrome. *Down Syndrome Research and Practice, 12,* 148–152.

Feeley, K.M., Jones, E.A., Blackburn, C., & Bauer, S. (2010). *Advancing imitation and requesting skills in toddlers with Down syndrome.* Manuscript submitted for publication.

Fey, M.E., Warren, S.F., Brady, N., Finestack, L.H., Bredin-Oja, S.L., Fairchild, M., et al. (2006). Early effects of responsivity education/prelinguistic milieu teaching for children with developmental delays and their parents. *Journal of Speech, Language, and Hearing Research, 49,* 526–547.

Fidler, D.J., Philofsky, A., Hepburn, S.L., & Rogers, S.J. (2005). Nonverbal requesting and problem-solving by toddlers with Down syndrome. *American Journal on Mental Retardation, 110,* 312–322.

Granpeesheh, D., Dixon, D.R., Tarbox, J., Kaplan, A.M., & Wilke, A.E. (2009). The effects of age and treatment intensity on behavioral intervention outcomes for children with autism spectrum disorders. *Research Autism Spectrum Disorders, 3,* 1014–1022.

Gray, S. (2003). Word-learning by preschoolers with specific language impairment: What predicts success? *Journal of Speech, Language, and Hearing Research, 46,* 56–67.

Hamilton, B.L., & Snell, M.E. (1993). Using the milieu approach to increase spontaneous communication book use across environments by an adolescent with autism. *Augmentative and Alternative Communication, 9,* 259–272.

Hancock, T.B., & Kaiser, A.P. (2002). The effects of trainer-implemented enhanced milieu teaching on the social communication of children with autism. *Topics in Early Childhood Special Education, 22,* 39–54.

Haring, T.G., Neetz, J.A., Lovinger, L., Peck, C., & Semmel, M.I. (1987). Effects of four modified incidental teaching procedures to create opportunities for communication. *Journal of The Association for Persons with Severe Handicaps, 12,* 218–226.

Hart, B.M., & Risley, T.R. (1974). Using preschool materials to modify the language of disadvantaged children. *Journal of Applied Behavior Analysis, 7,* 243–256.

Hart, B.M., & Risley, T.R. (1975). Incidental teaching of language in the preschool. *Journal of Applied Behavior Analysis, 8,* 411–420.

Holdgrafer, G., Kysela, G.M., & McCarthy, C. (1989). Joint action intervention and child language skills: A research note. *First Language, 9,* 299–305.

Hunt, P., Alwell, M., & Goetz, L. (1991). Interacting with peers through conversation turntaking with a communication book adaptation. *Augmentative and Alternative Communication, 7,* 117–126.

Johnson, J.W., & McDonnell, J. (2004). An exploratory study of the implementation of embedded instruction by general educators with students with developmental disabilities. *Education and Treatment of Children, 27,* 46–63.

Johnson, J.W., McDonnell, J., Holzwarth, V.N., & Hunter, K. (2004). The efficacy of embedded instruction for students with developmental disabilities enrolled in general education classes. *Journal of Positive Behavior Interventions, 6,* 214–227.

Johnston, S., Nelson, C., Evans, J., & Palazolo, K. (2003). The use of visual supports in teaching young children with autism spectrum disorder to initiate interactions. *Augmentative and Alternative Communication, 19,* 86–103.

Jones, E.A., Carr, E.G., & Feeley, K.M. (2006). Multiple effects of joint attention intervention for children with autism. *Behavior Modification, 30,* 782–834.

Jones, E.A., & Feeley, K.M. (2007). Parent implemented joint attention intervention for preschoolers with autism. *Journal of Speech-Language Pathology and Applied Behavior Analysis, 2,* 252–268.

Jones, E.A., Feeley, K.M., & Blackburn, C. (2010). A preliminary study of intervention addressing early developing requesting behaviours in young infants with Down syndrome. *Down Syndrome Research and Practice.* Advance online publication available at http://www.down-syndrome.org/research-practice

Kaiser, A.P., Hancock, T.B., & Nietfeld, J.P. (2000). The effects of parent-implemented enhanced milieu teaching on the social communication of children who have autism. *Early Education and Development, 11,* 423–446.

Kaiser, A.P., Hancock, T.B., & Trent, J. (2007). Teaching parents communication strategies. *Early Childhood Services: An Interdisciplinary Journal of Effectiveness, 1,* 107–136.

Koegel, L.K., Camarata, S.M., Valdez-Menchaca, M., & Koegel, R.L. (1998). Setting generalization of question-asking by children with autism. *American Journal on Mental Retardation, 102,* 346–357.

Koegel, L.K., Carter, C.M., & Koegel, R.L. (2003). Teaching children with autism self-initiations as a pivotal response. *Topics in Language Disorders, 23,* 134–145.

Koegel, R.L., Bruinsma, Y.E.M., & Koegel, L.K. (2006). Developmental trajectories with early intervention. In R.L. Koegel & L.K. Koegel (Eds.), *Pivotal response treatments for autism: Communication, social, and academic development* (pp. 131–140). Baltimore: Paul H. Brookes Publishing Co.

Koegel, R.L., & Koegel, L.K. (Eds.). (2006). *Pivotal response treatments for autism: Communication, social, and academic development.* Baltimore: Paul H. Brookes Publishing Co.

Koegel, R.L., Koegel, L.K., & Surratt, A. (1992). Language intervention and disruptive behavior in preschool children with autism. *Journal of Autism and Developmental Disorders, 22,* 141–153.

Leaf, R., & McEachin, J. (1999). *A work in progress: Behavior management strategies and a curriculum for intensive behavioral treatment of autism.* New York: DRL Books.

LeChago, S.A., & Carr, J.E. (2008). Recommendations for reporting independent variables in outcome studies of early and intensive behavioral intervention for autism. *Behavior Modification, 32,* 489–503.

Losardo, A., & Bricker, D. (1994). Activity-based intervention and direct instruction: A comparison study. *American Journal on Mental Retardation, 98,* 744–765.

Lovaas, O.I. (1981). *Teaching developmentally disabled children: The me book.* Austin, TX: PRO-ED.

Lovaas, O.I. (1987). Behavioral treatment and normal educational and intellectual functioning in young autistic children. *Journal of Consulting and Clinical Psychology, 55,* 3–9.

Luiselli, J.K., O'Malley, C.B., Cannon, B., Ellis, J.T., & Sisson, R.W. (2000). Home-based behavioral intervention for young children with autism/pervasive developmental disorder. *Autism, 4,* 426–438.

MacDuff, G.S., Krantz, P.J., MacDuff, M.A., & McClannahan, L.E. (1988). Providing incidental teaching for autistic children: A rapid training procedure for therapists. *Education and Treatment of Children, 11,* 205–217.

Maurice, C., Green, G., & Foxx, R.M. (Eds.). (2001). *Making a difference: Behavioral intervention for autism.* Austin, TX: PRO-ED.

Maurice, C., Green, G., & Luce, S.C. (Eds.). (1996). *Behavioral intervention for young children with autism: A manual for parents and professionals.* Austin, TX: PRO-ED.

McConnell, S.R., Rush, K.L., McEvoy, M.A., Carta, J.J., Atwata, J., & Williams, R. (2002). Descriptive and experimental analysis of child-caregiver interactions that promote development of young children exposed prenatally to drugs and alcohol. *Journal of Behavioral Education, 11,* 131–161.

McDonnell, J., Johnson, J.W., Polychronis, S., & Risen, T. (2002). Effects of embedded instruction on students with moderate disabilities enrolled in general education classes. *Education and Training in Mental Retardation and Developmental Disabilities, 37,* 363–377.

McEachin, J.J., Smith, T., & Lovaas, O.I. (1993). Long-term outcome for children with autism who received early intensive behavioral treatment. *American Journal on Mental Retardation, 97,* 359–372.

McGee, G.G., Almeida, C., Sulzer-Azaroff, B., & Feldman, R.S. (1992). Promoting reciprocal interactions via peer incidental teaching. *Journal of Applied Behavior Analysis, 25,* 117–126.

McGee, G.G., Krantz, P.M., & McClannahan, L.E. (1985). The facilitative effects of incidental teaching on preposition use by autistic children. *Journal of Applied Behavior Analysis, 18,* 17–31.

Pierce, K., & Schreibman, L. (1995). Increasing complex social behaviors in children with autism: Effects of peer-implemented pivotal response training. *Journal of Applied Behavior Analysis, 28,* 285–295.

Prizant, B.M., Wetherby, A.M., Rubin, R., Laurent, A.C., & Rydell, P.J. (2006). *The SCERTS® Model: A comprehensive educational approach for children with autism spectrum disorders: Vol. 1. Assessment.* Baltimore: Paul H. Brookes Publishing Co.

Reed, P., Osborne, L.A., & Corness, M. (2007). Brief report: Relative effectiveness of different home-based behavioral approaches to early teaching intervention. *Journal of Autism and Developmental Disabilities, 37,* 1815–1821.

Reichow, B., & Wolery, M. (2009). Comprehensive synthesis of early intensive behavioral interventions for young children with autism based on the UCLA Young Autism Project Model. *Journal of Autism and Developmental Disabilities, 39,* 23–41.

Rice, M., Oetting, J., Marquis, J., Bode, J., & Pae, S. (1994). Frequency of input effects on word comprehension of children with specific language impairment. *Journal of Speech and Hearing Research, 37,* 106–122.

Riches, N.G., Tomasello, M., & Conti-Ramsden, G. (2005). Verb learning in children with SLI: Frequency and spacing effects. *Journal of Speech, Language, and Hearing Research, 48,* 1397–1411.

Roark, T.J., Collins, B.C., Hemmeter, M.L., & Kleinert, H. (2002). Including manual signing as nontargeted information when using a constant time delay procedure to teach receptive identification of packaged food items. *Journal of Behavioral Education, 11,* 19–38.

Rogers-Warren, A., & Warren, S.F. (1980). Mands for verbalization: Facilitating the display of newly trained language in children. *Behavior Modification, 4,* 361–382.

Romski, M.A., Sevcik., R.A., & Pate, J.L. (1988). The establishment of symbolic communication in a person with severe retardation. *Journal of Speech and Hearing Disorders, 53,* 94–107.

Schepis, M.M., Reid, D.H., Behrmann, M.M., & Sutton, K.A. (1998). Increasing communicative interactions of young children with autism using a voice output communication aid and naturalistic teaching. *Journal of Applied Behavior Analysis, 31,* 561–578.

Schreibman, L., Stahmer, A.C., & Pierce, K.L. (1996). Alternative applications of pivotal response training: Teaching symbolic play and social interaction skills. In L.K. Koegel, R.L. Koegel, and G. Dunlap (Eds.), *Positive behavioral support: Including people with difficult behavior in the community* (pp. 353–371). Baltimore: Paul H Brookes Publishing Co.

Sheinkopf, S.J., & Siegel, B. (1998). Home-based behavioral treatment of young children with autism. *Journal of Autism and Developmental Disabilities, 28,* 15–23.

Sigafoos, J., Laurie, S., & Pennell, D. (1996). Teaching children with Rett syndrome to request preferred objects using aided communication: Two preliminary studies. *Augmentative and Alternative Communication, 12,* 88–96.

Smith, T. (2001). Discrete trial training in the treatment of autism. *Focus on Autism and Other Developmental Disabilities, 16,* 86–92.

Smith, T., Groen, A.D., & Wynn, J.W. (2000). Randomized trial of intensive early intervention for children with pervasive developmental disorder. *American Journal on Mental Retardation, 105,* 269–285.

Snyder-McLean, L.K., Solomonson, B., McLean, J.E., & Sack, S. (1984). Structuring joint action routines: A strategy for facilitating communication and language development in the classroom. *Seminars in Speech and Language, 5,* 213–28.

Sundberg, M.L., & Michael, J. (2001). The value of Skinner's analysis of verbal behavior for teaching children with autism. *Behavior Modification, 25,* 698–724.

Sundberg, M.L., & Partington, J.W. (1998). *Teaching language to children with autism or other developmental disabilities.* Danville, CA: Behavior Analysts.

Sundberg, M.L., & Partington, J.W. (1999). The need for both discrete trial and natural environment language training for children with autism. In P.M. Ghezzi, W.L. Williams, & J.E. Carr (Eds.), *Autism: Behavior analytic perspectives* (pp. 139–156). Reno, NV: Context Press.

Turnell, R., & Carter, M. (1994). Establishing a repertoire of requesting for a student with severe and multiple disabilities using tangible symbols and naturalistic time delay. *Australia and New Zealand Journal of Developmental Disabilities, 19,* 193–207.

Venn, M.L., Wolery, M., Werts, M.G., Morris, A., DeCesare, L.D., & Cuffs, M.S. (1993). Embedding instruction in art activities to teach preschoolers with disabilities to imitate their peers. *Early Childhood Research Quarterly, 8,* 277–294.

Warren, S.F., Fey, M.E., Finestack, L.H., Brady, M.C., Bredin-Oja, S.L., & Fleming, K.K. (2008). A randomized trial of longitudinal effects of low-intensity responsivity education/prelinguistic milieu teaching. *Journal of Speech, Language, and Hearing Research, 51,* 451–470.

Warren, S.F., Fey, M.E., & Yoder, P.J. (2007). Differential treatment intensity research: A missing link to creating optimally effective communication interventions. *Mental Retardation and Developmental Disabilities Research Reviews, 13,* 70–77.

Warren, S.F., & Kaiser, A.P. (1988). Research in early language intervention. In S.L. Odom & M.B. Karnes (Eds.), *Early intervention for infants and children with handicaps: An empirical base* (pp. 89–108). Baltimore: Paul H. Brookes Publishing Co.

Whalen, C., & Schreibman, L. (2003). Joint attention training for children with autism using behavior modification procedures. *Journal of Child Psychology and Psychiatry, 44,* 456–468.

Wolery, M., Anthony, L., Caldwell, M.K., Snyder, E.D., & Morgante, J.D. (2002). Embedding and distributing constant time delay in circle time and transitions. *Topics in Early Childhood Special Education, 22,* 14–25.

Wolery, M., Anthony, L., & Heckathorn, J. (1998). Transition-based teaching: Effects on transitions, teachers' behavior, and children's learning. *Journal of Early Intervention, 21,* 117–131.

Yoder, P., & Stone, W.L. (2006a). A randomized comparison of the effect of two prelinguistic communication interventions on the acquisition of spoken communication in preschoolers with ASD. *Journal of Speech, Language, and Hearing Research, 49,* 698–711.

Yoder, P., & Stone, W.L. (2006b). Randomized comparison of two communication interventions for preschoolers with autism spectrum disorders. *Journal of Consulting and Clinical Psychology, 74,* 426–435.

Yoder, P.J., & Warren, S.F. (1998). Maternal responsivity predicts the prelinguistic communication intervention that facilitates generalized intentional communication. *Journal of Speech, Language, and Hearing Research, 41,* 1207–1219.

Yoder, P.J., & Warren, S.F. (2001). Relative treatment effects of two prelinguistic communication interventions on language development in toddlers with developmental delays vary by maternal characteristics. *Journal of Speech, Language, and Hearing Research, 44,* 224–237.

Yoder, P.J., & Warren, S.F. (2002). Effects of prelinguistic milieu teaching and parent responsivity education on dyads involving children with intellectual disabilities. *Journal of Speech, Language, and Hearing Research, 45,* 1158–1174.

Monitoring Learner Performance

7

Kathleen M. Feeley and Emily A. Jones

▷ CHAPTER OVERVIEW

Interventionists monitor performance by recording information about the learner's demonstration of specific communication skills. **Monitoring performance** is a necessary component of effective intervention and an integral part of providing best practice augmentative and alternative communication (AAC) intervention.

▷ CHAPTER OBJECTIVES

After studying this chapter, readers will be able to

- Identify why and when to monitor learner performance
- Identify different measurement systems and when to use each of them
- Use measurement systems for monitoring learner performance
- Implement measurement of intervention integrity and response reliability

▷ KEY TERMS

- ▶ cumulative recording
- ▶ duration
- ▶ frequency
- ▶ frequency with limited opportunities
- ▶ interobserver agreement
- ▶ intervention integrity
- ▶ latency
- ▶ magnitude
- ▶ measurement system
- ▶ monitoring performance
- ▶ rate
- ▶ response reliability
- ▶ topography

THE IMPORTANCE OF MONITORING PERFORMANCE

Monitoring learner performance enhances the effectiveness of AAC interventions by

- Providing objective information (rather than memory or anecdotes) to make intervention decisions
- Providing a clear indication of when skills have been acquired, allowing for new, more advanced skills to be identified for intervention
- Increasing the likelihood interventions will be implemented correctly on a regular basis

WHEN SHOULD LEARNER PERFORMANCE BE MONITORED?

Learner performance should be monitored prior to implementing intervention, during intervention, and after intervention.

- Recording learner performance prior to intervention is referred to as *baseline* or *preintervention performance*. Baseline performance provides information about skills the learner already has in his or her repertoire, as well as those in need of change. Compare baseline performance with performance during and after intervention to determine intervention effectiveness. Obtain baseline performance in all settings where the learner will utilize the skill.

- Record learner performance while intervention is being implemented to determine whether the learner's performance is improving. Learner performance data will help guide changes in intervention strategies (e.g., prompting, consequence procedures) if performance is less than optimal.

- Monitor generalization of skills. Learners with severe disabilities may still fail to engage in generalized responding, even when intervention has adhered to best practice utilizing general case instruction. In addition, unanticipated contexts in which the use of the target skill is appropriate may be identified after intervention. For example, Jason was taught to use his communication wallet to request a break in a variety of environments, including school, home, and the homes of family members (i.e., his grandmother and aunt). Interventionists did not anticipate Jason attending an overnight field trip with his middle school class, however. Because intervention was not possible in this environment, generalized performance was monitored to determine the need for additional instruction. Systematically monitoring generalization allows for implementing intervention if generalization does not occur.

See Chapter 5 for information on general case instruction.

Steps for monitoring performance

Step 1: Write a behavioral objective.
Step 2: Choose a measurement system.
Step 3: Create a performance monitoring form.
Step 4: Display performance monitoring information.
Step 5: Analyze performance monitoring information.
Step 6: Develop procedures to monitor intervention integrity and response reliability.

- Many learners with severe disabilities have difficulty maintaining skills that are not regularly used. Therefore, ongoing monitoring of learner performance after acquisition (called *maintenance*) is important. If the learner does not maintain a skill, then additional intervention is required.

How Is Performance Monitored?

Monitoring learner performance involves observing the learner and documenting the extent to which he or she engages in specific communicative responses.

Step 1: Write a Behavioral Objective

To write a behavioral objective, identify

- The specific observable communicative behavior to be monitored

- The situations within which the behavior should occur

- With whom the behavior should occur

Be specific enough so that any interventionist can objectively determine whether the learner is engaging in that behavior. For example, "Mia will communicate" is a much too broad description of the behavior. "During free time in the classroom, Mia will initiate requests of her peers to play a game by pointing to a photograph of the game displayed on her eight-symbol communication board" is a more complete description.

Include criteria indicating the level of performance the learner should display. To complete the objective for Mia, criteria can be added about the number of times she should initiate a request during free play (e.g., "Mia will initiate requests at least four times during free play sessions"). The criteria can be stated in different ways but must correspond to the measurement system selected.

Step 2: Choose a Measurement System

Consider the following **measurement systems** (Alberto & Troutman, 2006; Cooper, Heron, & Heward, 2007):

1. A **frequency** measurement system involves counting the number of times a behavior occurs within a specific time period. For example, counting the number of times that a learner uses his or her communication system to interact with his or her peers during lunch.

When Should a Frequency Measurement System Be Used?
Use frequency to measure behavior that has a clear beginning and end. For example, touching a graphic symbol and forming the sign for HELP are behaviors with a clear beginning and end, appropriate for a frequency count.

Reporting the observation period is also important when measuring frequency. It is impossible to evaluate whether a given frequency count meets criteria for mastery without a specified time period. For example, performance indicates the learner initiated interactions with his peers five times; this may be sufficient if it occurred during an hour of playtime but not meet criteria if it spanned the entire day (e.g., 6 hours).

In addition, if observation length varies, then it must be accounted for in reporting frequency data. For example, if a communicative behavior occurred five times during two sessions, one lasting 10 minutes and the other 60 minutes, then the measurements of frequency in those two sessions have different meanings. Both the frequency count and the length of the observation period must be noted. This is referred to as the **rate** of a response.

In some instances, there are a limited number of opportunities for the behavior to occur (referred to as **frequency with limited opportunities** or controlled presentations). For example, opportunities are limited when a teacher presents questions to which the learner must respond. In this case, include the number of opportunities provided to the learner along with frequency. For example, reporting that a child used his or her communication system to respond to an adult's request for information on three occasions is only informative in the context of the number of times the caregiver requested information. This performance may meet criterion if there were 3 opportunities provided to the child (i.e., 100% correct performance). If the adult provided 10 opportunities, however, and the child only responded on 3 opportunities (i.e., 30%), then this may fall short of meeting criteria.

How Is Frequency Measured?
Record every occurrence of the target behavior during the observation period (e.g., make a tally mark on a data sheet). In addition, record the length of the observation period and number of opportunities presented when relevant.

☞ Helpful Hint

Pen and paper is often easy and readily accessible to record performance, but other ways of recording performance might be more easily implemented in some settings (e.g., on the playground) and might be less obvious than pen and paper. For example:

- Place a handful of small items (e.g., paper clips, marbles, plastic chips) in one pocket and transfer them to another pocket each time the behavior occurs

- Activate a small handheld tally counter each time the behavior occurs

- Transfer bracelets (e.g., rubber, medal, beaded) worn on one wrist to the other wrist each time the behavior occurs

Transfer the tally count (e.g., number of paper clips in a pocket) to a paper data sheet or graph following the observation period.

How Is Performance Reported in Terms of Frequency?
When observation periods are all of the same length, either report the total number of times the behavior occurred (e.g., three times during math, three times during science) or the average across time periods (e.g., average is one time per math session and one time per science session). Average is calculated using the following formula.

Average frequency per observation period =

$$\frac{\text{Total occurrences}}{\text{Number of observation periods}}$$

Report the **rate** of the response when observation periods vary in length. Rate converts the raw tally count information to a common denominator involving frequency per common time period (e.g., frequency per minute, frequency per day) using the following formula.

Rate =

$$\frac{\text{Number of times behavior occurred}}{\text{Length of observation period}}$$

CASE EXAMPLE

Monitoring Frequency

Charles often used his speech-generating device (SGD) while interacting one to one, but there was not a consensus among his teachers regarding the extent to which he used it during group class periods. The teaching assistant examined this by tallying each time Charles used the device in each of his 50-minute classes (see Figure 7.1; Form 7.1 is a blank version and is included on the accompanying CD-ROM).

Charles's interventionists observed that he participated in language arts class using his SGD at a much higher frequency (total of 27 times, average of 9 times per class session) than in his other classes (total for math, science, and social studies of 3, 3, and 6, and averages of 1, 1, and 2 times, respectively). Further inspection of these environments, as well as Charles's device, revealed a lack of vocabulary related to these subject areas (e.g., math, science, social studies). Consequently, Charles's interventionists added and taught the needed vocabulary while continuing to monitor his performance.

CASE EXAMPLE

Monitoring Rate

Jason had been taught to use his communication book to interact with peers during a number of structured activities (e.g., board game playing, paired reading). Interventionists observed Jason during morning preparation time, lunch, recess, and preparation to go home to examine his use of his communication book to interact with peers during unstructured periods at school. Jason's target behavior was "Selecting symbols from his communication book to communicate with peers during unstructured periods at school." The interventionists recorded a tally mark each time Jason selected a symbol using the performance monitoring form in Figure 7.2 (Form 7.2 is a blank version and is included on the accompanying CD-ROM).

Jason's interventionists calculated the rate at which he interacted with his peers using his communication book. The frequency with which he used his communication book (43 times) across the four observation periods, divided by the total number of minutes observed (80 minutes), revealed that Jason selected symbols to interact with his peers during unstructured time in school approximately 1 time every 2 minutes (rate = 43 times/80 minutes).

For frequencies with limited opportunities or controlled interactions, if the number of total opportunities is small and does not vary, then reporting raw frequency is appropriate (e.g., 2 out of 3 is more informative than 66%) for frequency with limited opportunities, or controlled presentations. Use the following formula, however, to report percentage when the number of opportunities provided to the learner varies across sessions.

Percent =

$$\frac{\text{Number of times behavior occurred}}{\text{Number of opportunities}} \times 100$$

If the learner responds correctly on 10 out of a total of 10 opportunities, then he or she is performing at 100% (10/10 × 100 = 100%). In contrast, if the learner responds correctly on only 10 out of 20 opportunities, then he or she is performing at 50% (10/20 × 100 = 50%).

CASE EXAMPLE

Monitoring Performance Using Frequency with Limited Opportunities

Jenn's interventionists have been implementing intervention strategies to increase her use of her SGD to respond to peers' questions. A

Learner's name: ___Charles___

Target behavior: ___Use of his communication device during academic instruction___

Interventionist: ___Kerry___

Circle one: (Baseline) Intervention   Maintenance   Generalization

Instructions: Fill in activity, time interval, and date. Indicate the number of times the target behavior occurred in the column corresponding to the interval in which observation occurred. Total the numbers in each row, indicating the total number of times per day the behavior occurred in the far-right column. Total the number of times per activity/time interval the behavior occurred and note it in the row labeled "Total." Calculate the average number of times the behavior occurred within each of the activities/intervals and record that number in the bottom row.

Activity →	Activity/time interval				
	Math	Science	Social studies	Language arts	
Time interval →	8:00–8:50	9:00–9:50	10:00–10:50	11:00–11:50	
Date ↓					Total
1/6	/	/	//	//// ////	12
1/7		/	//	//// //// ///	14
1/8	//	/	//	//// ////	13
Total	3	3	6	27	39
Average	1	1	2	9	13

Figure 7.1. Performance Monitoring Form illustrating the collection of frequency data for Charles. (*Note:* This is a filled-in version of Form 7.1, Performance Monitoring Form for Frequency Data. A blank, printable version appears on the accompanying CD-ROM.)

frequency count was used to monitor her performance. Jenn's performance was reported as a percentage because responding to a peer's question could only occur when a peer directs a question to Jenn (i.e., there are a limited number of opportunities), which varies each day. Figure 7.3 (Form 7.3 is a blank version and is included on the accompanying CD-ROM) displays performance information revealing that Jenn used her device an average of 46% of the opportunities across 3 days (50%, 43%, and 44% on each day). This information was used when her interventionists met to examine her performance and to develop additional strategies to increase the likelihood that Jenn would respond to questions from her peers.

2. **Duration** measures how long a learner engages in a particular behavior.

When Should a Duration Measurement System Be Used? Duration is useful when the concern is about the length of time a behavior occurs and intervention is intended to increase or decrease that length of time. For example, duration is appropriate to monitor the amount of time a learner sits during small-group instruction or the number of seconds required for a learner to complete a communicative utterance using a communication board.

How Is Duration Measured? Duration is measured by activating a stopwatch at the onset of the behavior and deactivating the stopwatch when the behavior ends. Record the time displayed on the stopwatch (see Figure 7.4; Form 7.4 is a blank version and is included on the accompanying CD-ROM). Alternatively, use a clock or watch and record

Learner's name: _Jason_ _____ Date: _7/15_ _____

Target behavior: _Selecting symbols from his communication book to communicate with peers_

during unstructured periods at school

Circle one: Baseline   Intervention   Maintenance   (Generalization)

Instructions: Fill in the interval, length of observation (to the nearest minute), and the frequency with which the target behavior occurred during that observation period. The rate of a response is calculated by identifying the total length of time the learner was observed divided by the number of times the behavior occurred.

Interval (activity, time)	Length of observation (in minutes)	Frequency	Rate
Morning preparation	10 minutes	ℳℐ	.5/minute
Lunch	30 minutes	ℳℐ ℳℐ ℳℐ ///	.6/minute
Recess	30 minutes	ℳℐ ℳℐ //	.4/minute
Preparation to go home	10 minutes	ℳℐ ///	.8/minute
Total	80 minutes	43	**Average rate** .54/minute or approximately once every 2 minutes

Figure 7.2. Performance Monitoring Form illustrating the collection of response rate data for Jason. (*Note:* This is a filled-in version of Form 7.2, Performance Monitoring Form Illustrating the Collection of Response Rate Data. A blank, printable version appears on the accompanying CD-ROM.)

both the time the behavior starts and the time it stops and then calculate the time that passed (see Figure 7.5; Form 7.5 is a blank version and is included on the accompanying CD-ROM).

✏ *Helpful Hint*

Make sure the behavior is defined with a clear beginning and end to indicate when to start and stop recording.

How Is Performance Recorded in Terms of Duration?   Report the average duration across opportunities using the following formula.

Average duration =

$$\frac{\text{Total duration across all responses}}{\text{Number of responses}}$$

CASE EXAMPLE

Monitoring Duration

Brianna's interventionists examined the length of time it took Brianna to formulate a message using her SGD. They used the performance monitoring form in Figure 7.4 (Form 7.4 on the accompanying CD-ROM) to monitor her performance (i.e., the selection of symbols to formulate a message on her communication device). Each time Brianna used her device, they recorded the message she selected as well as the number of seconds it took her to select the corresponding symbols.

The average duration of Brianna's message formulation was 12.25 seconds (5 + 20 + 5 + 19 seconds/4 episodes). Interventionists also noted a discrepancy between duration of question asking and question answering. The

Learner's name: __Jenn__

Target behavior: __Use of communication device in response to peers' questions__

Circle one: (Baseline)   Intervention   Maintenance   Generalization

Instructions: Fill in the date and circle the symbol corresponding to the learner's performance when he or she was provided an opportunity to perform the target behavior. Circle a plus (+) if the learner independently demonstrated the correct response or a minus (–) if the learner did not demonstrate the correct response or demonstrated an incorrect response. Calculate percent correct performance by dividing the number of opportunities during which the learner made a correct response by the number of opportunities presented and multiplying the number by 100. Fill in the percent and the interventionist's initials.

Date: 5/19	Response		Date: 5/20	Response		Date: 5/21	Response
⊕	–		⊕	–		+	⊖
⊕	–		+	⊖		⊕	–
+	⊖		⊕	–		+	⊖
+	⊖		+	⊖		⊕	–
⊕	–		+	⊖		+	⊖
+	⊖		⊕	–		+	⊖
+	⊖		+	⊖		⊕	–
⊕	–		+	–		+	⊖
+	–		+	–		⊕	–
+	–		+	–		+	–
Interventionist's initials: JP	Percent: 50%		Interventionist's initials: JP	Percent: 43%		Interventionist's initials: LB	Percent: 44%

Figure 7.3.   Sample Performance Monitoring Form illustrating the collection of frequency data with limited opportunities/controlled presentations. (*Note:* This is a filled-in version of Form 7.3, Performance Monitoring Form Illustrating the Collection of Frequency Data with Limited Opportunities/Controlled Presentations. A blank, printable version appears on the accompanying CD-ROM.)

average duration of Brianna's question asking was 5 seconds (5 + 5 seconds/2 episodes), but the average duration of her question answering was 19.5 seconds (20 + 19 seconds/2 episodes). Thus, Brianna used her device to ask a question much more quickly than she used it to answer a question. This information was used by her interventionists to modify Brianna's communication device, ensuring it was set up so that she could access a variety of symbols in a shorter amount of time and, thus, produce a response to a question more quickly.

3. **Latency** is a measure of the amount of time that passes between the cue for a

behavior to be emitted and the behavior's onset. For example, the time it takes for the AAC user to respond when someone says, "Hello," (e.g., 1, 2 , or more seconds) is the latency of the response.

When Should Latency Be Used to Measure Performance?   Latency data are useful when the concern is about the length of time it takes a learner to begin to emit a behavior. It might be desirable in some instances to decrease the latency of a communicative response. For example, it is desirable for the latency of the learner's response following a question (e.g., "Do you have the time?") to be relatively short. Therefore, decreas-

Learner's name: _Brianna_ _____ Date: _____

Target behavior: _The selection of one or more symbols to formulate a message on her speech-_
generating device _____

Interventionist: _Joe_ _____

Circle one: (Baseline)   Intervention   Maintenance   Generalization

Instructions: Activate the stopwatch at the onset of the behavior, and deactivate the stopwatch when the behavior stops. Record the time displayed on the stopwatch under the Length of Time column.

Episode	Length of time (in seconds)	Description of behavior
1	5 seconds	How are you?
2	20 seconds	I went to my friend Tammy's house.
3	5 seconds	What did you do this weekend?
4	19 seconds	We played video games.
Total:	49 seconds	**Average duration:** 12.25 seconds

Figure 7.4. Sample Performance Monitoring Form illustrating the collection of response duration data when using a stopwatch. (*Note:* This is a filled-in version of Form 7.4, Performance Monitoring Form Illustrating the Collection of Response Duration Data When Using a Stopwatch. A blank, printable version appears on the accompanying CD-ROM.)

ing a long latency to respond would be important.

Alternatively, the latency of some communicative responses may need to be increased. Consider a learner who is using an AAC system to request a break from an activity. Using latency will enable interventionists to monitor the time from the beginning of the activity to the learner's request for a break. If the length of time is short, then intervention can be implemented to increase this time interval, thus enabling the learner to engage in an activity for longer periods of time.

How Is Latency Measured?   Latency is measured by activating a stopwatch when the cue for the learner to emit the behavior occurs and by deactivating it when the learner begins to emit the behavior. Record the time displayed on the stopwatch (see Figure 7.6; Form 7.6 is a blank version and is included on the CD-ROM).

☞ *Helpful Hint*

Clearly define the behavior and the cue to which the AAC user should respond. For example, identify the point at which an activity begins or specific questions to which the learner should respond.

How Is Performance in Terms of Latency Reported?   Calculate the average latency of the target response across opportunities using the following formula.

$$\text{Average latency} = \frac{\text{Total latency across all responses}}{\text{Number of responses}}$$

CASE EXAMPLE

Monitoring Performance Latency

Rachel's AAC system consists of a multipage communication book. Her interventionist noticed that it required Rachel a long time to re-

Learner's name: _Sasha_ _____

Target behavior: _Responding to questions using a speech-generating device accessed_ via row _column scanning_ _____

Interventionist: _Maria_ _____

Circle one: (Baseline)   Intervention   Maintenance   Generalization

Instructions: Using a clock or watch, record the time the behavior starts under Start Time and the time the behavior stops under Stop Time. Then, calculate the amount of time that passed and record it under Duration.

Episode	Start time	Stop time	Duration
1	2:30	2:31	1 minute
2	3:24	3:25	1 minute
3	4:29	4:31	2 minutes
4	4:45	4:47	2 minutes
			Total duration: 6 minutes **Average duration:** 1.5 minutes

Figure 7.5. Sample Performance Monitoring Form illustrating the collection of response duration data recording both start and stop times. (*Note:* This is a filled-in version of Form 7.5, Performance Monitoring Form Illustrating the Collection of Response Duration Data When Recording Both Start and Stop Times. A blank, printable version appears on the accompanying CD-ROM.)

spond to others' communicative initiations on some occasions. Her interventionist evaluated this by observing Rachel's interactions and recording the time that elapsed between the end of her communication partner's utterance and the start of Rachel's symbol selection (on the Performance Monitoring Form in Figure 7.6).

Rachel's average latency to respond was 10 seconds (15 + 5 + 5 + 15 seconds/4 episodes) across types of responses. Her average latency to respond to a comment was 15 seconds (15 + 15 seconds/2 episodes), and her average latency to respond to a specific question was 5 seconds (5 + 5 seconds/2 episodes). Based on the information in Figure 7.6 (see also blank Form 7.6 on the accompanying CD-ROM), it took Rachel longer to respond to a comment than it did to respond to a specific question.

Rachel's interventionists developed intervention procedures to teach her strategies to better determine situations (i.e., when someone comments) that warrant a communicative exchange. Figure 7.7 illustrates how Rachel's performance improved. Responding to a comment began to occur as quickly as she responded to specific questions.

---

4. Form, or **topography,** refers to what a behavior looks like; for example, how a learner selects symbols on a communication board (e.g., using a closed fist or an isolated finger).

When Should Form Be Used to Measure Performance? Monitoring form is useful when replacing one response with another. For example, monitoring topography when replacing aggression with the use of a graphic symbol will enable the interventionist to determine the extent to which the replacement response is increasing and aggression is decreasing.

Form might also be used to describe behaviors that occur in a chain. For example,

Learner's name: _Rachel_

Target behavior: _Selecting symbols in her communication book_

Circle one: (Baseline)   Intervention   Maintenance   Generalization

Instructions: Record the date and describe the cue that occasioned the target behavior for each episode. Activate the stopwatch once the cue occurs, and deactivate the stopwatch when the target behavior is emitted. Record the time displayed on the stopwatch under Latency. Alternatively, use a clock or watch to record the time at which the cue occurred and when the behavior occurred. Then, calculate the time interval that passed.

Date	Episode	Cue: _Question or comment to which Rachel responded_	Latency (time prior to response in seconds)	Interventionist's initials
1/12	1	I saw a movie yesterday.	15 seconds	KL
1/12	2	What game do you want to play?	5 seconds	DT
1/12	3	What do you want for lunch?	5 seconds	EP
1/12	4	I love to play chess.	15 seconds	FW
			Total: 40 seconds	**Average latency:** 10 seconds

Figure 7.6.   Performance Monitoring Form illustrating the collection of response latency data during baseline. (*Note:* This is a filled-in version of Form 7.6, Performance Monitoring Form Illustrating the Collection of Response Latency Data Using a Stopwatch. A blank, printable version appears on the accompanying CD-ROM.)

sometimes challenging behavior escalates from mildly disruptive behaviors (e.g., whining) to those that are more disruptive (e.g., yelling) and possibly dangerous (e.g., throwing materials), creating a chain of behaviors. Interventionists may monitor the topography of responses that occur early in this chain (e.g., mildly disruptive whining) to determine the point at which a more appropriate communicative replacement can be prompted before the more serious behavior is emitted. For example, the interventionist can prompt an appropriate communicative response when the learner whines but has not yet engaged in a more severe challenging behavior (i.e., yelling), effectively avoiding the more serious form of challenging behavior.

How Is a Behavior's Form Measured?   The forms of behavior can be noted in separate

columns or recorded as codes (e.g., CF [closed fist], IF [isolated finger]; see Figure 7.8 and Form 7.7 on the accompanying CD-ROM).

How Is Performance Reported in Terms of a Behavior's Form?   Calculate the total and/or average occurrence of each form.

CASE EXAMPLE

Monitoring Topography

Mary is an adult who uses multiple modes to communicate, including gestures, facial expressions, a few verbalizations, and a communication book with several photographs depicting desired items and activities. Mary's interventionists decided to use topography to monitor which modes of communication

Learner's name: _Rachel_

Target behavior: _Selecting symbols in her communication book_

Circle one: Baseline (Intervention) Maintenance Generalization

Instructions: Record the date and describe the cue that occasioned the target behavior for each episode. Activate the stopwatch once the cue occurs, and deactivate the stopwatch when the target behavior is emitted. Record the time displayed on the stopwatch under Latency. Alternatively, use a clock or watch to record the time at which the cue occurred and when the behavior occurred. Then, calculate the time interval that passed.

Date	Episode	Cue: _Question or comment to which Rachel responded_	Latency (time prior to response in seconds)	Interventionist's initials
1/15	1	It's raining outside.	5 seconds	KL
1/15	2	What do you want to do tonight?	5 seconds	DT
1/15	3	What would you like to eat?	5 seconds	EP
1/15	4	This burger is delicious.	5 seconds	FW
			Total: 20 seconds	**Average latency:** 5 seconds

Figure 7.7. Performance Monitoring Form illustrating the collection of response latency data during intervention. (*Note:* This is a filled-in version of Form 7.6, Performance Monitoring Form Illustrating the Collection of Response Latency Data Using a Stopwatch. A blank, printable version appears on the accompanying CD-ROM.)

Mary used across each of three different environments (see Figure 7.8; Form 7.7 is a blank version and is included on the accompanying CD-ROM).

Mary used facial expressions an average of eight times across the three environments, her communication book an average of three times, verbalizations an average of eight times, and gestures an average of nine times. In fact, her communication book was used only at work, where it was used more often than verbalizations. Subsequent intervention involved teaching Mary to use communication forms she did not typically use in a given setting (to augment her existing communication), as well as teaching Mary's communicative partners about ways Mary tended to communicate in each environment (e.g., teaching Mary's roommates about specific gestures that Mary used to indicate her preferences).

5. **Magnitude** (force) refers to a behavior's strength or intensity. For example, magnitude can be used to measure the physical force of a response, volume of a communicative utterance, or intensity of a challenging behavior. Rating scales are often employed in practical applications to describe the magnitude of responses emitted by learners. Figure 7.9 shows a rating scale for volume.

When Should Magnitude Be Used to Measure Performance? Interventionists use magnitude when a qualitative change in the dimension of a behavior is desired. For example, use magnitude to monitor the volume at which a learner uses verbal communication, rated from "not audible" to "loud."

How Is Magnitude Measured? Develop a rating scale that reflects the key dimensions of the behavior of interest. For example, use a

Learner's name: _Mary_   Date: _____

Target behavior: _Mary's communication responses_

Circle one: (Baseline)   Intervention   Maintenance   Generalization

Instructions: List each of the behavior forms at the top of the columns under Responses. Record the setting in which observation took place in the column on the left, and note the interventionist's initials in the column on the right. Make a tally mark in the corresponding column each time a behavior form occurs. Record the total number of occurrences of the behavior within each setting and then calculate the total number of occurrences of each behavior form in the bottom row.

Setting	Responses				Interventionist's initials
	Facial expressions	Communi- cation book	Verbalizations	Gestures	
At home	✓✓✓✓✓ ✓✓✓✓✓ Total 10	✓ Total 0	✓✓✓✓✓ ✓✓✓✓✓ ✓✓✓✓ Total 11	✓✓✓✓✓ ✓✓✓✓✓ Total 14	BW
At work	✓✓✓✓✓ ✓✓✓ Total 8	✓✓✓✓✓ ✓✓✓✓✓ ✓ Total 11	✓✓✓✓ Total 4	✓✓✓✓✓ ✓✓✓✓✓ Total 10	SJ
Scrapbook club	✓✓✓✓✓ ✓✓ Total 7	Total 0	✓✓✓✓✓ ✓✓✓✓✓ ✓ Total 11	✓✓✓✓✓ Total 5	SH
Total	25	11	26	29	
Average	8.3	3.67	8.67	9.67	

Figure 7.8. Sample Performance Monitoring Form illustrating the collection of data describing behavior forms. (*Note:* This is a filled-in version of Form 7.7, Performance Monitoring Form Illustrating the Collection of Data Describing Behavior Forms. A blank, printable version appears on the accompanying CD-ROM.)

scale from *not fatigued* (1), to *somewhat fatigued* (2), to *very fatigued* (3) to describe the extent to which a learner who uses switch-activated scanning fatigues while communicating with his or her scanning device. Make sure to include clear and detailed descriptions of the points on the scale (see Form 7.8 on the accompanying CD-ROM).

How Is Performance Reported in Terms of Magnitude? Report the average magnitude of the target response using the following formula.

Average magnitude =

$$\frac{\text{Total magnitude across all responses}}{\text{Number of responses}}$$

Translate the average back to its corresponding qualitative label once an average magnitude is obtained. For example, if the average magnitude across several opportunities is 2 (e.g., $1 + 3 + 2/3 = 2$) on a scale from not fatigued (1) to somewhat fatigued (2) to very fatigued (3), then the average magnitude is somewhat fatigued.

CASE EXAMPLE

Monitoring Magnitude

Ann used some spoken language in addition to her SGD. Her verbalizations were often inaudible, making it imperative that she have her SGD available to her in environments where she could not be heard. Ann's interventionists monitored the volume of verbalizations via a rating scale ranging from *not audible* (1) to *loud*

1	2	3
Not audible	Audible	Loud
Interventionist could not hear	Interventionist could easily hear	Interventionist and others nearby could easily hear

Figure 7.9.   Rating scale for the volume of Ann's verbalizations

(3) to identify the environments in which Ann was inaudible (see Figure 7.9).

Ann's voice was inaudible on the playground (average 1), in classroom during structured acitivities (average 2), in classroom during unstructured activities (average 1.4), and in the school cafeteria (average 1) (see Figure 7.10; see also blank Form 7.8 on the accompanying CD-ROM). Using this information, interventionists made sure that Ann had her SGD with her in each of these environments.

☞ Helpful Hint

Each of these measurement systems may be used alone or in combination. For example, interventionists who are recording the topography of a response might also be interested in the frequency with which each topographical response occurs. Similarly, interventionists can simultaneously record both the magnitude and frequency of a behavior. Duration and latency can also easily be combined with a frequency count.

Step 3: Create a Performance Monitoring Form

Previous sections of this chapter provide examples of performance monitoring forms corresponding to each of the measurement systems. It is important to individualize forms to best suit the particular learner, communicative alternative, and situation (e.g., interventionists, setting). Make sure to include the following information.

- Identifying information

  The learner's name

  The interventionist(s) (and person recording performance information, if different from the interventionist)

  The behavioral objective

- An indication of whether performance is being monitored during baseline, intervention, maintenance, or generalization opportunities

- Performance information

  This section of a performance monitoring form describes the learner's performance. It should contain the date on which the information is being collected and a record of each occurrence or nonoccurrence of the behavior being monitored.

- Summary information

  Designate space on the performance monitoring form for reporting measurement data in summary form (as described within each measurement system). Summarizing performance information helps interventionists analyze the learner's performance and draw conclusions regarding the effectiveness of an intervention. For example, create a section on the form when monitoring the frequency with which a behavior occurs to document the total number of times the behavior occurred for a given observation period. If calculating the percentage of times the behavior occurred in relation to the number of opportunities, then include a section for the percent occurrence for each intervention session.

☞ Helpful Hint

Consider characteristics of the learner and available resources (e.g., number of available interventionists) when deciding how often to monitor performance.

Learner's name: _Ann_____ Date: _____

Target behavior: _The volume with which Ann emits verbal utterances_____

Circle one: (Baseline)   Intervention   Maintenance   Generalization

Instructions: Develop a rating scale that reflects the key dimensions of the behavior, providing clear and detailed descriptions of the points on the scale. Note a qualitative description of each of the points on the scale in the blank spaces under the Rating column. Note the environment in which the learner was observed, and rate the behavior during each episode. Record the total of the ratings in the Total column and calculate and record the average in the Average column.

1: _Not audible_____   2: _Audible_____   3: _Loud_____

Environments	Episode	Rating			Total	Average
		Not audible	Audible	Loud		
Playground	1	①	2	3	3	1
	2	①	2	3		
	3	①	2	3		
Classroom during structured activities	4	1	②	3	6	2
	5	1	②	3		
	6	1	②	3		
Classroom during unstructured activities	7	1	②	3	7	1.4
	8	①	2	3		
	9	①	2	3		
	10	1	②	3		
	11	①	2	3		
School cafeteria	12	①	2	3	4	1
	13	①	2	3		
	14	①	2	3		
	15	①	2	3		

Figure 7.10. Sample Performance Monitoring Form illustrating the collection of magnitude data. (*Note:* This is a filled-in version of Form 7.8, Performance Monitoring Form Illustrating the Collection of Magnitude Data. A blank, printable version appears on the accompanying CD-ROM.)

For example, if the learner acquires skills quickly, then frequent monitoring will enable interventionists to make adjustments to the intervention in a timely manner. In addition, be creative in utilizing resources for monitoring performance. Consider alternative frequency-counting devices (e.g., paper clips in your pocket) as well as alternative means of recording performance such as from video or audio recordings.

☞ *Helpful Hint*

Performance monitoring forms can include additional information such as

- Other behaviors (e.g., challenging behavior) related to the communicative behavior

- Environmental factors (e.g., other learners, location, materials)

- The extent to which the behavior was prompted (see Chapter 5)

Step 4: Display
Performance Monitoring Information

Graphing the data is an ideal way to display summary performance monitoring information. Graphically summarizing learner performance can be done in numerous ways. A line graph is used most often to show each time the behavior is measured. A graph is made up of two axes. The x axis is the horizontal axis and represents the passage of time. The y axis (drawn at the left-hand end of the horizontal axis) is the vertical axis and represents values of the behavior being monitored. Use a data point to indicate the amount of the target behavior (y axis) documented during a specific time interval (e.g., day, session; x axis). Figure 7.11 displays performance monitoring information for Jenn's use of her communication device to respond to peers' questions (data from the case example for frequency with limited opportunities/controlled presentations recorded on the performance monitoring form in Figure 7.3).

See Form 6.3 on the accompanying CD-ROM for a blank graph.

A cumulative record is another way to graph data in which a learner's performance during an observation is cumulated or added to the total of his or her previous performance and graphed. In this case, the value on the y axis is the total number of responses. If a response did not occur in an observation period, then a horizontal line is drawn on the graph with a data point plotted at the same y axis value as the previous data point (representing zero responses added to the cumulative record). A steep slope indicates a higher response rate, and a straight line indicates no response.

Cumulative recording is particularly useful

- For frequency data
- When the total number of responses is important (e.g., total number of new words learned)
- When only a few responses could occur in an observation period

Cumulative graphs clearly illustrate change more than a line graph of frequency when

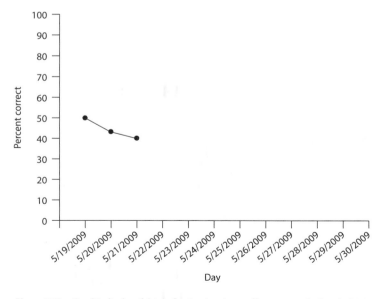

Figure 7.11. Graphic display of data reflecting Jenn's use of her communication device to respond to peers' questions.

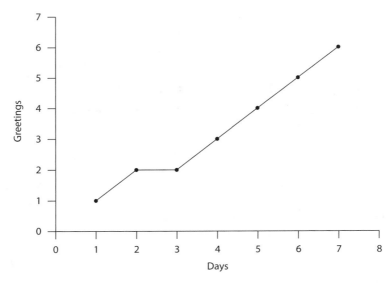

Figure 7.12.   Cumulative record of greetings using an SGD.

only a few responses occur in an observation. It can be difficult to see response rates for a given session, gradual rate changes, and differences between two high-response rates, when using cumulative recording.

Figure 7.12 depicts a learner's greeting of his teacher at the beginning of the school day. A cumulative record was used to depict changes in performance when his teacher introduced a new greeting symbol to his SGD because it was something that happened only once a day.

Step 5: Analyze Performance Information

Review performance information on a regular basis. Thorough and timely analysis of performance information enables interventionists to prevent ongoing implementation of ineffective interventions and extend the application of effective intervention procedures to new skills. Examine performance monitoring information for direction and variability of change.

- Change occurring in the desired direction suggests the intervention is effective in increasing/decreasing the communicative response. Figure 7.13 depicts graphs for different trends in perfor-

mance when intervention is introduced following a baseline period. Graph A depicts an increasing trend in the performance of a desired behavior following the introduction of intervention.

- Consider modifying intervention procedures if there is a plateau or considerable variability in performance. Graphs B and C (see Figure 7.13) depict no change and variable change, respectively, in performance following the introduction of intervention.

- Modify intervention procedures to enhance the effectiveness of the intervention if performance is changing in the opposite direction of that which is desired. Graph D (see Figure 7.13) depicts a change in performance; however, the desired direction is an increase in percent correct and, in this case, performance is decreasing.

How Often Should Performance Information Be Reviewed?   Review performance information more frequently

- When implementing a new intervention or following a change in intervention procedures

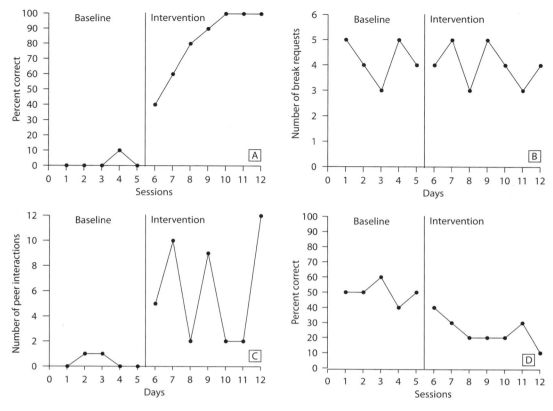

Figure 7.13. Graphic displays illustrating increasing trend in performance (A), no change in performance (B), variable performance (C), and an undesired decrease in performance (D) following the introduction of intervention.

- If a learner tends to acquire skills quickly
- When there have been errors in how the intervention has been implemented (see the sections regarding monitoring intervention integrity and response reliability, discussed shortly)

🏳 Helpful Hint

It is important in some instances to examine the actual data collected on the performance monitoring forms. For example, carefully examine the data during acquisition to ensure that the learner performed correctly on the first opportunity of the day/session. If the learner did not perform correctly on the first opportunity, then he or she may still have performed to criterion (e.g., 90%) based solely on the delivery of a prompt following that first incorrect response. Implement additional sessions to ensure

the learner demonstrates the skill in the absence of a prompted opportunity.

Step 6: Develop Procedures to Monitor Intervention Integrity and Response Reliability

Intervention procedures are intended to be implemented as written. Interventionists may interpret the procedures differently or incorrectly or forget to implement some steps, however. These types of unintentional mistakes alter the integrity of the intervention and put the effectiveness of the intervention at risk. **Intervention integrity** (sometimes called *treatment fidelity* or *procedural fidelity*) refers to the extent to which the intervention is implemented in the way it was intended.

Problems can also arise with the accuracy of the collection of performance monitoring information. One interventionist may score a learner's response as correct, whereas another scores it as incorrect. Such mistakes make evaluating learner performance and subsequent intervention program decisions difficult. **Response reliability**, or **interobserver agreement**, refers to the extent to which the interventionist's recorded performance data information matches that recorded by an observer or another interventionist.

Monitoring both intervention integrity and response reliability ensures that changes can be made if discrepancies arise, such as clarifying target behavior and training interventionist(s). Intervention integrity and response reliability should be monitored for approximately 25%–33% of the time performance is monitored (Cooper et al., 2007). It is important that intervention integrity and response reliability be monitored across sessions and conditions (i.e., during baseline, intervention, and maintenance) because interventionists' implementation of intervention and observation of learner responses can vary over time. This will also help ensure that interventionists continue to implement and monitor performance correctly.

Monitoring Intervention Integrity Identify the steps the interventionist should be following when implementing the intervention. Figure 7.14 (Form 7.9 is a blank version and is included on the accompanying CD-ROM) depicts a selection of information that might be collected while monitoring intervention integrity for an intervention that addresses teaching Brian to identify graphic symbols.

Once the interventionist(s) is determined, identify someone else (the observer) who will observe and record whether the intervention steps are being followed in the order and manner identified. The observer should be someone whose schedule allows for the collection of intervention integrity data on a regular basis. This can be done live or through video recording. Intervention integrity data should be collected more frequently when a new intervention is begun or following changes (e.g., a different or new interventionist begins to run the intervention) to an existing intervention plan.

The observer records whether the interventionist correctly implements each step of the intervention procedures (e.g., yes, no). Calculate the percentage of correctly implemented intervention procedures using the following formula.

$$\text{Percent intervention integrity} = \frac{\text{Number of correctly implemented opportunities}}{\text{Number of correctly and incorrectly implemented opportunities}} \times 100$$

☞ *Helpful Hint*

Give interventionists a copy of the form that will be used to monitor intervention integrity for review before they implement procedures and/or while implementing procedures. In fact, checking off the steps as they are implemented may help to ensure the integrity of implementation on an ongoing basis.

CASE EXAMPLE

Monitoring Intervention Integrity

Sarah was teaching Brian to identify symbols. Sarah's supervisor, Kelly, observed and recorded intervention integrity data while Sarah implemented the intervention with Brian.

Overall, Kelly's data indicated that Sarah was implementing the intervention procedures correctly 86% of the time (60 correctly implemented teaching opportunities/70 correctly plus incorrectly implemented teaching opportunities multiplied by 100). With respect to each of the components of intervention, Sarah's setup was implemented correctly 95% of the time (19/20 × 100), her use of prompting was implemented correctly 93% of the time (28/30 × 100), but her use of reinforcement was implemented correctly only 65% of the time (13/20 × 100). In fact, the errors in her use of reinforcement concerned the timing of delivery

Component of intervention	Date									
	10/2	10/2	10/2	10/2	10/2	10/2	10/2	10/2	10/2	10/2
Set up										
Are materials set up as noted?	(Y) N	(Y) N	(Y) N	Y (N)	(Y) N	(Y) N	(Y) N	(Y) N	(Y) N	(Y) N
Was the appropriate stimulus delivered?	(Y) N	(Y) N	(Y) N	(Y) N	(Y) N	(Y) N	(Y) N	(Y) N	(Y) N	(Y) N
Response										
Was sufficient time provided for a response?	(Y) N	(Y) N	(Y) N	(Y) N	(Y) N	(Y) N	(Y) N	(Y) N	(Y) N	(Y) N
Was the appropriate prompt delivered?	(Y) N	(Y) N	(Y) N	Y (N)	(Y) N	(Y) N	(Y) N	(Y) N	(Y) N	(Y) N
Was it delivered at the appropriate time?	(Y) N	(Y) N	(Y) N	(Y) N	(Y) N	(Y) N	Y (N)	(Y) N	(Y) N	(Y) N
Reinforcement										
Was the appropriate reinforcer provided?	(Y) N	(Y) N	(Y) N	Y (N)	(Y) N	(Y) N	(Y) N	(Y) N	(Y) N	(Y) N
Was it delivered at the appropriate time?	Y (N)	Y (N)	Y (N)	Y (N)	(Y) N	(Y) N	(Y) N	Y (N)	Y (N)	Y (N)
Interventionist	Sarah	Sarah	Sarah	Sarah	Sarah	Sarah	Sarah	Sarah	Sarah	Sarah
Observer	Kelly	Kelly	Kelly	Kelly	Kelly	Kelly	Kelly	Kelly	Kelly	Kelly

Figure 7.14. Intervention integrity monitoring form for Brian. (*Note:* This is a filled-in version of Form 7.9, Intervention Integrity Monitoring Form. A blank, printable version appears on the accompanying CD-ROM.)

of reinforcement (only 40% correct; 4/10 ×
100), whereas the choice of reinforcer was correct 90% of the time (9/10 × 100). Kelly met with
Sarah to clarify the timing of the delivery of reinforcement and then continued to monitor
Sarah's implementation of the intervention.

Monitoring Response Reliability Interventionists must have a good working definition
of the communicative skill being taught to
accurately record performance. The interventionist (as he or she would do anyway)
and an observer record learner performance
to examine response reliability. Recordings
can be made by the observer on the same
type of data sheet that the interventionist is
using to record performance, but should be
done independently of the interventionist.
The observer could also record response reliability and intervention integrity data simultaneously with a form that includes places to
document both types of information. Response reliability can also be recorded live
or from video recordings.

Calculate response reliability by comparing the interventionist's and the observer's
data for the learner's performance to obtain
a percentage for which they agree (referred
to as interobserver agreement). Figure 7.15
provides the formulas for calculating response reliability for each of the measurement systems described in this chapter.

CASE EXAMPLE

Monitoring Response Reliability

While Sarah implemented the intervention to
teach symbol identification to Brian and independently recorded performance information,
her supervisor, Kelly, observed and independently (i.e., on a separate performance monitoring form) recorded Brian's performance information. Figure 7.16 (Form 7.10 is a blank
version and is included on the accompanying
CD-ROM) shows Kelly's and Sarah's performance information side by side.

Sarah and Kelly compared their recordings at the end of the session. There were a
total of 10 opportunities, of which Sarah and

Measurement system	Percent agreement
Frequency data	$\dfrac{\text{Smaller count}}{\text{Larger count}} \times 100$
Rate	$\dfrac{\text{Smaller rate}}{\text{Larger rate}} \times 100$
Frequency data with limited opportunities	$\dfrac{\text{Number of agreements}}{\text{Number of agreements and disagreements}} \times 100$ *Note:* Agreements are defined by matching decisions about the learner's performance on each opportunity
Duration and latency	$\dfrac{\text{Shorter time}}{\text{Longer time}} \times 100$
Topography	$\dfrac{\text{Number of agreements}}{\text{Number of agreements and disagreements}} \times 100$ *Note:* Agreements are defined by matching decisions about the topography of a given occurrence of behavior
Magnitude	$\dfrac{\text{Number of agreements}}{\text{Number of agreements and disagreements}} \times 100$ *Note:* Agreements are defined by matching ratings on the magnitude scale

Figure 7.15.   Formulas for calculation of percentage agreement for each measurement system.

Name:	Brian							

Program: Symbol identification			**Program:** Symbol identification		
Target: Playing games or cards, watching video **Observer:** Kelly			**Target:** Playing games or cards, watching video **Interventionist:** Sarah		
Date: 10/2			**Date:** 10/2		
+	P	⊖	+	P	⊖
+	P	⊖	+	P	⊖
+	Ⓟ	–	+	P	⊖
+	Ⓟ	–	+	Ⓟ	–
+	Ⓟ	–	+	Ⓟ	–
+	Ⓟ	–	+	Ⓟ	–
⊕	P	–	⊕	P	–
⊕	P	–	⊕	P	–
⊕	P	–	⊕	P	–
⊕	P	–	⊕	P	–

+ = independent response

P = prompted response

– = learner made no response or incorrectly requested a break

Figure 7.16. Sample form for recording Kelly and Sarah's performance data used to examine response reliability. (*Note:* This is a filled-in version of Form 7.10, Sample Form for Recording Response Reliability Information Alongside a Copy of the Performance Information Recorded by the Interventionist. A blank, printable version appears on the accompanying CD-ROM.)

Kelly recorded the same response on 9 opportunities. They calculated percent agreement:

$$\frac{9 \text{ agreements}}{9 \text{ agreements plus } 1 \text{ disagreement}} \times 100 = 90\%$$

Sarah and Kelly agreed about Brian's performance 90% of the time—an acceptable level of reliability.

Evaluating Intervention Integrity and Response Reliability Intervention integrity and response reliability data must be analyzed regularly. Any discrepancy in implementation of intervention or recording of learner performance will be identified through regular examination. A general rule of thumb for acceptable response reliability and intervention integrity is 80% (Cooper et al., 2007). If discrepancies are identified, then interventionists must work together to clarify the intervention steps and/or definition of the target behavior. Continued monitoring of both intervention integrity and response reliability will ensure the accurate implementation of intervention and reliable documentation of learner performance.

SUMMARY

Monitoring learner performance is necessary to determine the effectiveness of intervention procedures. Monitoring learner performance involves defining relevant communicative behaviors and developing a way to measure the behavior. Careful and regular analysis of learner performance ensures reliance on objective information (rather than memory or anecdotes) to make intervention decisions and provides a clear indication of when skills have been acquired, allowing for new and more advanced skills to be identified for and addressed through intervention. It also increases the likelihood that in-terventions will be implemented correctly and on a regular basis.

REFERENCES

Alberto, P.A., & Troutman, A.C. (2006). *Applied behavior analysis for teachers* (7th ed.). Upper Saddle River, NJ: Merrill Prentice Hall.

Cooper, J.O., Heron, T.E., & Heward, W.L. (2007). *Applied behavior analysis* (2nd ed.). Upper Saddle River, NJ: Merrill Prentice Hall.

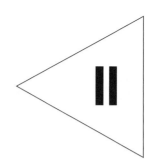

Establishing Functional Communication

Teaching Learners to Correspond Graphic Symbols to Objects and Events

8

Joe Reichle and Krista M. Wilkinson

▷ CHAPTER OVERVIEW

The ability to differentiate between and use specific symbols to reference specific real-world events depends on a number of skills. It is necessary to evaluate these skills when teaching initial symbol discriminations or when learners appear to make incorrect or seemingly random selections among symbols on a display to determine at what point the breakdown may be occurring. This chapter discusses practical methods for differentiating among the component skills, assessing children's performance on those skills, and, where necessary, intervening to teach the skill.

▷ CHAPTER OBJECTIVES

After studying this chapter, readers will be able to

- Differentiate between simple and conditional discriminations and describe how each is important to communication
- Describe levels of conditional discriminations involving matching to sample that enable individuals to use graphic symbols to represent real-world events
- Describe considerations in physically displaying graphic symbols
- Describe commonly encountered error patterns in matching-to-sample activities
- Describe procedures to address nonidentity matching
- Describe the importance of addressing conditional use of newly established communicative skills

▷ KEY TERMS

- ▶ conditional discrimination
- ▶ conditional use

- ▶ matching to sample
  - ▷ delayed matching to sample
  - ▷ identity
  - ▷ nonidentity

- ▶ oddity task
- ▶ simple discrimination
- ▶ stimulus fading
- ▶ stimulus shaping

IMPORTANT DISTINCTIONS IN DISCRIMINATIONS REQUIRED IN BECOMING A COMPETENT GRAPHIC MODE COMMUNICATOR

The chapter begins by reviewing some important concepts that relate to defining, identifying, and remediating component skills of learning graphic symbols.

Simple versus Conditional Discriminations

Two important skills necessary for a child to select specific symbols in reference to specific real-world items include

1. *Simple discrimination*—the ability to distinguish visually between symbols as well as distinguish between the actual items that are to be represented with symbols.

2. *Conditional discrimination*—the ability to choose a symbol under one set of conditions but select an alternative symbol (or refrain from selecting any symbol) under a different set of conditions. For example, the learner demonstrates a conditional discrimination when a ball is offered and he or she selects a matching ball rather than an apple (an alternative choice).

Conditional discriminations with respect to communication involve the ability to forge a one-to-one link between each symbol and its associated referent condition. That is, the learner selects the target symbol (and no other symbol) under some conditions and refrains from selecting the symbol (and may select an alternative symbol) when conditions do not call for the use of the target symbol. For example, requesting assistance with difficult problems to escape the frustration of difficult work but requesting a break from work that can be completed independently but has become tedious.

The ability to distinguish between items (**simple discrimination**) is a critical step in learning conditional discrimination. If a child cannot tell the difference between two symbols or two objects, then he or she will not be able to use symbols to represent events.

Reinforcing the selection of the same item from an array of choices whose position is randomized across selection opportunities is an example of a simple discrimination. For instance, a child needs to be taught to distinguish the color red from other colors. A red apple is presented during assessment. The child is directed to select the red apple. Selecting the apple is reinforced immediately. The interventionist introduces a second item that serves as a distractor (will not represent a correct choice). Once the learner consistently selects the red apple in the presence of other choices, regardless of their positions, the learner is on his or her way to engaging in a simple discrimination. For example, selecting a red apple in the presence of the other colored apples is the only response that results in reinforcement. If the learner maintains the correct selection of the red apple, regardless of the color of the distractors (or their position within the array), then he or she has shown simple discrimination of that color. The conclusion is that the learner can tell red from either yellow or green. It could not be concluded, however, that he or she could discriminate yellow from green. The learner knows which item to select as a result of the reinforcement history, which is sometimes referred to as *reinforcement control*. No instructional cue is required for the learner to demonstrate a simple discrimination.

Selecting a specific symbol from a choice array in response to a specific referent reflects conditional discrimination. This is demonstrated by selecting a specific stimulus (e.g., a picture of red cherries) conditionally on presentation of a specific sample (actual red cherries in this situation) and not on presentation of a different sample (e.g., a red apple). Functionally speaking, the choice item to be selected in a conditional discrimination can change from opportunity to opportunity, conditional on the sample item that is displayed. When the sample (e.g., a bowl of cherries) is presented, a reinforcer follows selection of a picture of cherries and not a picture of an apple; when an apple is presented, a reinforcer follows selec-

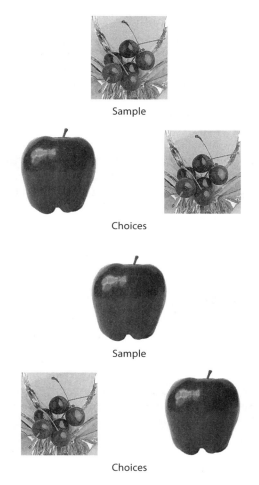

Sample

Choices

Sample

Choices

Figure 8.1. Simple two-real-picture identical matching-to-sample array.

contrast, the correct item on any given opportunity in conditional discrimination is determined by the sample being presented.

Conditional Discrimination and Matching to Sample in Aided Augmentative and Alternative Communication

The mechanics of learning to use a graphic mode communication system depend, in part, on a learner's ability to participate in a variety of conditional discriminations, which is often referred to as matching to sample. For example, a person using a communication board might see a bottle of Coke sitting on a countertop and decide that he or she would like to have it. The beverage would be provided after he or she touched a symbol representing Coca-Cola. The learner matched a real-object sample (i.e., Coke on the counter) and photographic choice (the symbol on the learner's communication board) in this sequence of events.

The previous example involved a specific type of **matching to sample** referred to as simultaneous matching. Both the sample and choices can be viewed at the same time during simultaneous matching. Alternatively, the sample and choice array are not concurrently available in delayed matching. For example, a learner may see a dog (sample) as it runs away. The sample is no longer available for reference when searching for the correct symbol choice (simultaneous/delayed distinction is discussed later in the chapter). Delayed matching is important to communicate about events that are not immediately visible in the learner's environment. A learner must be able to successfully participate in both simultaneous and delayed matching to be a competent communicator (e.g., Deacon, 1997; Romski, Sevcik, & Pate 1988; Savage-Rumbaugh, 1986). For example, consider a learner who might be thirsty. Even though there is no soft drink currently in sight, he or she knows that it is usually available. After seeking out a listener, he or she touches his or her photographic symbol of Sprite, bypassing the Coca-Cola symbol.

tion of a picture of an apple and not a bowl of cherries (see Figure 8.1).

The participant must choose a designated correct item from an array of at least two items in both tasks. Typically, the correct item in a simple discrimination is designated prior to the onset of the task (i.e., based on reinforcement history) and remains the same throughout. A sample is not necessary during a simple discrimination as it was in the conditional discrimination example. Simple discrimination tasks are useful to teach children how to produce a selection response as well as to test their ability to differentiate among choice stimuli. In addition, a simple discrimination task can be used to functionally assess vision acuity. In

Subsequently, if the learner selects the Sprite symbol rather than the Coca-Cola symbol when offered both beverages, then he or she is demonstrating behavioral consistency (and, thus, a conditional discrimination) with his or her original symbol production (choosing the referent that matches the symbol).

Sometimes, significant time elapses between when a communicator observes a sample and actually locates the symbol, which can happen when the user's symbol repertoire is too extensive to be housed on a single fixed display. For example, suppose a learner observes a peer requesting a Coke refill and decides that he or she would also like a refill. After looking at the first page of his or her communication wallet, he or she does not see a Coke symbol. Knowing that he or she has additional pages containing symbols, however, the learner locates the correct page and selects the symbol. Navigation between pages makes this a delayed match, which places an additional demand on attention and memory. The user must keep in mind the target symbol he or she seeks while also 1) inhibiting attention to

and selection of other (nontarget) symbols that appear on the display and 2) recalling on which specific page the symbol appears.

The learner must search through a number of symbols in simultaneous and delayed matching (inhibiting response to all nontarget symbols along the way). The continued availability of the sample in a simultaneous task allows the learner to remind him- or herself of the target at any point during the search. No such reminder prompt is available in delayed matching. Consequently, the learner must not only inhibit responses to potentially appealing nontargets in **delayed matching to sample,** he or she must also keep in mind the specific target being sought.

Describing Levels of Matching to Sample Involving Real Objects and Two-Dimensional Symbols

Keogh and Reichle (1985) described levels of visual matching that apply to both simultaneous and delayed matching (see Figure 8.2). Each level depends on the relationship between samples and choices. These levels

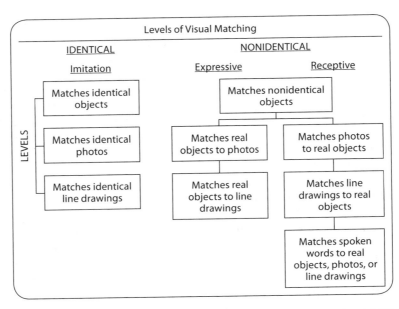

Figure 8.2. Levels of identical and nonidentical matching to sample. (From Reichle, J., York, J., & Sigafoos, J. [1991]. *Implementing augmentative and alternative communication: Strategies for learners with severe disabilities* [p. 205]. Baltimore: Paul H. Brookes Publishing Co.; reprinted by permission.)

separate into two major classes that include **identity** and **nonidentity** matching. Identity matching occurs when the sample and the correct choice are exactly the same. For example, a learner might be taught to match a real red apple sample to a real red apple choice in an array of items that include a red apple, a yellow apple, and a banana. When the learner makes a correct match (i.e., selects the red apple), he or she has engaged in identity matching. The term *identical matching to sample* can be used regardless of the specific form that actual materials take (e.g., pictures, line drawings, real objects). For example, matching a black-and-white line drawing of an apple to its duplicate line drawing in an array containing other black-and-white line-drawn symbol choices (e.g., representing apple, banana, and grape) also constitutes an identity match.

An individual may have learned to match an apple to an apple, a banana to a banana, and grapes to grapes; yet, the learner's selections are unreliable when presented with a new matching set (e.g., lemon to lemon). Such a pattern demonstrates that the learner has not yet acquired generalized identity matching concerning the underlying rule of "pick the one that is identical." Rather, he or she has learned just those specific relations taught (apple, banana, and grapes) through the direct reinforcement history associated with those specific items. Consequently, it is important to assess whether the learner extends his or her performance to previously untaught or new instances of matching. It is possible to begin learning faster and more vicariously from opportunities provided by a natural environment once a learner engages in generalized matching.

A nonidentical matching-to-sample task involves a sample item that differs functionally or perceptually from its choices. Matching an actual red apple sample to a color photographic choice of the same red apple in the presence of other choices that include color photographs of a banana and a grape is an example of nonidentity matching to sample (i.e., the sample apple is an object and the choice is a photograph). A learner

matching a real red apple sample to a real green apple that appeared in an array of choices that included a banana and a pear is another example of nonidentical matching. One (perhaps obvious) aspect of nonidentity matching is that there can be a range of ways in which the sample and the choices resemble or differ from one another. On the one hand, there may be few differences between the sample and the choice. On the other hand, the sample and choice may not resemble each other much. For example, when matching an actual red apple to a photograph of that red object, the two media clearly differ in dimension (the apple is a three-dimensional object, the photograph is a two-dimensional representation), but otherwise share features of physical form (e.g., color). Differences in dimension and color are apparent when matching a real red apple to a black-and-white photograph of that apple. More differences between sample and choices emerge when objects are matched to line drawings or icons, or when photographs and line drawings are matched (see Table 8.1).

Wilkinson and McIlvane (2002) summarized a range of physical differences between samples and choices that can be considered on a continuum, from no differences between sample and comparisons at all (identity matching, described previously), to the presence of some shared features (feature-based matching), to no shared features at all (arbitrary matching). Arbitrary matching tasks are familiar because all comprehension of spoken or written language involves an arbitrary match between a sample stimulus (a spoken or written word; for example, the spoken word *"dog"*) and a referent with which the stimulus shares no physical or other "featural" relation (e.g., the actual dog itself). Some research has suggested that stimuli with more shared features are more readily matched than those with fewer physical similarities (Bloomberg, Karlan, & Lloyd, 1990; Hurlbut, Iwata, & Green, 1982; Mizuko & Reichle, 1989).

It would be easier for the interventionist if all learners passed through similar de-

Table 8.1. Examples of two-dimensional nonidentical items

Sample	Corresponding choices
Color photograph of large red apple	Color photograph of small red apple
Black-and-white photograph of large apple	Color photograph of same-size large red apple
Black-and-white photograph of large apple	Black-and-white line drawing of large apple
Color photograph of large red apple	Color line drawing of large red apple
Color photograph of large red apple	Black-and-white line drawing of large apple
Photograph of large red apple	Photograph of large green apple
Photograph of large red apple	Photograph of small green apple
Photograph of sliced red apple	Photograph of whole red apple
Photograph of sliced red apple	Photograph of whole green apple
Photograph of shoe	Photograph of shoelaces
Photograph of shoe	Photograph of sock
Printed word *apple*	Line drawing of apple
McDonald's golden arches	Big Mac

velopmental sequences in mastering matching. Yet, available evidence addressing the physical similarity in matching suggests that the "hierarchy" is not universal—either across individuals of different social, cultural, or educational experiences or across individuals with and without disabilities (see Stephenson & Linfoot, 1996; Wilkinson & Hennig, 2007; Wilkinson & McIlvane, 2002). Consequently, an organized assessment strategy that samples the possible range of samples and choices should be considered. The next section assumes that a learner cannot match samples and choices at any level. In the next section, a repertoire of matching-to-sample skills is built from the bottom up, presenting intervention across a range of matching-to-sample skills. The procedures and skills can then be chosen and adapted to meet the unique pattern of each individual learner who might show differences in his or her pattern of acquisition of matching-to-sample skills.

ASSESSING SIMPLE DISCRIMINATIONS

A learner must be able to discriminate between different symbols placed on his or her communication display. This section begins with fundamental assessment steps and moves through increasingly more challenging steps.

The ability to discriminate underlies functional communication outcomes. The type of symbols that will be most beneficial is not clear to most learners, however. Early discrimination ability may best be evaluated in a noncommunicative environment using a variety of different potential two- and three-dimensional representations (e.g., product logos, photographs, line drawings [color or black and white]). Helpful steps in implementing a discrimination assessment are described in the following paragraphs.

Steps for assessing simple discriminations

Step 1: Establish a selecting response.
Step 2: Identify reinforcers.
Step 3: Verify the learner can distinguish between items.
Step 4: Implement concurrent assessments to compare the use of a variety of symbol types.

Step 1: Establish a Selecting Response

Evaluating and ensuring that the learner can select an offered choice is the first or perhaps most basic use of simple discrimination tasks. Thus, the interventionist should consider the types of selecting responses that may be available to the learner.

- Many learners will be able to reach for items directly.

- Other learners may only be able to direct eye gaze to an item.

- Some learners will not reach, pick up, or look at a desired item but will walk over and stand beside an item.

Placing the material on the communication board (without delivering any prompt) often results in the learner touching the symbol. If he or she does not initiate a selecting response, then the interventionist can determine the least amount of response prompt that is required to obtain a response approximation. For example, if the learner is directly selecting the symbols using a point, then the interventionist could move through the following prompting hierarchy until the learner responded.

- Point at the item.

- Tap the learner's hand.

- Lift the learner's hand off the table.

- Move the learner's hand in the direction of the item, but let go after a few inches.

- Continue to guide the learner's hand to the material.

If the preceding sequence is implemented across several opportunities, then it should become apparent which prompt is required to obtain learner participation. (See Chapter 5 for additional information addressing prompting strategies.) The interventionist should systematically reduce the prompting level across consecutive opportunities until the learner is responding independently. Reduce the prompt level used as quickly as possible with children who have autism because any prompt can be challenging to fade.

Step 2: Identify Reinforcers

The four-item reinforcer preference assessment sheet allows an instructor to determine which potential reinforcers are more or less preferred by a learner (see Form 8.1 on the accompanying CD-ROM). When various reinforcers are presented repeatedly and in different combinations, the percentage of opportunities on which the learner chooses each one can be calculated.

Step 3: Verify the Learner Can Distinguish Between Items

Once the learner is selecting an item independently, the interventionist can determine if he or she continues to make the same choice in a slightly larger array of two- or three-choice options. The assessor should arrange the two or three items randomly across assessment opportunities while carefully recording the learner's selections as shown on the data sheet in Figure 8.3.

Conducting a discrimination assessment also allows flexibility in the nature of the reinforcing feedback presented. In these initial steps, a reinforcer that is not directly tied to the content of the simple discrimination itself may be used. That is, reinforce a learner's selection of the target item with social reinforcers such as praise ("great job") or tangible reinforcers that are not represented by the symbol. This is different from the kind of feedback provided if the interventionist's goal was to teach a requesting communicative function. In that event, the interventionist would want to be fairly cer-

Trial	Left choice	Right choice
1		
2		
3		
4		
5		
6		
7		
8		

Figure 8.3. Data sheet depicting arrangement of choices in simple discrimination (circled item represents choice selected by learner).

tain that the item offered is actually highly preferred. Treating the learner's selection as a request, however, can complicate the introduction of the second symbol in a conditional discrimination (or matching-to-sample activity). Suppose, for example, that the learner was selecting the initial target item, which confirmed a discrimination skill. To ensure that the learner was able to discriminate based on history of reinforcement, switching the reinforcement so that the selection of what had been the distractor as the new correct response can be difficult unless that item has reinforcement value that is equal to the original target item (i.e., is equally preferred to the learner). This problem can be avoided by using a variety of reinforcers that indicate that the learner has produced a correct response. The process just described is referred to as a reversal. Teaching a learner to be able to switch his or her selection of responses as a function of reinforcement history assists in moving toward teaching conditional discriminations that will be required for a learner to successfully engage in matching to sample.

It may be necessary to once again provide prompts when initially demonstrating the expectations of a reversal to the learner. Once desired responses are produced, the goal is often to maintain the discrimination under more challenging circumstances while at the same time reducing support that may have been required to initially produce the behavior (see Chapter 5 for more information on prompting and prompt lessening).

Step 4: Implement Concurrent Assessments to Compare the Use of a Variety of Symbol Types

It is always challenging to determine which type of symbol to utilize with a beginning communicator (e.g., color photographs, black-and-white photographs, color line drawings). The prospective interventionist can implement concurrent simple discrimination assessments for different symbol types to facilitate the process of identifying

the optimal symbol type. In so doing, one can compare a learner's performance with each of several types of symbols. For example, black-and-white line-drawn symbols could be used in a simple discrimination game during one activity. The game could be played using color photographs during a different time of day. The activity could use color line drawings at another time during the day. By concurrently implementing these activities, the learner's data can be used to make decisions regarding choice of symbol type to use in representing referents instead of making arbitrary choices about which type of symbol to use during intervention opportunities. The simple discrimination worksheet provides the instructor with a model for how to structure an assessment of simple discrimination by the learner (see Form 8.2 on the accompanying CD-ROM). Interventionists can first assess whether the learner can tell the difference between the item and the *foil* or distractor (an item that is displayed in the symbol array that does not represent a response option for the learner) by reinforcing the selection of a target item in the presence of one or more foils. Evaluating the potency of the reinforcement history for altering behavior occurs by implementing reversal. The worksheet offers a model for how to counterbalance the placement of the items.

TEACHING SIMPLE DISCRIMINATIONS

This section outlines a sequence of activities for which there is an evidentiary base supporting their merit in establishing a beginning graphic mode communicative repertoire.

Steps for teaching simple and conditional discriminations

Step 1: Use evidence-based strategies to teach simple discriminations.
Step 2: Use of an oddity (stimulus fading) procedure as a troubleshoot.

Step 1: Use Evidence-Based Strategies to Teach Simple Discriminations

- The interventionist could place an item close to the learner's hand.

- If the learner selects the item across successive correct responses, then the interventionist could systematically move the item further from the learner's hand (requiring an increased effort on the learner's part).

- A correct response would occur during repeated opportunities if the learner chooses the same item that he or she selected during the original opportunity, regardless of the position of the target object and a second object (a distractor that has been added to the array).

- After several opportunities, the interventionist should observe whether the learner has selected the same object consistently (regardless of position). If not, further intervention is required. When the learner reaches toward the incorrect choice, then he or she is immediately interrupted—his or her hand is returned to its starting point. After a brief pause in which there is no opportunity to make a selection, the least intrusive prompt that is required to ensure that the learner selects the target object should be delivered. Subsequently, a reinforcer should be provided immediately.

- The interventionist might choose to refrain from delivering a reinforcer for a prompted response once the learner produces correct choices without a prompt for a prespecified criterion (e.g., during greater than 75% of the opportunities). Ensure that powerful reinforcers are available during this phase of intervention.

- It is important to randomize the placement of the two target items across instructional opportunities.

Some children may not be successful with simple discrimination, even when implemented systematically. For example, the learner could have a significant visual impairment. Alternatively, the reinforcer might not be sufficiently powerful to make it worth engaging in a discriminative response. Finally, the task may not be sufficiently clear to allow the learner to acquire the discrimination, in spite of what seems like small discriminable steps in the implemented procedure. Interventionists must consider these possibilities and assess them directly in children who fail to show reliable simple discrimination learning.

After the learner consistently selects the same item that has been associated with reinforcement regardless of its placement, the interventionist can begin applying the reinforcer to the selection of a different item in the array. This is done to begin to ensure that selections are based on the association of reinforcement with a particular item. Often learners with more severe disabilities have difficulty making this transition. Once the learner has shifted to selecting the new item associated with reinforcement, the interventionist may switch the reinforcer back so that it is once again associated with the original item. These "reinforcement reversals" are aimed at ensuring learner attention to surrounding contingencies and also ensure that learners are less likely to perseverate in the same selection.

Step 2: Use of an Oddity (Stimulus Fading) Procedure as a Troubleshoot

The interventionist might consider using an **oddity task** as an alternative to the strategy in Step 1. The learner selects the one stimulus that is unlike all of the others during an oddity task. For instance, a child might be presented with eight balls and a butterfly (see Figure 8.4). The butterfly is the "odd" stimulus presented within a set of balls. The hypothesis is that the structure of the stimulus array itself should prompt the viewer's attention to the odd outstanding (target) stimulus. Eight butterflies and one ball would be delivered during the next instructional opportunity.

After arranging the symbols, the interventionist would deliver an instruction such as "find it." It may be necessary the first several times to deliver a more intrusive prompt to assist in demonstrating to the learner his or her role in participating in the task. Try to minimize the use of prompts, however, and allow the learner enough time to make an independent selection without the need for a prompt.

In our example in Figure 8.4, the location of the butterfly within the array would vary across opportunities, and the learner's role would be to locate that same butterfly every time. Across consecutive opportunities, the position of the target item within the array is randomized across consecutive opportunities. The advantage of randomizing the location of choice stimuli during simple discrimination is that it avoids the learner attending to the position of the choices as a cue for responding.

The interventionist should systematically begin reducing the number of identical choices (see Figure 8.5) once the learner is consistently selecting the correct item, regardless of position or the actual choice involved. Initially, one duplicate choice should be removed, leaving seven identical symbols and the target symbol. If the learner continues to make correct selections, then one item should be removed at a time until there are only three symbols remaining—the target symbol and two of the other choice symbols. If the learner continues to respond correctly, then he or she is on his or her way to discriminating between the two objects.

> ### What Does the Research Say?
> #### Oddity Procedures
>
> Soraci, Deckner, Baumeister, and Carlin (1990) described work in which there were repeated failures of typically developing preschool-age children as well as individuals with intellectual disabilities to perform correctly on oddity reversals when three elements were presented (two butterflies and a ball or two balls and a butterfly). Soraci et al. (1987, 1990) argued that this failure might be related to a lower sensitivity on the part of chronologically and developmentally younger individuals to contrast the necessary features (in shape, in this case). This argument was supported by studies in which the number of identical nonodd stimuli was increased from two to eight (Soraci, Alpler, Deckner, & Blanton, 1983; Soraci et al., 1987). This structural alteration to the stimulus display was designed to enhance the perceptual salience of the odd stimulus. Children who had failed to perform oddity or oddity reversals when there were three elements (i.e., one odd, two nonodd) showed reliable oddity-based selections when there were nine elements (i.e., one odd, eight non-odd). Furthermore, many children showed successful oddity performance when they were subsequently presented with the smaller array of three elements. It appeared that the increased salience of the odd stimulus under the nine-element condition allowed transfer of oddity performance back to the original format.

Oddity tasks have been used to teach matching to sample but, for the most part, have not been reported as a

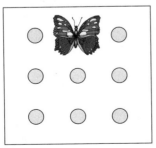

Simple vs. conditional discrimination

Figure 8.4.   Oddity stimulus fading task.

Opportunity 1   Opportunity 2

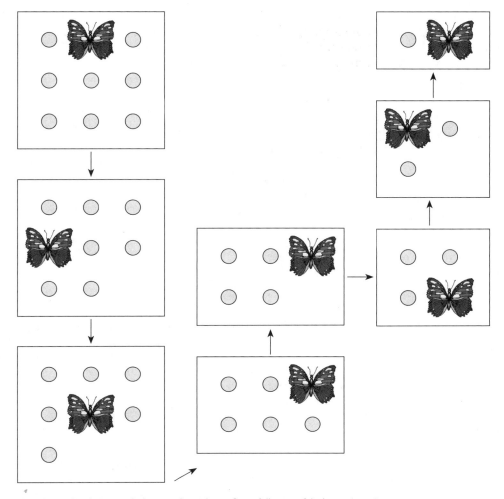

Figure 8.5. Displaying symbols across the grids to reflect a full range of the learner's motion.

CONDITIONAL DISCRIMINATION: IDENTITY MATCHING

The interventionist can begin introducing symbol choices whose selection is conditional on a particular sample after a learner is successful with simple discrimination tasks. For example, when the learner sees a sample photograph of a cat, an opportunity is created to select an identical photograph of a cat displayed in an array of choices. When the learner sees a sample consisting of a photograph of a dog, he or she should select the identical photograph of a dog displayed among available choices.

Moving from Simple Discrimination to Conditional Discrimination: Adding a Sample

Thus far the learner has been engaging in a simple discrimination between two or three items. This next step is intended to teach the learner that it is necessary to obtain the instructional cue from the sample in a matching-to-sample task in order to determine which choice to select. Eventually, the samples, as well as the choices, should be presented randomly. It might be helpful to begin with a variation on this randomization, however, with learners who find this task difficult.

Adding a Sample to the Oddity Task

The oddity task can be implemented to teach conditional discrimination in children who may have a history of failing with more traditional instructional strategies. It is important to note that on some occasions the butterfly (from our previous example) would serve as the sample with an array of multiple balls and one butterfly as choices. During other opportunities, the ball would be the sample with an array of a single ball and multiple butterflies as the choices.

☞ *Helpful Hint*

The following option may be helpful with learners who struggle with the randomization of samples across instructional opportunities.

- Instead of randomizing both samples and choices, randomize only the choices in the array. The same sample should be used during each of the first three instructional opportunities.

- The remaining item should be used as the sample during the next three opportunities. This presentation format is referred to as blocking. The sample object should be placed in front of the learner when presenting an instructional opportunity. Once the learner has looked at it, the two choice objects can be placed between the learner and the sample. Then, attention can be directed to the sample (i.e., by pointing) with the instruction, "Find one like this."

- If the learner begins to reach for an incorrect choice, then his or her response should be interrupted and his or her hands returned to the starting position.

- Impose a delay after an incorrect response to attempt to avoid the learner getting into a chained response pattern in which the learner selects one choice on some irrelevant basis. If incorrect, he or she immediately selects the remaining choice.

    Subsequently, the least intrusive prompt that is required to have the learner select the correct choice can be delivered, followed by delivery of a reinforcer.

    The response prompt can be faded systematically across opportunities.

The interventionist can systematically move from blocking to an increasingly random presentation pattern of choices once the learner is performing consistently in the blocked condition. The interventionist may choose not to reinforce prompted instructional opportunities once the learner is performing independently at a level above chance.

In addition to an oddity task, errorless instructional strategies relying on stimulus prompts can be utilized (see Chapter 5). Several of those prompting strategies will be briefly summarized next.

ADDRESSING NONIDENTITY MATCHING TO SAMPLE

A learner engages in nonidentity matching to sample when he or she sees an item of interest in the natural environment and subsequently selects a symbol that represents it. If an explicit symbol had been introduced in the previous procedure, then the learner would have needed to be able to engage in nonidentity matching to sample to be successful. The real item in which the learner indicated interest would become the sample. The choice array would be the array of symbols on the learner's graphic mode communication display. Correspondingly, suppose that a learner requested using the MILK symbol. Subsequently, his or her mother brought milk and orange juice, and the learner selected the milk. In this example, the learner engaged in nonidentity matching. Nonidentity matching can occur with either objects (e.g., red apple/green apple), with objects and two-dimensional items (e.g., red apple and photograph of red apple), or with two-dimensional items (e.g., photograph of red apple and photograph of green apple). A wide variety of nonidentity matching options exist (e.g., photograph of red apple, black-and-white line drawing of apple) because there are many types of two-dimensional representations. Of course, the most important nonidentity match for a beginning communicator involves real-object samples and the type of symbol that is to be used to represent symbol choices for that individual learner. The following assessment process is useful in teaching the learner to successfully engage in nonidentity matching. Assume the learner has mastered identity matching using a wide variety of two- and three-dimensional items.

Determining Whether the Learner Can Generalize from Identity to Nonidentity Matching

Samples in this assessment consist of two different examples used in an identity-matching program that the learner successfully completed. The choice array could consist of two items that correspond to each of the samples selected. They should represent stimuli associated with a different level of matching, however. For example, if the samples are real objects, then the choices might be color photographs. The interventionist should remember that the primary objective during a non–identity-matching task is to determine whether the learner can match a real object to its representation. The position of the items in the choice array and the presentation of samples will be randomized during the assessment. Participation will be reinforced during this assessment, but no feedback will be given for correctness of response.

If the learner was unsuccessful in the assessment just described, then the interventionist may wish to consider implementing non–identity-matching intervention using items for which the differences between the sample and the choices is not as dramatic. For example, suppose that a real red apple was used as the sample item and a photograph of a small green apple served as the corresponding choice. If the learner was unsuccessful, then the interventionist may wish to repeat the assessment using the same real red apple and an equal-size high-quality colored photograph of the red apple instead of a photograph of a small green apple. In addition to teaching the use of photographs as

graphic symbols, the interventionist may concurrently teach the learner to match real objects to line-drawn symbols, given that many commercially available symbol dictionaries utilize color or black-and-white line drawings.

If the learner did well matching real objects to line drawings, then the interventionist may determine whether the learner can engage in matching symmetry, in which samples and choices are juxtaposed. For example, the learner touches a symbol representing "apple" in self-initiating a communicative request. Symmetry is important in providing the learner the flexibility in not only producing graphic symbols but also comprehending them. In addition, it may be an important parameter in verifying that the learner is matching symbols to objects when the learner initiates the use of graphic symbols. For example, assume that a request has been made at a family style snack time with apples, oranges, and banana slices in the center of the table. Having selected the apple symbol, the interventionist responds, "Go ahead and take some." In this scenario, the symbol serves as the sample and the real objects serve as choices (a reversal of the matching task during assessment). Some learners with significant developmental disabilities have difficulty with matching symmetry. Sometimes they appear to produce more accurate responses when the more abstract representation serves as a choice compared with it serving as a sample. Consequently, it may be helpful to ensure matching symmetry in order to ensure initiated communicative production using symbols.

The conditional discrimination worksheet with symmetry testing offers a model of how to conduct an assessment of conditional matching-to-sample performance (see Form 8.3 on the accompanying CD-ROM). The sheet demonstrates the counterbalancing of the positions of the choices in the initial block and then the reversal of the positions of the samples and the choices in the symmetry trials. This model can be extended to provide more trials, where necessary. When using this worksheet to address simple discriminations, remember that no samples are presented—only choices.

Stimulus shaping is one option for teaching nonidentity matching that involves serial changes made to the target or correct stimulus. This application of stimulus shaping is much like an animated "morphing," in which the matching task initially starts out as an identity-matching task. The physical features of the target choice (but not the sample) are gradually altered over a series of steps. Correct matching should be maintained if the alteration is systematically accomplished in small incremental steps. Carr, Wilkinson, Blackman, and McIlvane (2000) described the successful use of such a shaping procedure to establish relations between line drawings and written word symbols in individuals with significant intellectual disabilities.

ADDRESSING RESPONSE BIASES THAT CAN EMERGE IN SIMPLE AND CONDITIONAL DISCRIMINATION TASKS

Position and item biased response patterns are two of the more common error patterns produced by beginning communication system users. Each pattern will be briefly described, followed by some potential troubleshooting ideas to implement should problems occur.

Position Bias Responding Pattern

Position bias responding occurs when the learner selects a symbol choice based on its position rather than on its functional and/or perceptual characteristics with reference to the sample. Guessing will result in the learner being correct half of the time in a two-choice symbol array that has been used in the examples. If the learner simply chooses to touch the same location and the interventionist is doing a good job of randomizing the symbol choices, then he or she will be positively reinforced during 50% of the teaching opportunities. Depending on how powerful the reinforcer happens to be, a schedule of reinforcement that, on average, pays off every second opportunity may be sufficient to maintain a position bias response strategy. Here are several strategies to eliminate it.

For example, suppose that the learner has been consistently selecting the choice on the right.

- One option is to move a proportionately greater number of the correct choices to the position opposite the learner's position bias. The interventionist can begin to equalize the array as soon as the learner begins to make choices independently to the side opposite his or her bias.

- A second strategy is for the interventionist to make the position bias response strategy not pay off as handsomely. By significantly decreasing the magnitude of reinforcement for each correct response, the learner may become less interested in selecting only choices on the right. That is, the learner may need to focus on a more efficient strategy than position bias to obtain more frequently delivered reinforcement.

- A third strategy involves increasing the number of symbol choices resulting in a leaner schedule of reinforcement. For example, a position bias response strategy in a four-choice array will result in obtaining the reinforcer during 25% of the instructional opportunities.

The interventionist should do the following each time the learner begins to make a selection in accordance with his or her position bias with any of the strategies described.

- Interrupt the incorrect response as soon as possible and return the learner to a starting position.

- Impose a brief waiting period.

- Deliver the least intrusive prompt that is required for the learner to select the matching symbol. Prompted opportunities should not be reinforced.

- Impose another brief waiting period after this teaching opportunity.

- The sample or choice should not be re-randomized for the very next opportunity (which is actually error correction on the incorrect teaching opportunity). Instead, the teaching opportunity should be repeated to see if the learner can respond independently on the second correction opportunity.

- The interventionist could randomize the choices and proceed to the next opportunity once the learner receives reinforcement for a nonprompted response.

- The latency between a prompted and a repeated opportunity should be increased across opportunities to promote more independent responding.

- Alternatively, the magnitude of the response prompt should be reduced systematically during prompted opportunities.

Item Bias Responding Pattern

An item bias response pattern occurs when the learner consistently selects the same item in a choice array, regardless of the sample. Item bias responses often develop in the initial phases of intervention programs designed to teach the learner to request desired objects. The interventionist often selects the most preferred item to use in teaching an initial requesting response. Subsequently, the learner continues to select the initial item taught when the second symbol to be introduced is not as reinforcing as the first. Several strategies can be implemented to decrease the probability of an item bias responding pattern emerging.

- Implement teaching opportunities for less preferred items after the learner has become satiated on the most powerful reinforcer. Although challenging to implement, this will result in other items and activities being relatively more reinforcing during this period of satiation. Unfortunately, it may be relatively

challenging to provide sufficient access to result in satiation, depending on the learner's preference for the item. Consequently, it is important to have other strategies available.

- Mark the symbol to make it more discriminable to the learner during particular times, even if the learner selects the symbol. For example, selecting a highly preferred symbol in some contexts will never be reinforced, whereas selecting it will be fairly consistently reinforced in other contexts. For example, requesting a pudding at snack time will be reinforced, but selecting it during an academic activity will never be reinforced. Many learners come to discriminate the context in which selecting the pudding symbol pays off as well as learning the contexts in which selecting the same symbol will not pay off.

Ensuring that the learner can match symbols to a sample (instructional cue) once he or she can discriminate between symbols is the basis for using a graphic mode communication system (the learner sees an object or event in the environment [sample] and selects a symbol [choice] to use to communicate with a social partner). Demonstrating graphic symbol comprehension and production requires that the learner engages in conditional discriminations.

What follows is a description of how to get the process of nonidentity matching started in the context of a beginning program to teach an initial symbol selection in the presence of a nonidentical symbol choice using stimulus building and stimulus fading.

Instructional Procedures that Rely on Stimulus Prompts

Instructional strategies that will likely reduce errors and corresponding frustration are available for children who have difficulty learning to match to sample. These strategies represent stimulus prompting strategies in which the goal of the procedure is to establish discrimination (simple or conditional) under a simple set of circumstances and maintain the discrimination as it becomes increasingly more challenging in the absence of errors.

Stimulus Shaping

Stimulus shaping is one primary technique used in stimulus prompting procedures. The goal in stimulus shaping (sometimes referred to as *stimulus building*) is to begin by making the selection of a choice easy. The interventionist systematically increases the challenge provided by distractors once that response has been established.

Figure 8.6 depicts an example of a choice array during the implementation of a stimulus-shaping procedure. In this example, the distractor (symbol that the learner should refrain from selecting) is gradually built while the placement of the two symbols in the choice array is randomized.

Stimulus Fading

The goal in **stimulus fading** is for the symbol to change in appearance without decreasing the probability that the learner would select it in response to the presentation of a nonidentical sample. Stimulus building is being applied to the car while stimulus fading is concurrently applied to the pineapple in Figure 8.6. These two strategies can be combined with response prompts in teaching a learner a beginning requesting skill. The steps for this procedure follow.

- Place three reinforcing objects on a tray.
- A single two-dimensional graphic symbol (e.g., for "want") should be placed in front of the learner with no other symbols in the array. This symbol should be between the tray of items and the learner. A large symbol containing the printed word *want* can be used. This word should be maximally discriminable from any graphic chosen to subsequently represent specific items.

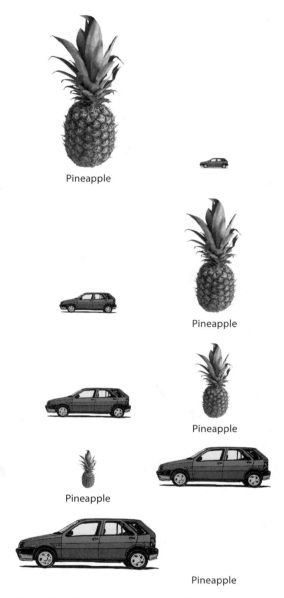

Pineapple

Pineapple

Pineapple

Pineapple

Pineapple

Figure 8.6. Example of choice array used in a stimulus-shaping procedure.

- Begin to move the tray to the learner. As he or she reaches for the tray, deliver a response prompt so that his or her hand contacts the symbol.
- Release the learner's hand as the tray is moved closer, allowing him or her to select the item of his or her choice.

- Fade the level of response prompt used across successive opportunities to ensure that he or she touches the symbol (see Chapter 5 for a discussion of the range of response prompts).

- The placement of the symbol should be randomized so that sometimes it is directly in front of the learner and sometimes it is positioned to his or her right or left (to avoid position bias). In addition, the positions of the items on the tray that is offered should be randomized.

- A distractor can be introduced once the learner is independently selecting the target symbol. Across successive opportunities, it can be systematically made more challenging via stimulus building to become increasingly more competitive with the target symbol for the learner's attention.

- More explicit symbols can be added to the array once the learner is selecting the target symbol. For example, as the distractor grows larger (stimulus building), the target symbol which, originally, was substantially enlarged, can grow smaller (stimulus fading).

- If a more explicit symbol was initially chosen to implement, then the tray of items from which the learner was shown in the first step of the procedure would have been eliminated. Instead, the learner would have been allowed to sample each of several desired items. The item for which the learner showed the most interest would have been selected. A symbol representing that item would have been made available. At this point, the initial step of the procedure described at the beginning of this section would be implemented.

- Stimulus fading on the target symbol and stimulus building on the distractor would continue to proceed across successful opportunities. If two symbols were taught concurrently, then each of the two different symbols and corresponding referents used in the matching task would have been implemented.

ENSURING CONDITIONAL USE OF SYMBOLS

Numerous situations exist in which conditional uses of symbols are important (see Chapter 1 for additional discussion of conditional use of communicative behavior). For example, a learner should request assistance only when he or she has encountered a situation that he or she cannot competently address on his or her own. If the learner overused a communicative intent such as an assistance request, then it could jeopardize his or her opportunity to learn to perform more independently. Suggestions to address when learners fail to use newly acquired communicative skills conditionally follow.

Consistently Deliver Consequences for Symbol Selection

Interventionists must be consistent in consequating the learner's symbol use. If there are contexts where it is unacceptable to deliver reinforcers, then it is important that the learner refrains from selecting the corresponding symbols. Suppose that a learner has the book and yogurt symbols on his or her aided communication display. Selecting the book symbol during mealtime would result in the book not being delivered, whereas selecting the yogurt symbol would result in the delivery of yogurt. In this context, the learner should refrain from selecting the book symbol because requesting yogurt would represent a viable response option. Even though books are more powerful reinforcers than yogurt, the yogurt symbol is more likely to be selected during mealtime because, in effect, the book symbol "does not work" during meals. Alternatively, the learner should be consistently reinforced for choosing the book symbol in situations where it is appropriate to use the book symbol (e.g., playtime, free time).

Provide a Differential Signal that a Symbol Selection Will Not Be Reinforced During Specified Activities

There are times and places where certain items can't be made available. For example, one cannot smoke in a "no smoking" section of a restaurant or eat a candy bar in the middle of a religious service. Unfortunately, some learners have difficulty self-regulating their behavior to refrain from gaining access to reinforcers at socially unacceptable times or places. This problem may be exacerbated when a visual representation of the reinforcer is displayed on a learner's aided communication system. One strategy is to make the availability or unavailability of a reinforcer reflected in the status of symbols that are available to the learner. The symbol could be displayed on the learner's symbol array during activities in which it is acceptable to request a particular item or event. Alternatively, a line may be placed through the symbol indicating that its use cannot be honored during a particular activity.

Intervention strategies addressing the conditional use of new communicative forms and functions represent a topic that has not been addressed extensively in the communication intervention literature. Combined with generalization, however, conditional discrimination represents an extremely important skill that influences whether the learner can functionally use newly acquired communication skills across a range of naturally occurring contexts. This topic is addressed in other chapters with respect to establishing specific communicative functions (see Chapters 9, 10, and 11 for additional procedural information).

CONSIDERATIONS IN PHYSICALLY DISPLAYING GRAPHIC SYMBOLS ONCE A SIMPLE DISCRIMINATION HAS BEEN ESTABLISHED

Numerous concerns must be considered in teaching the initial discriminations required to use graphic symbols, including symbol size, the space required between symbols on a display, the surface area that can be used in a fixed-symbol display, whether the learner can open a booklike fixed display, and bias in responding patterns. Consider the symbol arrangement on the display once the learner has demonstrated that he or she is capable of discriminating between symbols.

Determining the Size of Each Symbol on the Display

Learners should be evaluated by a competent ophthalmologist to determine ocular health and vision acuity. Other tasks can be implemented, however, to glean some general information regarding the size of symbol that might be required for the learner to discriminate among symbols successfully. Initially, present simple discrimination tasks with very large choices that rest approximately 10–12 inches from the bridge of the learner's nose. The size of the entire array of symbols can be decreased systematically across successive successful opportunities until significantly more errors are produced than when the symbols were at their largest size. The interventionist can gain a rough idea of the size of symbol from which the learner might benefit by using a copy machine that systematically reduces the size of symbols.

Determining the Space Required Between Symbols on a Display

Determining the optimal symbol size from which the learner may benefit is helpful, but this alone is not sufficient to determine symbol placement. If the learner has a precise pointing response, then it may be possible to place the symbols edge to edge. The symbols may need to be placed further apart when the learner tends to produce a less precise point (of course, an alternative is using an orthotic). The following steps are useful in determining the placement of symbols once the optimal size has been identified.

- Place six symbols edge to edge. The size of each symbol is dictated by the preceding assessment.

- Provide the learner with an opportunity to select the target symbol. Carefully note the learner's response.

  Is there any ambiguity in his or her pointing or touching the target symbol?

  Would an individual who is unfamiliar with the learner have any difficulty determining which symbol had been selected?

If the answer to these questions is yes, then the interventionist should move the symbols apart so that there is slightly more space between each symbol and repeat the opportunity. This process should continue until the symbols are sufficiently far apart that it is easy to determine which symbol the learner selected.

Determining the Surface Area That Can Be Used in a Fixed-Symbol Display

The interventionist can explore the surface area that may be available to display symbols once the size and the spacing of symbols have been addressed. This will help the interventionist determine how many symbols can be displayed before considering implementing a more dynamic symbol display. Assuming that the learner has completed the size and spacing of symbols tasks, the following steps are useful in determining the surface area to be used in setting up a fixed-symbol display.

- The interventionist should place each of the six symbols that were used in the previous assessment in one of the nine equal areas that cover the range of the available surface area on the display being considered.

- Each area within the grid should be sampled. Initially, the six symbols should be sequentially placed in each of the nine locations with the learner asked to find one or two symbols in each of the nine areas. Subsequently, the interventionist

should compare the learner performance across the areas of the display.

Determining Whether the Learner Can Open a Book-like Fixed Display

Creating a communication display that can be open to display two pages rather than one (i.e., like a book) is one strategy to increase the surface area for a fixed-symbol display. The following can be used to determine whether the learner can 1) open a larger display and 2) can use displays in which pages are sequentially displayed.

- Create a sequential two-page display of the communication aid that you have selected for the learner.

- Obtain the learner's attention and allow him or her to see the potential reinforcer placed inside the folded display. Next, offer the closed display to the learner to see if he or she can open the display. Sometimes learners have difficulty getting their fingers under the page to open it. If this is the case, then "page fluffers" (inserts between pages) may allow the learner to get his or her hand under the page to open it without having to use a pincer grasp.

Reichle and Brown (1986) described a procedure to teach a learner to sequentially turn pages in a communicative display.

FINAL CONSIDERATIONS

An important rule for interventionists is to avoid making unwarranted assumptions, such as the following two myths:

- *Myth:* It does not matter which material serves as the sample and which material serves as the choice array (symmetry of matching) in matching to sample.

In fact, research has demonstrated that learning can be facilitated or disrupted depending on the choice of sample and comparison stimulus sets. Brady and Saunders (1998) reported a study with one participant with severe intellectual disabilities learning relations between objects and abstract visual-graphic symbols called lexigrams. Visually, lexigrams are composed of specific features (e.g., circles, rectangles, horizontal lines) superimposed on one another. The participant did not demonstrate behavior consistent with learning when a lexigram served as the sample and objects were the choices. Learning proceeded readily, however, when the lexigrams were the choices and the object served as sample. Brady and Saunders' work would suggest that initially presenting the less discriminable (i.e., more difficult) stimuli as choices facilitates learning, perhaps because the learner can examine the visually difficult stimuli together (i.e., simultaneously). The advantages of simultaneous discrimination over successive presentation for learning have received empirical support for quite some time (see, e.g., Saunders, Williams, & Spradlin, 1996).

- *Myth:* If a learner associates a spoken word and an object and the spoken word and a symbol (e.g., photograph, line drawing), then he or she will naturally demonstrate understanding that the symbol and the object relate to one another (i.e., transitivity of relations learned through matching to sample).

Although perhaps surprising, some individuals with developmental disabilities (and even young children who are typically developing) sometimes fail to demonstrate either simple symmetric relation and/or transitivity relations (cf. Pilgrim & Jackson, 2000). Consequently, the interventionist should test for these untaught relations directly to confirm their emergence. Wilkinson and McIlvane (2001) argued that these emergent relations serve to demonstrate simple forms of early categories and, thus, are important evidence on an individual basis that a learner is not simply producing rote-learned associative behaviors. It can be argued that the learner has acquired simple word categories with the demonstration of such symmetric and transitive relations.

SUMMARY

This chapter covered a wide-ranging set of concepts concerning the relationships between different kinds of stimuli, including graphic stimuli used on a communication board. The chapter introduced important terminology, particularly the notions of simple and conditional discriminations between stimuli, and offered practical hints for assessing and teaching relevant skills. Although some learners will effortlessly demonstrate the constituent skills that were covered in this chapter, others may struggle with some or all of them. For those learners, breaking the communication task into small constituent parts can be a productive means by which challenges are identified.

The chapter reviewed the ways in which a communicative event relies on matching behaviors; for instance, a learner must be able to match the symbol representation on his or her display with the real-world item being referenced in order to use a graphic symbol to successfully request or comment on a specific item. This seemingly simple behavior actually involves a fairly complex matching task in which the symbol representation and the real-world referent do not share many, if any, physical attributes. Such a match is called either a feature match (if some attributes are shared) or an arbitrary match (if no attributes are shared). If a learner fails to demonstrate reliable symbol use in this way, then identify the source of the challenge by assessing whether the learner understands the relationships involved. The chapter identified variables involved in the learner's ability to produce a reliable response, engage in simple discrimination of the stimuli him- or herself, and discriminate among stimuli conditionally on the presence of a sample (conditional discrimination) or under appropriate contextual conditions (conditional use).

Initially, a simple discrimination task was addressed as a way to establish a learner's single response to a specified target in order to receive reinforcement. Simple discrimination tasks are also useful to determine the psychoperceptual capabilities of learners.

Focus on conditional discrimination abilities once simple discriminations are assessed and/or taught because these make up the bulk of communication acts. Practical means for assessing and teaching conditional discrimination among stimuli were reviewed. Simply teaching the production of symbols is not sufficient, however, as the learner must also become aware of the contextually appropriate times for those productions. A variety of stimulus prompting techniques were addressed. Finally, problems that can occur in establishing simple and conditional discriminations and possible troubleshoots for these challenges were discussed.

Establishing visual discriminations represents the crux of the challenge in teaching beginning communicators to effectively use aided communication systems. This chapter addressed a number of strategies that can be helpful in better equipping interventionists to establish these skills, even among the most challenging to teach learners.

REFERENCES

Bloomberg, K., Karlan, G.R., & Lloyd, L.L. (1990). The comparative translucency of initial lexical items represented in five graphic symbol systems and sets. *Journal of Speech and Hearing Research, 33,* 717–725.

Brady, N., & Saunders, K. (1998). Considerations in the effective teaching of object to symbol matching. *Augmentative and Alternative Communication, 7,* 137–151.

Carr, D., Wilkinson, K.M., Blackman, D., & McIlvane, W.J. (2000). Equivalence classes in individuals with minimal verbal repertoires. *Journal of the Experimental Analysis of Behavior, 74,* 101–115.

Deacon, T. (1997). *The symbolic species the co-evolution of language and the brain.* New York: Columbia University Press.

Hurlbut, B., Iwata, B., & Green, J. (1982). Nonvocal language acquisition in adolescents with severe physical disabilities: Bliss symbol versus iconic stimulus formats. *Journal of Applied Behavior Analysis, 15,* 241–258.

Keogh, W., & Reichle, J. (1985). Communication intervention for "difficult to teach" severely handicapped. In S. Warren & A. Rogers-Warren (Eds.), *Language intervention: Vol. IX. Teaching functional language: Generalization and maintenance of language skills* (pp. 157–194). Baltimore: University Park Press.

Mizuko, M., & Reichle, J. (1989). Transparency and recall of symbols among intellectually handicapped adults. *Journal of Speech and Hearing Disorders, 54,* 627–633.

Pilgrim, C., & Jackson, J. (2000). Acquisition of arbitrary conditional discriminations by young normally developing children. *Journal of the Experimental Analysis of Behavior, 73,* 177–193.

Reichle, J., & Brown, L. (1986). Teaching the use of a multi-page direct selection communication board to an adult with autism. *Journal of The Association for Persons with Severe Handicaps, 11,* 68-73.

Reichle, J., York, J., & Sigafoos, J. (1991). *Implementing augmentative and alternative communication: Strategies for learners with severe disabilities.* Baltimore: Paul H. Brookes Publishing Co.

Romski, M., Sevcik, R., & Pate, J. (1988). Establishment of symbolic communication in persons with severe retardation. *Journal of Speech and Hearing Disorders, 53,* 94–107.

Saunders, K.J., Williams, D.C., & Spradlin, J.E. (1996). Derived stimulus control: Are there differences among procedures and processes? In T.R. Zentall & P.M. Smeets (Eds.), *Stimulus class formation in humans and animals* (pp. 93–109). New York: Elsevier Science.

Savage-Rumbaugh, S. (1986). *Ape language: From conditioned response to symbol.* New York: Columbia University Press.

Soraci, S., Alpler, V., Deckner, C., & Blanton, R. (1983). Oddity performance and the perception of relational information. *Psychologia, 26,* 175–184.

Soraci, S., Deckner, C., Baumeister, A., & Carlin, M. (1990). Attentional functioning and relational learning. *American Journal on Mental Retardation, 95(3),* 304–315.

Soraci, S., Deckner, C., Haenlein, M., Baumeister, A., Murata-Soraci, K., & Blanton, R. (1987). Oddity performance in preschool children at risk for mental retardation: Transfer and maintenance. *Research in Developmental Disabilities, 8,* 137–151.

Stephenson, J., & Linfoot, K. (1996). Pictures as communication symbols for students with severe intellectual disability. *Augmentative and Alternative Communication, 12,* 244–256.

Wilkinson, K.M., & Hennig, S. (2007). State of the art and current recommended practice in augmentative and alternative communication. *Mental Retardation and Developmental Disabilities Research Reviews, 13,* 58–69.

Wilkinson, K.M., & McIlvane, W.J. (2001). Methods for studying symbolic behavior and category formation: Contributions of stimulus equivalence research. *Developmental Review, 21,* 355–374.

Wilkinson, K.M., & McIlvane, W.J. (2002). Considerations in teaching graphic symbols to beginning communicators. In D. Beukelman & J. Reichle (Series Eds.) & J. Reichle, D.R. Beukelman, & J.C. Light (Vol. Eds.), *AAC series: Exemplary practices for beginning communicators: Implications for AAC* (pp. 273–322). Baltimore: Paul H. Brookes Publishing Co.

Gaining Access to Desired Objects and Activities

Susan S. Johnston and Joan Schumann

▷ CHAPTER OVERVIEW

In addition to providing a way to obtain preferred and needed objects/activities, requesting provides a method of exerting control over the environment. This chapter builds on the information provided in previous chapters by focusing on procedures that are effective for establishing functional communication to gain access to desired objects/activities. Procedures are described for teaching requests to obtain and maintain contact with objects/activities, establish or maintain engagement in activities, and obtain assistance. A summary of the research related to teaching these functions to individuals with severe disabilities illustrates the evidence base supporting each procedure, and case studies illustrating the application of these procedures are discussed.

▷ CHAPTER OBJECTIVES

After studying this chapter, readers will be able to

- Identify whether an augmentative and alternative communication (AAC) user might benefit from interventions designed to teach the variety of **requests for objects/activities, requests for continued engagement** in an activity, and **requests for assistance**

- Describe strategies for teaching AAC users with severe disabilities to use a variety of requests

- Describe the evidence base supporting the implementation of strategies described to teach AAC users with severe disabilities to request objects/activities, continued engagement, and assistance

▷ KEY TERMS

- conditional use of communication
- general case instruction

- request for assistance
- request for continued engagement

- request for objects/activities

WHY TEACH AAC LEARNERS TO GAIN ACCESS TO DESIRED OBJECTS AND ACTIVITIES?

It is necessary to understand why it is important to teach requesting before describing strategies and procedures for teaching AAC users with severe disabilities to gain access to desired objects/activities (via requests for objects/activities, assistance, or continued engagement). Reichle and Sigafoos (1991) suggested that teaching requesting

- Provides a way to obtain access to preferred objects/activities

- Provides a way to obtain access to needed objects/activities

- Provides a way to exert a measure of control over the environment

- Incorporates the receipt of preferred items/activities into the intervention (which may facilitate the success of future interventions)

- Replaces existing access- or attention-motivated challenging behaviors

Requests for objects/activities are often one of the first social-communicative functions taught to AAC users with severe disabilities.

TEACHING COMMUNICATION TO REQUEST ACCESS TO NEEDED OBJECTS/ACTIVITIES

Consider when it will (and will not) be acceptable and/or feasible to honor (reinforce) the request when teaching individuals with severe disabilities to request objects/activities; this teaches the learner to use the communication conditionally (e.g., teaching an individual when he or she should and should not engage in the requesting behavior). The interventionist should consider using strategies that better assist the learner in self-regulating his or her own behavior in contexts in which it is not appropriate to reinforce a request (see Reichle & Johnston, 2006, and Johnston & Reichle, 1993, for a discussion of strategies for teaching learners to self-regulate).

If it is possible to honor (reinforce) the request, then an intervention strategy designed to teach the AAC user to request can proceed. Once a decision has been made to teach an AAC user to request, the next question concerns which specific requesting function(s) to teach. Table 9.1 summarizes the communicative acts that may be appropriate for a given situation.

Numerous studies have demonstrated the effectiveness of requesting intervention strategies using AAC. Participants ranged from preschoolers to adults, had a variety of identified disabilities, and utilized a variety of AAC devices. The majority of the research has been implemented in school settings. The effective use of procedures, however, has also been demonstrated in home and community settings. Although most research has been implemented to teach requests for objects/activities, effective strategies for teaching requests for assistance and continued engagement have also been documented.

What Does the Research Say?

Teaching Requests

A significant body of research has demonstrated effective strategies to teach requesting using AAC. A range of modes have been taught, including gestures (e.g., Johnson & Mc-
(continued)

Table 9.1.   Determine the most appropriate communicative response to teach a learner to request access to desired objects/activities

If the learner	Then
Attempts to pursue objects/activities in the environment using a form that is not easily understood	A request for objects/activities may be appropriate.
Engages in socially unacceptable behaviors as a way to obtain objects/activities	A request for objects/activities may be appropriate.
Attempts to persist in an activity using a form that is not easily understood	A request for continued engagement may be appropriate.
Engages in behaviors that are socially unacceptable as a way to maintain participation in desired activities	A request for continued engagement may be appropriate.
Attempts to obtain assistance to leave or finish a less desired activity or to gain access to a more desired activity that he or she cannot successfully accomplish on his or her own using a form that is not easily understood	A request for assistance may be appropriate.
Engages in behaviors that are socially unacceptable as a way to obtain assistance	A request for assistance may be appropriate.

Donnell, 2004; Keen, Sigafoos, & Woodyatt, 2001; Reichle & McComas, 2004); no-tech aided AAC such as eye gaze communication boards and graphic symbols (e.g., Grunsell & Carter, 2002; Keen et al., 2001; Reichle, Drager, & Davis, 2002; Reichle et al., 2005; Sidener, Shabani, Carr, & Roland, 2005); and speech-generating devices (SGDs) with voice output (e.g., Cosbey & Johnston, 2006; Sigafoos et al., 2004; Sigafoos, Penned, & Versluis, 1996).

This research has involved both children (e.g., Cosbey & Johnston, 2006; Grunsell & Carter, 2002; Johnson & McDonnell, 2004; Reichle & McComas, 2004; Sidener et al., 2005) and adults (e.g., Reichle et al., 2002, 2005; Sigafoos et al., 2004) with a variety of disabilities (e.g., cerebral palsy, Pierre Robin syndrome, autism, Rett syndrome, severe intellectual disability). Intervention has been conducted in home (e.g., Reichle et al., 2002, 2005; Sidener et al., 2005), school (e.g., Keen et al., 2001; Reichle & Johnston, 1999), and community (e.g., Durand, 1999; Sigafoos et al., 2004) settings.

Studies have taught individuals to request objects (e.g., Cosbey & Johnston, 2006; Keen et al., 2001; Sidener et al., 2005; Sigafoos et al., 2004), request assistance (Durand, 1999; Johnson & McDonnell, 2004; Reichle et al., 2002, 2005; Reichle & McComas, 2004), and request continued engagement (e.g., Gee, Graham, Goetz, Oshima & Yoshioka, 1991; Grunsell & Carter, 2002), each of which are reviewed in the corresponding sections of this chapter.

☞ Helpful Hint

Interventionists are encouraged to complete the intervention planning form (Form 6.1 on the accompanying CD-ROM) when selecting intervention strategies to teach requests to obtain or maintain access to objects/activities or to obtain assistance. Completing the intervention planning form will ensure that the intervention procedures are well documented, increasing the likelihood of accurate and reliable implementation.

TEACHING REQUESTS FOR OBJECTS/ACTIVITIES

Requests for objects/activities can be made prior to encountering the preferred object/activity (e.g., a preschool-age child can indicate his or her desire to play with the blocks as the daily schedule is being presented during opening circle time) as well as at the point that preferred objects are presented or offered to the learner (e.g., when blocks are offered as an activity choice during free playtime).

Who Might Benefit from Learning to Request Objects/Activities?

Teaching requests for objects/activities provides individuals with severe disabilities with a strategy for communicating a desire to gain access to preferred objects or activities. Individuals with severe disabilities often make some effort to pursue novel or desired objects/activities in their environments. The form of intentional communication directed to a social partner may be marginal or unacceptable (e.g., biting a peer who has a desired toy) or difficult to interpret (e.g., subtle change in body posture when a desired object is presented), however. Teaching a request for items/activities in these situations can be beneficial to the learner as well as his or her communication partners.

What Is the Evidence Base?

Although the specific procedures vary across studies, features that are common across all studies include 1) creating an opportunity, 2) prompting communication to request the desired object/activity, and 3) providing access to the desired object/activity.

What Does the Research Say?
Teaching Requests for Objects/Activities

Research demonstrating successful strategies for teaching individuals to request desired objects/activities reveals that there are a variety of ways to create opportunities to request.

- Placing high-interest items in view but out of reach (e.g., Cosbey & Johnston, 2006; Reichle & Johnston, 1999; Sigafoos et al., 2004)

(continued)

- Utilizing existing opportunities that occur in the participant's environment (e.g., Durand, 1993, 1999; Kratzer & Spooner, 1993)

- Creating and embedding opportunities for the participant to request (e.g., Keen et al., 2001; Sigafoos, Penned, et al., 1996)

- Presenting an array of high-interest items from which the participant can choose (Kozleski, 1991; Sigafoos, Laurie, & Pennell, 1996)

- Presenting materials for an activity with incorrect, broken, or inoperative items (Romer & Schoenberg, 1991; Sigafoos & Couzens, 1995)

In addition to creating opportunities, a variety of successful prompt and prompt-fading procedures have been used in studies designed to teach individuals to request. Successful prompt and prompt-fading procedures include the following:

- Models (e.g., Keen et al., 2001; Sigafoos, Couzens, Roberts, Phillips, & Goodison, 1996)

- Physical prompts (e.g., Cosbey & Johnston, 2006; Durand, 1999; Reichle & Johnston, 1999; Sigafoos et al., 2004; Sigafoos, Laurie, et al., 1996)

- Verbal prompts (e.g., Derby et al., 1997; Durand, 1999; Keen et al., 2001; Reichle & Johnston, 1999; Sigafoos et al., 2004)

- Stimulus prompts (e.g., Reichle, Dropik, Alden-Anderson, & Haley, 2008; Reichle & Johnston, 1999; see Chapter 5)

- Time delay (e.g., Cosbey & Johnston, 2006; Keen et al., 2001; Sigafoos & Couzens, 1995; Sigafoos, Penned, & Versluis, 1996)

Finally, all successful strategies for teaching individuals to request desired objects/ activities have provided the learner with access to the desired object/activity contingent on engagement in the desired behavior (e.g., Cosbey & Johnston, 2006; Derby et al., 1997; Durand, 1999; Keen et al., 2001; Reichle & Johnston, 1999; Sigafoos et al., 2004).

Using Evidence-Based Strategies to Teach Requests for Objects/Activities

There are a number of strategies available to teach requests for objects, Unfortunately, not all have been experimentally validated. The steps below represent experimentally validated strategies to implement a program to teach a learner to request desired objects/ activities.

Steps for teaching requesting

Step 1: Identify situations.
Step 2: Identify the communicative behavior.
Step 3: Identify intervention strategies to teach requesting.
Step 4: Implement intervention, and monitor learner performance.

Step 1: Identify Situations

Identify the preferred objects/activities that will be used in the context of instruction in order to create opportunities for an individual to request objects/activities.

What Objects/Activities Should Be Used? Implementing a functional assessment is one strategy for identifying objects/activities. Individuals with severe disabilities often already make an effort to pursue objects/activities in their environments. The form of their effort may be socially unacceptable or difficult to interpret, however. A functional assessment may be helpful in this case in identifying these existing communicative intents.

Information regarding identifying items/ activities likely to be requested can be found in Chapter 5.

Using preference assessments and/or ecological inventories is another strategy for identifying objects/activities. It is unclear in some cases which objects/activities in an environment are being pursued by a learner. This may be due to ambiguous findings from the functional assessment, unique features of the environment (e.g., limited range of objects/activities), and/or characteristics of the AAC user (e.g., learned helplessness, inconsistent use of behaviors to signal the pursuit of objects/activities). Using strategies for identifying preferences is warranted in this case.

How Will There Be Sufficient Opportunities to Request the Identified Objects/Activities? Identify naturally occurring opportunities by examining existing activities and routines to identify situations when requests for objects/activities are warranted. Create opportunities for the AAC user to request objects/activities. For example,

- Place desired objects in view but out of reach (e.g., storing desired DVDs on a high shelf).

- Withhold one or more of the items needed for completion of an activity (e.g., withholding glue during construction of a model airplane).

- Provide only limited quantities of a desired item (e.g., only a small amount of juice during snack time).

How Can the Learner Acquire the Conditional Use of Communication? The learner is taught the conditional use of communicative behaviors when both positive and negative teaching examples are included in instruction. That is, learners are taught when they should (positive teaching examples) and should not (negative teaching examples) engage in a particular communicative act.

The **conditional use of communication** to request objects/activities can be established by using **general case instruction**. General case instruction (O'Neill & Reichle, 1993) ensures that intervention opportunities are carefully selected to sample the range of response forms and situations in which the learner should (and should not) demonstrate target communi-

> Information regarding the conditional use of communication and general case instruction is discussed in Chapter 5.

cation skills so that both acquisition and generalization of skills occur concurrently.

Step 2: Identify the Communicative Behavior

Interventionists must consider the form of the communicative behavior, as well as the level of specificity of the vocabulary taught to request objects/activities, when teaching requesting. The interventionist must determine the following when identifying the target behavior:

- The mode of communication

- The specific AAC system features

- How the AAC user's skills/abilities (e.g., hearing, vision, motor ability) will be addressed

- How specific environmental factors (e.g., the physical and social environment) will influence decisions

- The type of symbol that will be used if the AAC user will utilize graphic symbols

- How specific the vocabulary will be and how the vocabulary will be displayed

A request can involve vocabulary that is general with regard to what is desired (e.g., "I want to play") or vocabulary that is explicit (e.g., "I want to play with the red ball"). General requests may be advantageous because

- The form of the AAC user's behavior remains the same across all objects/activities. Thus, generalized requests are efficient from the AAC user's perspective.

- They provide an immediately useful means for requesting a variety of desired objects/activities across a variety of situations

- They provide a greater number of learning opportunities because the general request can be used with a variety of objects/activities

> Information regarding issues to consider when identifying appropriate communicative alternatives is provided in Chapter 3.

- They may increase the likelihood of generalization across situations

The listener must determine the specific object/activity that the learner is requesting when using general requests, however, resulting in an increased burden on the communication partner. As a result, interventionists may choose to teach more explicit vocabulary. More explicit requests may be advantageous because they

- Clearly indicate to the listener what the learner is seeking, which may result in fewer requests for clarification

- May be more easily understood by unfamiliar communication partners

- May be particularly useful for learners with few and relatively stable preferences

- May be useful for learners who acquire vocabulary fairly quickly

- May be acquired more quickly by some learners because they are associated with a specific response/reinforcer

The interventionist can define the target behavior once these issues have been considered. In addition to the issues stated previously, ensure that the target behavior is observable, measurable, will be understood by others, and is socially appropriate.

☞ Helpful Hint

If the target behavior involves using graphic symbols, then make extra copies of the symbols so that they are available in case a symbol is lost or destroyed.

Step 3: Identify Intervention Strategies to Teach Requesting

See Chapter 5 for a discussion of choosing intervention strategies, including prompting, reinforcement, and error correction procedures. Interventionists should consider the following when identifying intervention strategies to teach requesting:

- The type of prompt that will be used to instruct both the positive and the nega-

tive teaching examples (e.g., verbal, gestural, physical)

- The plan for promoting skill generalization

- How prompts will be faded over time (e.g., gradually decreasing the intrusiveness of the prompts, time delay)

- The consequences that will be provided for an incorrect response (e.g., no access to the preferred item/activity followed by a new opportunity to request)

- Strategies for promoting skill maintenance

- The criterion for mastery

☞ Helpful Hint

Consider issues related to response efficiency when designing and implementing interventions (see Chapter 1).

Step 4: Implement Intervention and Monitor Learner Performance

The next step is to implement the intervention and monitor learner performance. It is important to note that the interventionist must reinforce the communicative behavior when the learner appropriately requests the desired object/activity by providing the learner with access to the object/activity. Use a performance monitoring form to monitor learner performance (see Form 6.6 on the accompanying CD-ROM).

☞ Helpful Hint

Following some requests, consider presenting an array of items that include the requested item and allowing the AAC user to independently take the item (rather than always handing the requested item to the AAC user). This provides an opportunity to check for correspondence (e.g., Does the item requested correspond with the item chosen from the presented array?).

CASE EXAMPLE

Reichle and Johnston (1999)

Reichle and Johnston (1999) taught two beginning AAC users with severe disabilities to conditionally use communicative requests to obtain desired snack items in an elementary school setting. The learners were taught to directly reach for desired items when they were proximally near. Alternatively, the learners were taught to point to a graphic symbol to request that the item be delivered when items were in the possession of another person (teacher, peer) or proximally distant. Results revealed that the students did not automatically engage in the most efficient strategy. Efficient and conditional use was successfully acquired, however, after fairly brief periods of intervention, which maximized the immediacy of reinforcement.

The following case example further illustrates how each of these steps was utilized in teaching a student with autism to request objects/activities.

CASE EXAMPLE

Requesting for Objects

Shakina is a 13-year-old female student with autism. Although Shakina had access to an SGD, she rarely used it. Instead, Shakina physically manipulated familiar adults in order to express her wants and needs. For example, when she wanted something out of reach, she pulled on her teacher's arm until he followed Shakina over to the object. Then, Shakina moved her teacher's arm in the direction of the object until he knew what she wanted. If Shakina was in an unfamiliar environment, then she did not communicate at all, remaining helpless, because most people were unresponsive to her unique communicative behavior.

Shakina's intervention team included her father, speech-language pathologist, special education consultant, and general education teacher. The team designed an intervention during an initial meeting to address Shakina's needs. The team decided to teach her to request desired objects/activities because this was the most pervasive issue in her middle school classroom. The team also programmed her SGD to include vocabulary representing desired objects/activities. See Figure 9.1 for Shakina's intervention planning form.

Shakina's general education teacher agreed to create opportunities for Shakina to learn the conditional use of communicative requests. Specifically, the teacher created some opportunities when it was necessary for Shakina to make requests during daily free choice time (e.g., by moving Shakina's favorite materials out of reach but in sight from her desk) as well as some opportunities when Shakina did not need to communicate in order to gain access to desired objects/activities (e.g., by sometimes placing favorite materials directly on her desk).

The special education consultant, who served as the primary interventionist, stayed near Shakina in the early stages of intervention in order to physically prompt her to request using her device or to independently gain access to materials. The consultant provided a physical prompt before Shakina had an opportunity to emit an error response (i.e., start pulling on the teacher's arm). The requested item was immediately delivered along with specific praise, contingent on a correct response. The prompts were faded over time (see Figure 9.2).

Shakina soon began independently requesting objects during daily free choice time (and refrained from requesting objects when objects were within reach). The team documented an increased number of requests during the 30 minutes of free time each day (see Figure 9.3). Shakina became skillful in making requests for objects using her AAC device over time, and now the team has moved on to teaching Shakina to use additional communicative functions.

Teaching learners to request objects/activities allows them to obtain preferred

Learner's name: _Shakina_   Start date: _2/6_

Setting (circle one):   HOME   (SCHOOL)   COMMUNITY   WORK

Communication skill/function: _Requesting desired objects using a speech-generating device (SGD)_
with black-and-white line drawings representing desired objects/activities

Opportunities

When: _Free choice time_   Where: _General education classroom_

Minimum opportunities per day/session: _6 per day_

Context for instruction: _Embedded within free choice time in class_

Set up: _Teacher tells class it is free choice time_

Materials: _Preferred objects (i.e., checkers, smelly markers, playdough, race cars, water twirler), SGD_

Target Behavior

Mode: _SGD with black-and-white line drawings_

Augmentative and alternative communication system features: _Digitalized speech, all items appear on one_
screen

Vocabulary: _Object symbol with spoken phrase I WANT ___ PLEASE (e.g., checkers symbol for I WANT_
THE CHECKERS PLEASE)

Instructional Strategies

Skill sequence/steps: _1) Shakina's teacher says, "It's time for free choice"; 2) peers make choices;_
3) teacher observes Shakina's eye gaze to see what object is desired; 4) teacher physically
prompts Shakina to ask for desired object using SGD; 5) Shakina receives the object immedi-
ately following a correct response.

Prompts: _Use physical assistance to touch symbol on SGD._

Consequences

    Correct response: _For primary reinforcement, use immediate provision of the requested object._
For secondary reinforcement, offer verbal praise.

    Incorrect response (no response or error response): _For no response, give a verbal reminder followed by a_
physical prompt as needed. For error response, wait 5 seconds, begin a new opportunity, and
provide a more intrusive physical prompt for the next opportunity to ensure a correct response.

Prompt fading: _Use a 5-second time delay before providing a physical prompt._

Generalization: _Create opportunities in home and community_

Maintenance: _When Shakina has reached her goal, collect data one day each week in order to_
assess maintenance.

Criterion for Mastery

Shakina will independently request desired objects using her SGD at least 5 opportunities per
day for 3 consecutive days.

Performance Monitoring

The team—Max (dad), June (speech-language pathologist), Chiara (special education
teacher), and Jake (general education teacher)—will meet every week to evaluate progress.
Graphs, data tables, prompting, and prompt fading will be discussed and revised as needed.

Figure 9.1. Intervention Planning Form for Shakina. (*Note:* This is a filled-in version of Form 6.1, Intervention Planning Form. A blank, printable version appears on the accompanying CD-ROM.)

Dates	Monday	Tuesday	Wednesday	Thursday	Friday	Notes
2/6–2/10	FP FP PP PP I	PP PP I PP I	PP I I I I	I I PP I I	I I PP P I I	
2/13–2/17	I I I PP I I I	I I I PP PP I	I PP I I I I	I I I I I	I I I I I	Mastered 2/17
2/20–2/24			I I I I I I			

Figure 9.2. Shakina's performance using her speech-generating device to request objects. (*Key*: FP, full physical prompt; I, independent; PP, partial physical prompt.)

and needed objects/activities while simultaneously providing a way to exert control over their environment. Sometimes, learners engage in activities that they enjoy but do not have to request in order to participate (e.g., recess and leisure time that occur as part of the learner's daily schedule). Teaching a learner to request continued engagement in an activity is appropriate in this case.

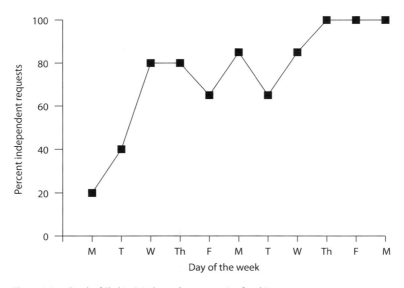

Figure 9.3. Graph of Shakina's independent requesting for objects.

TEACHING REQUESTS FOR CONTINUED ENGAGEMENT

Teaching requests for continued engagement in an activity provides individuals with severe disabilities with a strategy for communicating a desire to persist in doing something that they enjoy (e.g., continue swinging on a swing set, continue playing a video game). It may be easier in some cases to teach a request for engagement than to teach a request for objects/activities because the activity itself acts as part of the cuing mechanism for the target behavior.

What Is the Evidence Base?

Researchers have demonstrated successful strategies for teaching individuals with severe disabilities to request continued engagement.

What Does the Research Say?

Teaching Requests for Continued Engagement

Gee et al. (1991) taught three individuals with severe disabilities (ages 5–10 years) to activate a call device to request continued engagement with desired objects/activities. Researchers conducted interviews and observations in order to identify routines for interruption. Requesting was taught by 1) interrupting routines, 2) waiting for the participant to indicate a desire to continue the routine through nonsymbolic behaviors (e.g., change in body tone/position, change in affect), and 3) physically prompting the student to activate the call device. Reinforcement for engaging in the target behavior was immediate continued engagement in the interrupted routine. Prompts were faded using time delay, and results revealed that all three participants learned to request continued engagement as a result of the intervention.

Grunsell and Carter (2002) taught four individuals with moderate to severe disabilities (ages 7–8 years) to touch a graphic symbol to request continued engagement with desired objects/activities. Routines that were identified for interruption included music, leisure skills, and mealtime. Interruption strategies embedded into these routines included opportunities when items were visible but out of reach as well as opportunities when required items were absent. Physical prompts and time delay were used to teach the requesting behavior. Results revealed that all four participants learned to request continued engagement

---

as a result of intervention. Furthermore, the participants' ability to request continued engagement was maintained for up to 18 weeks following acquisition, and the skills generalized to untaught routines.

Using Evidence-Based Strategies to Teach Requesting Continued Engagement with an Activity

Steps for teaching requests for continued engagement

Step 1: Identify situations.
Step 2: Identify the communicative behavior.
Step 3: Identify a strategy for creating an opportunity to request.
Step 4: Identify intervention strategies to teach requesting.
Step 5: Implement intervention, and monitor learner performance.

The existing research relative to teaching individuals with severe disabilities to request continued engagement in an activity provides interventionists with an opportunity to utilize evidence-based practices in their work. The following sections provide procedures for teaching requests for continued engagement. The procedures for teaching requests for continued engagement in many cases are similar to the previously identified procedures for teaching requests for objects/activities. These similarities will be noted. Differences in teaching these functions do exist, however, and those differences will be highlighted.

Step 1: Identify Situations

Interventionists will need to identify opportunities during which it is appropriate to request continuation. Hunt and Goetz (1988) suggested that selected routines should

• Occur daily

• Already exist in the environment

• Consist of at least three steps

• Be able to be performed independently by the learner

Step 2: Identify the Communicative Behavior

Identify the communicative behavior to be taught in the routine that represents communicative obligations and/or opportunities for the learner. The issues to consider in choosing the target behavior for requesting continued engagement are the same as the previously discussed issues for identifying the target behavior for requesting objects/activities.

Step 3: Identify a Strategy for Creating an Opportunity to Request

There are several ways to create opportunities to request continued engagement:

- Utilize existing opportunities by identifying activities that occur in the participant's environment (e.g., singing songs during preschool circle time) and include natural breaks (e.g., at the end of each song). Then, the AAC user can be prompted to request continued engagement when each natural break occurs.

- Embed opportunities by creating activities that include the need for requests for continued engagement (e.g., modifying the activities at recess to include time for playing on the swings). The AAC user can be prompted to request continued engagement when each opportunity occurs (e.g., after the swing stops moving following an initial push).

- Use chain interruption, which involves intentionally interrupting or preventing continuation of a familiar routine. The AAC user will begin a desired activity (e.g., playing a video game) and then the interventionist will terminate the activity after a predetermined amount of time (e.g., 5 minutes) or number of times completing the activity (e.g., 1 game). Terminating the activity interrupts the activity, thereby creating an opportunity for the AAC user to request continuation.

> Detailed procedures for implementing a chain interruption strategy are discussed in Chapter 5.

Step 4: Identify Intervention Strategies to Teach Requesting

See Chapter 5 for a discussion on choosing intervention strategies, including prompting, reinforcement, and error correction procedures. The issues to consider in developing a teaching strategy are the same as the previously discussed issues for developing a strategy for teaching an individual to request items/activities.

Step 5: Implement Intervention and Monitor Learner Performance

The next step is to implement the instructional strategy and collect data to monitor effectiveness. The issues to consider in implementing the strategy and collecting data to monitor effectiveness for teaching an individual to request continued engagement are the same as the previously discussed issues for teaching an individual to request objects/activities.

CASE EXAMPLE

Requesting Continued Engagement

Patrick is a 32-year-old man with mild cerebral palsy and a moderate cognitive delay who lives in a group home for adults with developmental disabilities. Prior to intervention, Patrick communicated using mostly idiosyncratic behaviors along with some common gestures such as pointing. Patrick would often grunt or shake his hands repeatedly when he wanted to continue a desired activity. People around him learned over time to understand these unique behaviors as requests. This was problematic, however, during community outings and interactions with people who were unfamiliar with Patrick's communicative attempts.

Several staff and family members designed and implemented an intervention strategy (see Figure 9.4). The team noticed that Patrick often displayed these idiosyncratic communicative requests for continued engagement during leisure or recreation time in his home. Based on assessment data and previous successful history with sign language, the team decided

Learner's name: _Patrick_   Start date: _1/12_

Setting (circle one): (HOME)   SCHOOL   COMMUNITY   WORK

Communication skill/function: _Requesting continued engagement in activities using the sign MORE_

Opportunities

When: _Leisure and recreation time_   Where: _Game room_

Minimum opportunities per day/session: _6 per day_

Context for instruction: _Embedded within free time at home_

Set up: _Patrick is engaged in the desired recreation activities of playing cards and watching television_

Materials: _Activity materials (playing cards, television set)_

Target Behavior

Mode: _Sign language_

Augmentative and alternative communication system features: _N/A_

Vocabulary: _Sign for MORE_

Instructional Strategies

Skill sequence/steps: _1) Patrick is engaged in a leisure activity of playing cards or watching television; 2) a staff member waits for 3 seconds and then provides a physical prompt to sign MORE at the end of a card game or 30-minute television show; 3) Patrick is allowed to continue the activity._

Prompts: _Physical assistance to sign MORE_

Consequences

     Correct response: _For primary reinforcement, immediately allow Patrick to continue the activity. For secondary reinforcement, offer verbal praise such as, "Great, let's play some more."_

     Incorrect response (no response or error response): _For no response, provide a full physical prompt if no response after 3 seconds. For error response, wait 10 seconds, begin a new opportunity, and provide a full physical prompt for one trial to ensure the correct response._

Prompt fading: _Use 10-second time delay after 2 consecutive days of 80%–100% accuracy with full physical prompt_

Generalization: _Create opportunities to request continued engagement at the city park and library._

Maintenance: _After reaching criteria, collect data once per month to monitor maintenance of the skill._

Criterion for Mastery

Patrick will independently sign MORE to request continued engagement for 5 out of 6 opportunities across 3 consecutive days.

Performance Monitoring

The team—Jake (staff member), Ann (staff member), Carl (staff member), and Mark (Patrick's brother)—will meet weekly to discuss Patrick's progress. The team will look at graphs, data forms, prompts, and prompt fading and make changes as needed.

Figure 9.4. Intervention planning form for Patrick. (*Note:* This is a filled-in version of Form 6.1, Intervention Planning Form. A blank, printable version appears on the accompanying CD-ROM.)

Dates	Monday	Tuesday	Wednesday	Thursday	Friday	Notes
1/12–1/19	− FP − FP − FP − PP + +	− FP − PP + + + − PP	− PP − PP + + + +	− PP + + + + +	+ − PP + + + +	
1/20–1/27	− PP − PP + + + +	+ + + − PP + +	+ + + + + +	+ + + + + +	+ + + + + +	

Figure 9.5. One week of data for teaching Patrick to request continued engagement. (*Key:* FP, full physical prompt; I, independent; PP, partial physical prompt; +, correct response; −, incorrect response.)

to teach Patrick to sign MORE in order to request continued engagement in an activity.

The team selected card games and television routines (Patrick usually played five to six card games or watched two to three sitcoms at one sitting) as the context for instruction in order to create opportunities to request. Specifically, Patrick was prompted to sign MORE at the end of each card game or 30-minute television show. Initially, full physical prompts were used to assist Patrick to sign MORE. This physical assistance was faded across time until Patrick was independently signing MORE to request continued engagement (see Figure 9.5).

Patrick was successful in learning to request continued engagement (see Figure 9.6). After reaching criterion during leisure time, his

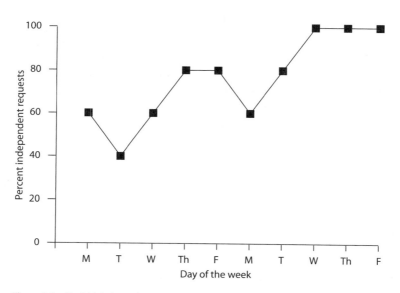

Figure 9.6. Patrick's independent requests for continued engagement.

team began to intervene during daily community outings. After noticing very limited generalization to the community, more community outings were arranged to help Patrick practice.

Requesting objects/activities and requesting continued engagement in activities provide a way for learners to obtain access to desired object and activities. Being able to request assistance is another important skill. Requesting assistance can be used when learners want to escape/avoid an activity (e.g., cleaning up toys after an afternoon of play) as well as when learners need help in order to successfully engage with desired objects and/or participate in desired activities (e.g., completing a puzzle, inserting a new CD into the player).

> Detailed procedures for teaching learners to request assistance to escape/avoid are discussed in Chapter 10.

TEACHING REQUESTS FOR ASSISTANCE

Teaching a request for assistance provides individuals with severe disabilities with a strategy for obtaining help or support in an activity that they cannot independently execute. Individuals with severe disabilities may already make some efforts to obtain assistance. Communicative forms produced may not be easily understood (e.g., unintelligible vocalizations when experiencing difficulty completing a puzzle), however, or may be socially unacceptable (e.g., challenging behaviors such as throwing a box of candy that is difficult to open).

What Does the Research Say?

Teaching Requests for Assistance

Reichle et al. (2005) taught a 40-year-old man with autism and severe intellectual disability to use a graphic symbol representing HELP to request assistance with difficult tasks as well as to complete work tasks independently. Opportunities for instruction were embedded into a vocational task of connecting pipes with nuts and washers. Interventionists implemented a backward chaining method to teach pipe assembly. Intervention to teach the use of the graphic symbol to request assistance utilized a most-to-least prompting hierarchy. Providing assistance in completing the task was the consequence for correctly using the graphic symbol. A brief work break during which the participant was allowed access to a preferred edible item was the consequence for assembling the pipe. Results revealed that the participant learned to request assistance independently as well as to complete the assembly task independently. Furthermore, the participant's use of the request assistance symbol decreased as his ability to independently complete the assembly task increased.

As part of a study involving five participants, Durand (1999) taught two students with disabilities to use their SGD to request assistance with their work. Opportunities to request assistance (I NEED HELP) occurred in the classroom setting and were based on data obtained from functional analyses. Interventionists taught the use of the SGD through verbal and physical prompts. Providing assistance was the consequence for correctly using the SGD. Results revealed that the participants learned to request assistance as a result of the intervention.

As part of a study involving three participants, Johnson and McDonnell (2004) implemented an intervention designed to teach an 11-year-old student with Down syndrome to request assistance by signing HELP. The student's general and special education teachers identified five tasks that the student could not complete independently (e.g., using a tape recording, using a computer, obtaining materials needed for task completion) as opportunities for instruction. The participant's general education teacher implemented the intervention using verbal prompts, models, and physical prompts. Time delay was used to fade prompts. Providing assistance was the consequence for correctly using the sign for HELP. Results revealed that the participant learned to request assistance as a result of the instruction.

Reichle and McComas (2004) examined the conditional use of communication when they taught a 12-year-old child who experienced a severe behavior disorder to request assistance during the completion of math worksheets by raising his hand as an alternative to engaging in challenging behavior that functioned to escape difficult tasks. The new communicative behavior was acquired quickly, and challenging behaviors were eliminated. Investigators noted, however, that there was not an increase in

(continued)

independent solution of math problems. Thus, the participant was taught the math skills during didactic sessions utilizing errorless instruction without allowing the learner to request assistance. Although the participant acquired the math skills, the learner continued to request assistance by raising his hand during the worksheet activity. In order to increase math worksheet performance, the investigators provided the participant with more immediate reinforcement contingent on independent problem solving than when he requested assistance. Results revealed that this change resulted in the learner beginning to solve problems with increasing independence.

Using Evidence-Based Strategies to Teach Requests for Assistance

The procedures for teaching requests for assistance in many cases are similar to the previously identified procedures for teaching requests for objects/activities. These similarities will be noted; however, the important differences for teaching these two functions do exist, and these differences will be highlighted.

Steps for teaching requests for assistance

Step 1: Identify situations.
Step 2: Identify the communicative behavior.
Step 3: Identify the point at which to prompt a request for assistance.
Step 4: Identify intervention strategies to teach requesting.
Step 5: Implement intervention and monitor learner performance.

Step 1: Identify Situations

Identify the activities during which assistance is needed in order to create opportunities for an individual to request assistance. These activities will then be used as the context for instruction. Opportunities to request assistance are sometimes already present in the environment. Other times, however, the opportunities for an individual to request assistance are infrequent or unclear. It may be

necessary in this case to create opportunities for the individual to request help or support when engaged in an activity. This can be accomplished in a variety of ways, including withholding the provision of assistance in situations where assistance is usually provided (e.g., not helping a child to put on his or her coat even though you have done so in the past) or putting desired objects in transparent containers with lids that the user is unable to open (e.g., putting desired candy in a glass jar with the lid screwed on tight). It is important to teach the conditional use of requests for assistance through the use of general case instruction in which both positive and negative teaching examples are included in instruction.

Step 2: Identify the Communicative Behavior

It is necessary to select the target behavior after identifying situations. The issues to consider in identifying the target behavior for requesting assistance are the same as the previously discussed issues for identifying the target behavior for requesting objects/activities.

Step 3: Identify the Point at Which to Prompt a Request for Assistance

Interventionists are encouraged to observe the learner engaging in the difficult task across several opportunities and note the point at which the learner experiences difficulty in order to determine the point at which the learner needs assistance. Interventionists will be able to identify the common point(s) across opportunities that are difficult for the learner after several observations. Intervention should be implemented at this point(s).

Step 4: Identify Intervention Strategies to Teach Requesting

See Chapter 5 for a discussion of choosing intervention strategies, including prompting, reinforcement, and error correction procedures. The issues to consider in developing a teaching strategy are the same as the previously discussed issues for developing a strategy for teaching an individual to request items/activities. Reinforcement will involve providing assistance.

Step 5: Implement Intervention and Monitor Learner Performance

Next, implement the instructional strategy and collect data to monitor effectiveness. The issues to consider in implementing the strategy and collecting data to monitor effectiveness for teaching an individual to request assistance are the same as the previously discussed issues for teaching an individual to request objects/activities.

CASE EXAMPLE

Requesting Assistance

Rosa was a 6-year-old student with severe cognitive and communication delays. Rosa's primary form of communication was to throw toys/objects across the room. Outcomes of a functional assessment revealed that the function of her aggressive behavior was to gain assistance with difficult tasks, and, therefore, Rosa's team decided to teach Rosa to request assistance using a single-switch SGD as a replacement for her aggressive behavior (see Figure 9.7).

The team chose to intervene during activities that required cutting with scissors because this was an area of difficulty for Rosa. The team also selected this task because the classroom routine already included several opportunities to engage in cutting activities throughout the day. Observation revealed that Rosa had a tendency to throw her scissors about 5 seconds after the presentation of the task. Therefore, the team decided that they would prompt her 3 seconds after the presentation of a difficult task.

The team used a full physical prompt (which was faded over time) to help Rosa activate her SGD, which was programmed to say I NEED HELP, PLEASE. The instructional strategy for

teaching Rosa was posted on the wall near the art table so everyone could easily refer to it as needed. Rosa had at least three opportunities each day to request assistance with using scissors to cut paper, and the team recorded the prompting level that was used on a chart located next to the summarized procedures (see Figure 9.8). Posting the intervention procedures, implementation schedule, and data sheets in close proximity to the intervention area made it easy to stay consistent in intervention efforts and to keep track of Rosa's progress.

After one week of intervention, the interventionists waited 5 seconds rather than 3 seconds prior to prompting the request for assistance. After that point, the team was able to gradually fade all prompts (see Figure 9.9).

SUMMARY

Communicating to obtain access to desired objects/activities is a powerful skill. In addition to providing learners with a way to obtain preferred and needed objects/activities, it also provides a way for learners to exert control over the environment. This chapter focused on procedures that are effective for establishing functional communication to gain access to desired objects/activities. Specifically, information was provided in order to assist readers in 1) identifying whether an AAC user might benefit from interventions designed to teach requests for objects/activities, continued engagement in an activity, and assistance; 2) delineating the procedures for teaching AAC users with severe disabilities to request objects/activities, continued engagement in an activity, and assistance; and 3) understanding the ways in which the research related to teaching AAC users with severe disabilities to request objects/activities, continued engagement, and assistance can be used to support evidence-based practice.

Learner's name: _Rosa_   Start date: _5/9_

Setting (circle one):   HOME   (SCHOOL)   COMMUNITY   WORK

Communication skill/function: _Requesting assistance during cutting activities using a speech-generating device (SGD)_

Opportunities

When: _Cutting with scissors_   Where: _Small table in classroom_

Minimum opportunities per day/session: _3 per day_

Context for instruction: _Embedded in school activity_

Set up: _During activities involving cutting_

Materials: _Paper, scissors, SGD_

Target Behavior

Mode: _SGD_

Augmentative and alternative communication system features: _Direct selection to access a switch that produces the utterance_ I NEED HELP, PLEASE _when pressed_

Vocabulary: _HELP symbol stands for_ I NEED HELP, PLEASE

Instructional Strategies

Skill sequence/steps: _1) Rosa is presented with a cutting task; 2) the teacher waits the predetermined time delay; 3) the teacher physically prompts Rosa to press the switch; 4) Rosa is immediately given teacher assistance with the cutting task._

Prompts: _Physical prompt to access SGD_

Consequences

    Correct response: _For primary reinforcement, provide immediate assistance with the task. For secondary reinforcement, give verbal praise (e.g., "Sure, I'll help!")._

    Incorrect response (no response or error response): _For no response, provide a full physical prompt (after the time delay). For error response, wait 5 seconds, begin a new opportunity, and provide an immediate full physical prompt for one trial to ensure correct response._

Prompt fading: _Use a 5-second time delay after 2 consecutive days of 80%–100% accuracy with a full physical prompt._

Generalization: _All staff members will provide assistance with the cutting task each day. Create opportunities to request help in other settings (e.g., opening milk carton during lunch)._

Maintenance: _When Rosa reaches her goal, check periodically (e.g., once every 2 weeks) to make sure that skills are maintained._

Criterion for Mastery

Rosa will independently request assistance using the SGD within 5 seconds on 3 out of 3 daily opportunities for 3 consecutive days.

Performance Monitoring

The team—Michelle (mom), Carlos (dad), Jane (general education teacher), Jack (special education teacher), Cindy (aide), Juan (occupational therapist), and Charlotte (speech-language pathologist)—will meet each week to discuss Rosa's progress. Because Rosa's dad cannot come to every weekly meeting, he will join the team every other week to talk about Rosa's use of this skill at home. The team will review the graphs, data tables, prompting, and prompt fading and will make changes to the plan as needed and record them in the team binder.

Figure 9.7. Intervention Planning Form for Rosa. (*Note:* This is a filled-in version of Form 6.1, Intervention Planning Form. A blank, printable version appears on the accompanying CD-ROM.)

Dates	Monday	Tuesday	Wednesday	Thursday	Friday	Notes
5/9–5/13	FP FP FP	FP PP I	PP PP I	I PP PP	I I PP	
5/15–5/19	I I PP	I I I	I PP I	I I I	I I PP	
5/22–5/26	I I I	I I I	I I I			Mastered 5/24

Figure 9.8. Rosa's performance using her speech-generating device to request assistance. (*Key*: FP, full physical prompt; I, independent; PP: partial physical prompt.)

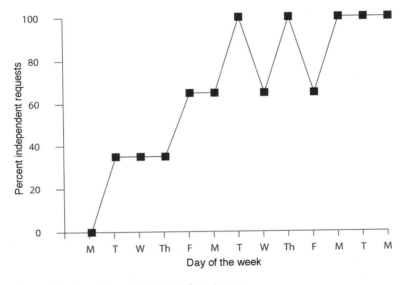

Figure 9.9. Rosa's independent requests for assistance.

REFERENCES

Cosbey, J.E., & Johnston, S. (2006). Using a single-switch voice output communication aid to increase social access for children with severe disabilities in inclusive classrooms. *Research and Practice for Persons with Severe Disabilities, 31,* 144–156.

Derby, K.M., Wacker, D.P., Berg, W., DeRaad, A., Ulrich, S., Asmus, J., et al.(1997). The long-term effects of functional communication training in home settings. *Journal of Applied Behavior Analysis, 30,* 507–531.

Durand, M.V. (1993). Functional communication training using assistive devices: Effects on challenging behavior and affect. *Augmentative and Alternative Communication, 9,* 168–176.

Durand, M.V. (1999). Functional communication training using assistive devices: Recruiting natural communities of reinforcement. *Journal of Applied Behavior Analysis, 32,* 247–267.

Gee, K., Graham, N., Goetz, L., Oshima, G., & Yoshioka, K. (1991). Teaching students to request the continuation of routine activities by using time delay and decreasing physical assistance in the context of chain interruption. *Journal of The Association for Severely Handicapped, 16,* 154–167.

Grunsell, J., & Carter, M. (2002). The behavior chain interruption strategy: Generalization to out-of-routine contexts. *Education and Training in Mental Retardation and Developmental Disabilities, 37,* 378–390.

Hunt, P., & Goetz, L. (1988). Teaching spontaneous communication in natural settings using interrupted behavior chains. *Topics in Language Disorders, 9,* 58–71.

Johnson, J., & McDonnell, J. (2004). An exploratory study of the implementation of embedded instruction by general educators with students with developmental disabilities. *Education and Treatment of Children, 27,* 46–63.

Johnston, S., & Reichle, J. (1993). Designing and implementing interventions to decrease challenging behaviors. *Language, Speech, and Hearing Services in Schools, 24*(4), 225–235.

Keen, D., Sigafoos, J., & Woodyatt, G. (2001). Replacing prelinguistic behaviors with functional communication. *Journal of Autism and Developmental Disorders, 31,* 385–398.

Kozleski, E.B. (1991). Expectant delay procedure for teaching requests. *Augmentative and Alternative Communication, 7,* 11–19.

Kratzer, D.A., & Spooner, F. (1993). Extending the application of constant time delay: Teaching a requesting skill to students with severe multiple disabilities. *Education and Treatment of Children, 16,* 235–255.

O'Neill, R., & Reichle, J. (1993). Addressing socially motivated challenging behaviors by establishing communicative alternatives. In S.F. Warren & M.E. Fey (Series Eds.) & J. Reichle & D.P. Wacker (Vol. Eds.), *Communication and language intervention series: Vol. 3. Communicative alternatives to challenging behaviors: Integrating functional assessment and intervention strategies* (pp. 205–235). Baltimore: Paul H. Brookes Publishing Co.

Reichle, J., Drager, K., & Davis, C. (2002). Using requests for assistance to obtain desired items and to gain release from nonpreferred activities: Implications for assessment and intervention. *Education and Treatment of Children, 25,* 47–66.

Reichle, J., Dropik, P.L., Alden-Anderson, E., & Haley, T. (2008). Teaching a young child with autism to request assistance conditionally: A preliminary study. *American Journal of Speech-Language Pathology, 17,* 231–240.

Reichle, J., & Johnston, L. (2006). *Early Childhood Behavior Project.* Minneapolis: University of Minnesota.

Reichle, J., & Johnston, S. (1999). Teaching the conditional use of communicative requests to two school-aged children with severe developmental disabilities. *Language, Speech, and Hearing Services in Schools, 30,* 324–334.

Reichle, J., & McComas, J. (2004). Conditional use of request for assistance. *Disability and Rehabilitation, 26,* 1255–1262.

Reichle, J., McComas, J., Dahl, N., Solberg, G., Pierce, S., & Smith, D. (2005). Teaching an individual with severe intellectual delay to request assistance conditionally. *Educational Psychology, 25,* 275–286.

Reichle, J., & Sigafoos, J. (1991). Establishing an initial repertoire of requesting. In J. Reichle, J. York, & J. Sigafoos (Eds.), *Implementing augmentative and alternative communication: Strategies for learners with severe disabilities* (pp. 89–114). Baltimore: Paul H. Brookes Publishing Co.

Romer, L.T., & Schoenberg, B. (1991). Increasing requests made by people with developmental disabilities and deaf-blindness through the use of behavior interruption strategies. *Education and Training in Mental Retardation, 26,* 70–78.

Sidener, T.M., Shabani, D.B., Carr, J.E., & Roland, J.P. (2005). An evaluation of strategies to maintain mands at practical levels. *Research in Developmental Disabilities, 27,* 632–644.

Sigafoos, J., & Couzens, D. (1995). Teaching functional use of an eye gaze communication board to a child with multiple disabilities. *British Journal of Developmental Disabilities, 41,* 114–125.

Sigafoos, J., Couzens, D., Roberts, D., Phillips, C., & Goodison, K. (1996). Teaching requests for food and drink to children with multiple disabilities in a graphic communication mode. *Journal of Developmental and Physical Disabilities, 8,* 247–262.

Sigafoos, J., Drasgow, E., Halle, J.W., O'Reilly, M., Seely-York, S., Edrisinha, C., et al. (2004). Teaching VOCA use as a communicative repair strategy. *Journal of Autism and Developmental Disorders, 34,* 411–422.

Sigafoos, J., Laurie, S., & Pennell, D. (1996). Teaching children with Rett syndrome to request preferred objects using aided communication. *Augmentative and Alternative Communication, 12,* 88–96.

Sigafoos, J., Penned, D., & Versluis, J. (1996). Naturalistic assessment leading to effective treatment of self-injury in a young boy with multiple disabilities. *Education and Treatment of Children, 19,* 101–123.

Escaping and Avoiding Objects and Activities

10

Emily A. Jones and Christopher E. Smith

▷ CHAPTER OVERVIEW

Everyone communicates to escape or avoid. Some people pass on the asparagus at dinner (**reject/ protest**), asking for the green beans instead (**request for alternative**). Others excuse themselves for a few moments when the dinner conversation becomes boring (**request for break**). After dinner, it is not unusual to seek help washing the dishes (**request for assistance**). A growing body of empirically demonstrated interventions that address communication alternatives that can be used to escape or avoid common daily events has been experimentally scrutinized for individuals with developmental disabilities (e.g., Reichle, Dropik, Alden-Anderson & Haley, 2008; Reichle & McComas, 2005; Sigafoos et al., 2004; Sigafoos, O'Reilly, Drasgow, & Reichle, 2002).

▷ CHAPTER OBJECTIVES

After studying this chapter, readers will be able to

- Decide whether socially acceptable communication to express a desire to escape/avoid can be reinforced in a particular situation

- Identify which specific communicative function (e.g., obtain assistance, take a break) best matches the reason for the learner's motivation to escape/avoid

- Develop intervention procedures to teach communication to escape/avoid, including rejecting, requesting an alternative, requesting a break, and requesting assistance

- Evaluate learner performance of the communication being taught

▷ KEY TERMS

- ▶ choices
- ▶ critical point
- ▶ high-probability request sequence
- ▶ preferred item as distractor
- ▶ reject/protest
- ▶ request for alternative
- ▶ request for assistance
- ▶ request for break
- ▶ tolerance for delay of reinforcement

WHAT IS COMMUNICATION TO ESCAPE OR AVOID OBJECTS OR ACTIVITIES?

Both escape and avoidance involve negative reinforcement (i.e., removing or terminating an object/activity that is aversive or non-preferred). They result from different experiential histories, however. Avoidance refers to taking action to prevent contact with an object/activity (e.g., pass on the asparagus at dinner). In contrast, escape refers to situations in which the learner takes action to

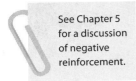

See Chapter 5 for a discussion of negative reinforcement. separate him- or herself from the situation after experiencing the object or activity (e.g., leaving when the conversation becomes boring). Several types of communicative alternatives serve an escape or avoidance function.

- Rejecting or protesting allows the learner to completely avoid a nonpreferred object or activity.

- Requesting an alternative allows the learner to both avoid/escape one option and obtain another object or activity.

- Requesting a break allows the learner to temporarily escape a nonpreferred activity (with the expectation of reengagement in the activity).

- Requesting assistance allows escape from one or more aspects of an activity because of the learner's difficulty completing it.

The situations that give rise to different types of communication to escape/avoid are sufficiently different that learning one type of escape/avoidance response may not generalize to the others, so each may need to be explicitly addressed during intervention (Sigafoos et al., 2002, 2004). For example, learning to reject a nonpreferred object may not generalize to requesting a break from a nonpreferred activity.

The same communicative act that serves the social function of escape/avoidance (i.e., that results in negative reinforcement) can simultaneously serve the function of obtaining other desired objects/activities (i.e., positive reinforcement). Learners who request a break often gain access to preferred objects/ activities during the break (e.g., leaving the dinner table to escape the boring conversation [negative reinforcement], finding what is for dessert [positive reinforcement]).

Requesting alternatives and requesting assistance can also serve the function of obtaining objects or activities, as described in Chapter 9.

Learners who request alternatives avoid the nonpreferred object or activity (negative reinforcement) and obtain a more preferred one (i.e., the alternative [positive reinforcement]). Learners who request assistance escape the difficult task (negative reinforcement) and obtain help in completing the task (positive reinforcement).

The same communicative act can serve one function in one situation and another function in another situation. For example, a request for assistance can function to gain access to an object (e.g., help getting the cookies off the high shelf; see Chapter 9) or escape a nonpreferred activity (e.g., help completing nonpreferred homework), as is discussed in this chapter. Generalization across functions may not occur spontaneously; therefore, both functions should be addressed in intervention.

WHY TEACH LEARNERS WHO USE AAC TO ESCAPE OR AVOID OBJECTS OR ACTIVITIES?

Communication used to escape or avoid is one of the first functions of communication in typically developing children (Carpenter, Mastergeorge, & Coggins, 1983; Crais, Douglas, & Campbell, 2004). Learners may use forms of communication that are not widely understood by others or use challenging behavior when they do not have an appropriate means of escaping or avoiding nonpreferred objects or activities. The importance of teaching communication to escape or avoid has been perhaps most extensively documented in teaching communicative replacements for challenging behavior (e.g., Carr et al., 1999; Durand, 1993; Steege et al., 1990). Socially acceptable ways to escape or avoid allow learners to indicate preference and exert control over their environment (Sigafoos et al., 2002).

TEACHING COMMUNICATION TO ESCAPE/AVOID

Consider the acceptability and feasibility of reinforcing a communication act to escape or avoid.

- Is it appropriate to escape or avoid the object or activity (e.g., excuse oneself from a leisure activity for a moment when it becomes boring) or not (e.g., during an academic lesson)?

- Is the activity one in which the learner must engage (i.e., obligatory; e.g., taking medication) or not (i.e., nonobligatory; e.g., watching an extra television show)?

on several opportunities, and the interventionist gradually increased the delay (e.g., "Do two more.") before delivering reinforcement (i.e., removing the worksheet). Increase the delay by increasing the number of steps the learner must complete or the amount of time the learner engages with the nonpreferred task/activity (e.g., 1 minute, 2 minutes).

What Does the Research Say?

What to Do If It Is Not Possible to Reinforce Communication to Escape or Avoid

If it is not possible to allow the learner to escape or avoid the situation (i.e., it is not possible to reinforce appropriate communication), even on a temporary basis, then do not proceed with teaching communication to escape or avoid those objects or activities. Instead, use strategies to establish the learner's involvement with the undesired object or activity. Antecedent strategies can be used to decrease the aversiveness of the situation. Present the nonpreferred object or activity in conjunction with a **preferred item as a distractor** (e.g., Davis, Reichle, & Southard, 2001). For example, Shawn watched a video (preferred activity) while getting his hair cut (nonpreferred activity). Present the learner with **choices** about the nonpreferred item or activity (e.g., Dunlap, Kern-Dunlap, Clarke, & Robbins, 1991; Dyer, Dunlap, & Winterling, 1990; Romaniuk et al., 2002). For example, Shawn's mother also gave him a choice about sitting or standing during his haircut. Offering several choices (e.g., two to three) (e.g., Shawn's mother asked, "Do you want to sit or stand for your haircut?") is better than open-ended questions such as, "Do you want to get your hair cut?" (to which the likely answer is a resounding "no"). Offer options that are safe and appropriate and for which the materials and resources are available to honor the learner's choice.

Gradually increase the learner's **tolerance for delay of reinforcement;** that is, the ability to wait for reinforcement (Carr et al., 1999). In a situation in which the learner desires to escape or avoid an activity or object, gradually increase the learner's exposure to and/or engagement with the object or activity by gradually delaying the withdrawal of that object or activity (i.e., reinforcement). For example, the interventionist initially presented a nonpreferred worksheet and said, "Do one more. Then, we are done." The learner successfully completed the one problem

If it is possible to allow the learner to escape or avoid the object or activity (i.e., reinforce appropriate communication to escape or avoid the object or activity), then proceed with instruction of appropriate communication skills to escape/avoid. The general instructional sequence for teaching communication to escape or avoid is 1) present the nonpreferred object or activity, 2) prompt communication to escape or avoid (prior to the occurrence of challenging behavior if the situation is associated with challenging behavior), and 3) withdraw the object or activity (i.e., negative reinforcement) contingent on appropriate communication. Table 10.1 summarizes which escape or avoid response to consider teaching in a given situation.

REJECTING

Rejecting refers to communication used to escape/avoid an object or activity altogether. Rejections can be made prior to encountering the nonpreferred object or activity. For example, the learner rejected asparagus as the choice of vegetable as plans were being made for dinner. Rejections can also be made at the point when the nonpreferred object is presented or offered to the learner. For example, the learner rejected the asparagus when it was offered during dinner (either verbally [e.g., "Would you like some asparagus?"] or visually [e.g., being passed the bowl of asparagus]). Rejections can also occur once the learner has the item. For example, the learner tasted the asparagus and then rejected it (e.g., because the learner disliked the preparation).

Table 10.1. Appropriate communicative responses to teach a learner to escape or avoid

If	Then
The learner actively avoids the object or activity before it is even presented	A rejection or request for alternative may be appropriate
The learner does not engage with the object or activity for any amount of time before desiring to escape or avoid	A rejection may be appropriate
The learner seeks a different activity from the one in which he or she is currently engaged	A request for alternative may be appropriate
The learner does not want an object or activity because a better option is available	A request for alternative may be appropriate
The learner engages with the object or activity for some amount of time before behavior to escape or avoid	A break request may be appropriate
The learner engages in behavior to escape or avoid a task/activity because it is difficult	A request for assistance may be appropriate
The task/activity is something in which the learner would likely continue to engage with assistance	A request for assistance may be appropriate
The learner engages in behavior to escape or avoid an object or activity in addition to seeking attention	A request for assistance may be appropriate

Who Might Benefit from Learning a Rejecting Response?

Rejecting allows the learner to avoid the onset/presentation of the object or activity altogether, protect him- or herself from another's inappropriate requests (e.g., partner suggests "Let's go outside" during a blizzard), and regulate his or her own behavior (e.g., communicating, "I don't want more cake," after having already consumed one piece) (Sigafoos & Reichle, 1991). If the nonpreferred object or activity is associated with challenging behavior, then appropriate ways to reject, prior to any contact with the nonpreferred object or activity, are particularly important.

What Does the Research Say?

Rejecting

Research demonstrates learners have been taught to reject objects or activities using manual signs and gestures, speech-generating devices (SGDs), and speech (see Sigafoos et al., 2004, for a review). In several studies, interventionists created opportunities to reject using the "wrong item" format in which an object was presented to the learner that he or she did not select when given a choice. For example, an adult provided a banana when the child asked for a cookie. Offering the wrong item creates an opportunity to teach socially appropriate forms of rejecting.

Sigafoos and Roberts-Pennell (1999) used the wrong item format to teach socially appropriate forms of rejecting to a pair of 6-year-old boys with severe intellectual disabilities. Shaking the head side to side gesturing "no" was taught to one child, and using an SGD to indicate "no" was taught to the other child. The interventionist presented a most and a least preferred object (identified from a preference assessment; see Chapter 5) and asked each child, "Which one?" On some opportunities, the interventionist provided the item for which the child reached; on other opportunities, the interventionist offered the other object (the one for which the child did not reach). Interventionists prompted rejecting using verbal instructions, models, and physical guidance faded with a least-to-most prompting strategy in conjunction with a time delay. Appropriate rejecting responses resulted in praise and removal of the wrong item. In the multiple baseline across participants design, one child began to show some independent rejecting during baseline, but the other child did not show any correct rejections during baseline. Both children increased appropriate rejecting that generalized to novel interventionists and maintained over periods of 3–4 months.

Duker and Jutten (1997) examined similar types of opportunities to teach three women with intellectual dis-

(continued)

abilities gestural requests (e.g., clapping their hands two to three times) and rejections (e.g., moving their hands back and forth two to three times). Once the learner requested a particular object or activity, the interventionist presented either that object or activity or the wrong one and asked, "Do you want this one?" The interventionist prompted using a most-to-least prompt hierarchy (from verbal model and physical assistance to verbal only). All three women acquired requesting and rejecting gestures, establishing conditional use of the rejecting response.

Duker and Jutten (1997) and Sigafoos and Roberts-Pennell (1999) taught general rejections (e.g., a general "no") in response to a verbal offer of a nonpreferred object or activity. Consider teaching more explicit rejecting responses (e.g., "no juice") as well as sampling the range of nonpreferred objects or activities (highly and less highly nonpreferred), situations (e.g., normally preferred objects that are not preferred because the individual is satiated), and ways to offer objects or activities (e.g., verbal offer, giving gesture) (Sigafoos & Reichle, 1991) when developing interventions to teach rejecting.

Using Evidence-Based Strategies to Teach Rejecting

When it is socially acceptable for a learner to escape or avoid engaging in an activity, a rejecting communicative act may represent the best communicative match to meet an individual's communicative needs. The following represent steps in implementing a rejecting strategy that are supported in the empirical literature.

Steps for teaching rejecting

Step 1: Identify situations.
Step 2: Identify the communicative alternative.
Step 3: Identify the critical point at which to prompt a rejection.
Step 4: Identify intervention strategies to teach rejecting.
Step 5: Implement intervention and monitor learner performance.
Step 6: Build tolerance for delay of reinforcement.

Step 1: Identify Situations

Identify situations associated with avoidance in which appropriate rejections can result in reinforcement.

What Objects or Activities Should Be Used to Teach Rejecting?

- Identify objects that were never selected or actively avoided (e.g., learner pushed the item away) in a preference assessment. It is likely these will function as negative reinforcers such that their removal, contingent on rejection, will increase the rate of that response.

- Identify and create a hierarchy of positive teaching examples; that is, all specific objects or activities that are regularly avoided and acceptable for the learner to avoid. Rank the objects or activities from those that are highly nonpreferred, followed by less highly nonpreferred, then those that are usually preferred, but not in a given situation (e.g., learner is satiated, ill). Typically, intervention begins with highly nonpreferred objects or activities.

- Identify negative teaching examples, including 1) obligatory objects or activities the learner will not be allowed to avoid and 2) preferred objects or activities that the learner should not reject. Begin intervention with

 Highly preferred objects or activities as negative teaching examples so that they are maximally different from the positive teaching examples (i.e., highly nonpreferred and highly preferred objects or activities).

 Objects or activities that are neither highly distressing nor associated with significant challenging behavior (because challenging behavior may make it difficult to prompt appropriate communication).

Helpful Hint

The most nonpreferred objects or activities may produce a high level of challenging behavior for some learners. If challenging behavior occurs in some of the identified teaching situations, then intervention should begin with situations that are less problematic so that the interventionist can more easily prompt appropriate communicative responses. Even if the new socially acceptable communicative behavior does not generalize to the more problematic situations, it may require a lower dose of intervention.

How Are Opportunities Created to Teach Rejecting?
Opportunities for rejecting may occur when

- A nonpreferred object is likely to be offered to the learner (e.g., interventionist is coming with a work task) or a nonpreferred activity is about to begin (e.g., reading is the next scheduled activity).

> See Chapter 6 for general procedures about identifying and creating teaching opportunities.

- The learner is offered a nonpreferred object (e.g., gesturally, verbally).
- The learner is offered a preferred object or activity but an even more preferred object or activity is available (e.g., crackers are offered at snack time but there are also cookies).

- The learner becomes satiated with a preferred object or activity (i.e., the learner's interaction with a preferred object or activity decreases because of his or her continued contact with or consumption of that object or engagement in that activity).

- A normally preferred object is unappealing (e.g., food is rancid; favorite attire is a short-sleeve shirt, but it is a cold day).

- There is a need for the learner to self-regulate or engage in self-control (e.g., when offered a second piece of cake).

- The learner is offered the wrong object or activity following a request (e.g., when offered a cracker after requesting a cookie), as in the wrong item format (Sigafoos & Roberts-Pennell, 1999).

Helpful Hint

If the interventionist's only interactions with the learner involve the presentation of nonpreferred objects or activities, then the learner may begin to associate the interventionist with the nonpreferred objects or events and avoid the interventionist. Interventionists must ensure they also present preferred objects or activities to the learner so that the interventionists are also associated with the delivery of preferred objects or events and, hence, someone to approach, not avoid.

Step 2: Identify the Communicative Alternative

Consider the form of the communicative behavior (e.g., communication mode, system features; see Chapter 2) as well as the level of specificity of the vocabulary taught to reject objects or activities. The learner may already show socially acceptable forms of rejecting that occur inconsistently and simply need consistent reinforcement. Pay attention to indicators of rejection (e.g., turning away) that can be expanded to more sophisticated communication. Sigafoos and Reichle (1991) recommended teaching a general rejection (e.g., "no") first to beginning communicators, followed by a more explicit rejection (e.g., "no juice"). An explicit rejection is necessary when there is insufficient context for the listener to easily infer the object or activity being rejected. Although often taught after first teaching a more general rejection, explicit rejections or a combination of general and explicit rejections can be taught from the outset. For example, explicit rejections could be taught for highly disliked objects and a more general rejection for moderately nonpreferred objects. Advantages and disadvantages of teaching general and explicit rejections are outlined in Table 10.2.

Helpful Hint

After first teaching a general rejection, chain the general rejection (e.g., "no") to a label for a specific object or activity (e.g., "work") to teach an explicit rejection (e.g., "no work"). See Chapter 5 for information about chaining.

Table 10.2.   Advantages and disadvantages of teaching general and explicit rejecting responses

	Advantages	Disadvantages
General rejection	Provides an immediately useful means for rejecting a variety of nonpreferred objects in a variety of situations Provides a greater number of opportunities (because it applies to a variety of objects and activities) Increases the likelihood of generalization across additional objects and activities Reduces the need to teach numerous additional or specific vocabulary items	Places the burden on the listener to determine what is being rejected (e.g., when a learner signs NO in response to the offer of juice, the learner may be rejecting the juice, but could be rejecting a drink altogether or the cup that contains the juice)
Explicit rejection	Clearly indicates what is being rejected May be clearer to a novel listener May be particularly useful for situations in which the learner desires to avoid specific objects or activities and/or engages in challenging behavior	Requires learning multiple response forms, which may be prohibitive as an initial target for some learners May require a number of teaching opportunities for each situation because a different rejection is taught for each

Step 3: Identify the Critical Point at Which to Prompt a Rejection

To teach appropriate rejections, deliver a prompt just prior to the point that the learner anticipates the presentation of a nonpreferred object or activity (referred to as the **critical point**). To determine this point,

- Observe the learner across several days.

- Measure the point at which the learner anticipates the presentation of a nonpreferred object or activity (e.g., as indicated by challenging behavior) by

  The distance at which the object can be introduced before the learner shows avoidance behavior (e.g., caregiver holding the asparagus at the doorway, placing it on the table as close as possible to the learner)

  The discrete event that occurs just prior to the onset of the nonpreferred object or activity (e.g., the interventionist terminates free time by asking the class to clean up [the next activity is reading, a nonpreferred activity]) or presents the wrong item

- Identify the greatest distance or the predictively occurring discrete event to examine the point at which the learner anticipates the nonpreferred object or activity.

> Use a performance monitoring form (e.g., Form 10.1 on the accompanying CD-ROM) to record the point at which the learner desires to avoid the nonpreferred object or activity. A blank version (Form 10.1a) as well as a filled-in sample (Form 10.1b) are provided on the accompanying CD-ROM.

- The interventionist will be implementing the intervention (i.e., prompt a rejection) just prior to the greatest distance or discrete event.

Step 4: Identify Intervention Strategies to Teach Rejecting

Choose prompting, reinforcement, and error correction procedures (see Chapter 5). Reinforcement procedures must include negative reinforcement; that is, withdrawing the object or activity the learner rejected.

> Use the Intervention Planning Form (Form 6.1 on the accompanying CD-ROM) to document intervention strategies.

Step 5: Implement Intervention and Monitor Learner Performance

Use a performance monitoring form such as Form 10.2 on the accompanying CD-ROM.

Step 6: Build Tolerance for Delay of Reinforcement

As the learner acquires communication skills to reject objects or activities, he or she will likely use the response repeatedly and regularly. This situation may be acceptable on a temporary basis, but it may not always be possible to reinforce a rejection, or it may be necessary to involve the learner with the rejected activity or object to increase instructional opportunities for other skills. For example, although teaching an appropriate means of rejecting math work is important to replace dangerous challenging behavior, repeated avoidance of math work then results in missing important instructional opportunities.

Tolerating a delay in reinforcement in situations that involve rejecting means waiting (in the absence of challenging behavior) for the removal of the object or activity that has been rejected. Introduce a *tolerance cue* when the learner rejects the object or activity or just prior to the learner's usual point of rejection in order to build tolerance. To illustrate, after Eva signed NO when offered a bite of peas, her father said, "Just one small bite." Alternatively, just prior to offering the peas, he could have said, "Let's eat just one small bite" and offered the peas. When the delay passes (i.e., Eva ate the small bite of peas), the interventionist delivers another cue to release the learner from the situation (a safety signal or release cue) and withdraws the object or activity. Once Eva ate the small bite, her father said, "Okay, you are all done," and removed the peas. As the learner consistently tolerates small, short delays, gradually increase the delay (e.g., time, amount) before delivering the tolerance cue or between the tolerance and release cues. As Eva ate one bite of peas, her father said, "Okay, eat two small bites, and then you are done," at the next meal.

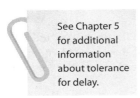

See Chapter 5 for additional information about tolerance for delay.

CASE EXAMPLE

Rejecting

Mark, a 7-year-old boy with autism who used manual signs to communicate, was enrolled in an inclusive classroom at his local elementary school. Mark usually screamed on the playground at recess when asked to play by one of his peers. A functional behavioral assessment indicated Mark's screaming served to avoid interacting with his peers. (See filled-in sample Form 10.1b on the accompanying CD-ROM.) Baseline data indicated that Mark never appropriately rejected interaction with his peers. Intervention involved teaching Mark to sign NO when approached by a peer to play.

Intervention began with two peers (Justin and Molly). As one of the peers asked Mark to play, the paraprofessional used hand-over-hand physical assistance to prompt Mark to emit the sign for NO. The paraprofessional praised Mark's communication once he produced the sign, directed the peer to say, "Maybe next time," and told Mark that he did not have to play. Intervention procedures are described in detail on the intervention planning form in Figure 10.1 (Form 6.1 is a blank version and is included on the accompanying CD-ROM). Mark's paraprofessional recorded his performance on the form in Figure 10.2 (Form 10.2 is a blank version and is included on the accompanying CD-ROM). Once Mark successfully signed NO to avoid interactions with Justin and Molly, additional peers (Craig and Sarah) were involved to further ensure Mark's generalized use of the sign NO.

Mark's interventionists also wanted to increase Mark's successful interactions with his peers because social skills are important. Therefore, intervention also focused on increasing Mark's interactions before he terminated the interaction. When Mark signed NO, his paraprofessional said, "You can play by yourself, but first play with [name of peer] until the timer goes off." The paraprofessional then set a timer for a specified interval (initially, a brief interval [i.e., 1 minute]). If Mark stayed with his peers for the interval, then his paraprofessional de-

Learner's name: _Mark_   Start date: _1/11_

Setting (circle one):   HOME   (SCHOOL)   COMMUNITY   WORK

Communication skill/function: _Mark will be taught to appropriately reject (i.e., sign NO) to avoid_
interacting with his peers when they ask him to play at recess.

Opportunities

When: _Recess time_   Where: _On the playground_

Minimum opportunities per day/session: _One opportunity per day_

Context for instruction: _Opportunities will be dictated by Mark's peers asking him to play._

Set up: _A peer approaching Mark and verbally inviting him to play_

Materials: _None_

Target Behavior

Mode: _Manual sign_

Augmentative and alternative communication system features: _None_

Vocabulary: _Sign for NO_

Instructional Strategies

Skill sequence/steps: _1) Peer invites Mark to play; 2) paraprofessional prompts Mark to sign NO;_
3) peer ends interaction.

Prompts: _Use full physical assistance (hand over hand) or partial physical (touching the wrist)_
assistance.

Consequences

     Correct response: _Provide praise (e.g., "Nice signing NO"), and terminate interaction with the_
peer.

     Incorrect response (no response or error response): _Immediately increase the prompt level._

Prompt fading: _Use most-to-least prompt fading._

Generalization: _Following mastery with the target peers (Justin and Molly), direct other peers_
(Craig and Sarah) from Mark's class to ask Mark to play. Following mastery in generalization,
increase the time Mark interacts with peers in 1-minute increments up to 10 minutes

Maintenance: _Monitor Mark's use of the new skill weekly_

Criterion for Mastery

Mark will independently reject interaction with each of the peers for each opportunity across
3 consecutive days.

Performance Monitoring

Document Mark's response on each opportunity.

Figure 10.1. Intervention Planning Form for teaching socially appropriate rejecting to Mark. (*Note:* This is a filled-in version of Form 6.1, Intervention Planning Form. A blank, printable version appears on the accompanying CD-ROM.)

Learner's name: __Mark__

Condition (circle one): (Baseline)   Intervention   Maintenance   Generalization

Correct response: __Mark will sign NO when approached by a peer and asked to play__

Instructions: Provide the date and the learner's performance of a rejecting response (e.g., a plus [+] for an independent response, a *P* for a prompted response, and a minus [–] for an incorrect response). Record whether the learner engaged in challenging behavior (e.g., "yes" if the learner engaged in challenging behavior, "no" if the learner did not). Record the initials of the interventionist, and use the Notes column to record any information relevant to learner performance (e.g., record the point at which the learner desires to avoid the nonpreferred object or activity during baseline observations). This performance monitoring form was developed for a learner's appropriate rejection of interactions with his peers. A column is included to record the peer who was the communicative partner. A column (delay) is also included to record the amount of time the learner engages with the peer before rejecting further interaction during tolerance building.

Date	Rejection	Challenging behavior (yes/no)	Delay	Interventionist's initials	Peer	Notes
1/11	FP	No	0 minutes	AE	Justin	Intervention
1/14	FP	No	0 minutes	AE	Molly	Intervention
1/15	FP	No	0 minutes	AE	Justin	Intervention
1/16	PP	No	0 minutes	AE	Justin	Intervention
1/17	PP	No	0 minutes	AE	Molly	Intervention
1/18	PP	No	0 minutes	AE	Molly	Intervention
1/21	I	No	0 minutes	AE	Justin	Intervention
1/22	I	No	0 minutes	AE	Justin	Intervention
1/23	I	No	0 minutes	AE	Molly	Intervention
1/24	I	No	0 minutes	AE	Craig	Generalization
1/25	I	No	0 minutes	AE	Sarah	Generalization
1/28	I	No	0 minutes	AE	Craig	Generalization
1/29	I	No	1 minute	AE	Justin	Tolerance building
1/30	I	No	1 minute	AE	Molly	Tolerance building
1/31	I	No	1 minute	AE	Craig	Tolerance building
2/1	I	No	2 minutes	AE	Sarah	Tolerance building
2/4	I	No	2 minutes	AE	Justin	Tolerance building
2/5	I	No	2 minutes	AE	Justin	Tolerance building
2/6	I	No	3 minutes	AE	Craig	Tolerance building
2/7	I	No	3 minutes	AE	Sarah	Tolerance building
2/8	I	No	3 minutes	AE	Justin	Tolerance building

Figure 10.2. Performance Monitoring Form for recording Mark's communications to avoid. (*Key:* FP, full prompt [hand over hand]; I, independent [no prompt]; PP, partial prompt [touching Mark's wrist].) (*Note:* This is a filled-in version of Form 10.2, Performance Monitoring Form for Recording Rejecting Responses. A blank, printable version appears on the accompanying CD-ROM.)

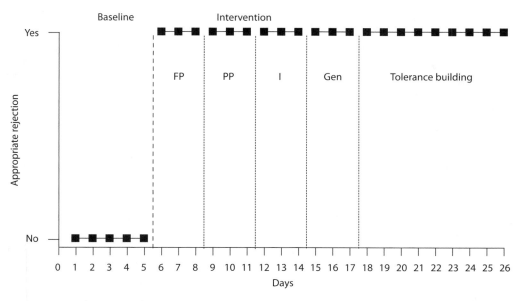

Figure 10.3.   Mark's rejection of peer's invitation to play during intervention, generalization, and tolerance building. (*Key*: FP, full prompt; Gen, generalization; I, independent; PP, partial prompt.)

livered reinforcement (praise and the opportunity to terminate the peer interaction). The data in Figure 10.2 indicate Mark tolerated 3-minute interactions with his peers; tolerance building will continue until Mark tolerates a 10-minute interaction with his peers. Graphic presentations of Mark's performance, both acquisition of

appropriate rejecting and increases in the time he interacted with peers, are presented in Figures 10.3 and 10.4, respectively.

Many learners who express a desire to avoid an object or activity may also be seek-

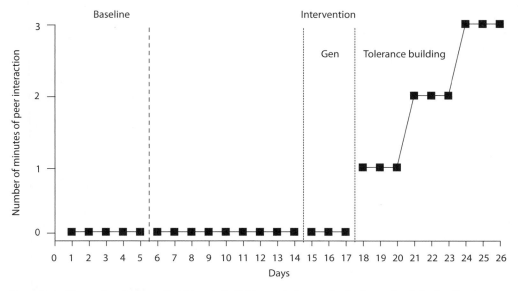

Figure 10.4.   The number of minutes Mark interacted with his peers before terminating interaction during baseline, intervention, generalization, and tolerance building. (*Key*: Gen, generalization)

ing an alternative they would like to gain access to instead. If Mark's baseline and functional assessment had revealed that he preferred playing only select games with peers, then requesting an alternative (discussed next) following a peer's invitation to play a nonpreferred game would have been more appropriate.

REQUESTING AN ALTERNATIVE

Requesting an alternative involves not only escape/avoidance of one object/activity, but also access to another, presumably more preferred, object/activity. For example, when offered a nonpreferred food item such as asparagus, requesting the other available vegetable (e.g., pointing to the graphic symbols for GREEN BEANS and PLEASE) would be appropriate.

> Procedures to teach requesting an alternative are similar to those for teaching other requesting responses (see Chapter 9).

Who Might Benefit from Learning to Request an Alternative?

Generalization to a situation involving requesting an alternative to avoid a nonpreferred object or activity is not guaranteed, even if requesting objects or activities is part of the learner's repertoire. That is, even if a learner can request blocks at the beginning of free play when he or she is given a choice, he or she will not necessarily request them when given a toy car (a less preferred toy). Learning to request an alternative can be particularly important to help learners obtain that specific object or activity when they have specific preferences (e.g., blocks).

What Does the Research Say?
Requesting an Alternative

Requesting an alternative has most often been taught in conjunction with requesting and rejecting responses. Sigafoos and Roberts-Pennell (1999) taught one participant to

reject the offer of an item that had not been requested by pressing a button to activate a message saying NO, THANKS. I WANT THE OTHER ONE—rejecting one item and requesting an alternative. After teaching requesting access, Duker, Dortmans, and Lodder (1993) found that participants (14- to 31-year-olds with intellectual disabilities) took the object provided even if it was not the one they requested (i.e., as in the wrong item format when the interventionist provides the item the learner did not choose). Subsequently, when the learner accepted the wrong object, the interventionist prompted the learner to repeat the initial gestured request as a rejection of the wrong item and a request for an alternative to that wrong item.

Yamamoto and Mochizuki (1988) encountered a similar situation with three 10- to 11-year-old children with autism. When the wrong object was presented during intervention, the interventionist verbally modeled, "That's not it" (rejection) and then "Give me ___" (request for alternative). Once the learner imitated, the interventionist offered the requested object. Learners acquired requesting an alternative and showed a high percentage of correct responses with a second offer of the nonrequested object and offers of nonrequested objects in a different situation.

Using Evidence-Based Strategies to Teach Requesting an Alternative

When there is an alternative object or activity that would lessen or eliminate an individual's need to escape or avoid a situation, requesting an alternative represents a viable communicative function to establish. For example, suppose that a child would rather use a blue marker than the red marker he or she is given. The child may attempt to escape or avoid the activity because it is aversive when the child cannot use a preferred marker. Re-

> Steps for teaching requesting an alternative
>
> Step 1: Identify situations.
> Step 2: Identify the communicative alternative.
> Step 3: Identify the point at which to prompt a request for an alternative.
> Step 4: Develop intervention strategies.
> Step 5: Implement intervention, and monitor performance.
> Step 6: Build tolerance for delay.

questing an alternative represents a viable option to escape when the interventionist who is monitoring the activity has not given the child a choice of markers.

Step 1: Identify Situations

Consider situations in which rejection would be appropriate:

- When there is a a better option available

- An array of options are available, some more preferred and some less preferred

- The wrong object is provided following a learner's request (i.e., wrong item format)

Step 2: Identify the Communicative Alternative

Requesting an alternative may involve an explicit request for a specific object or activity or a rejection followed by a request for an alternative (e.g., Sigafoos & Roberts-Pennell, 1999). If a rejection is already in the learner's repertoire, then a request for an alternative can be taught by chaining the rejection to the request.

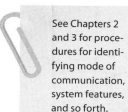

See Chapters 2 and 3 for procedures for identifying mode of communication, system features, and so forth.

Step 3: Identify the Critical Point at Which to Prompt a Request for an Alternative

- Observe the learner across several days.

- Note the point at which the learner avoids the situation (e.g., as indicated by challenging behavior) and attempts to gain access to an alternative.

- Identify the common point across opportunities.

- Implement intervention just prior to this point—the critical point.

Use a performance monitoring form, such as Form 10.3 provided on the accompanying CD-ROM, to record the step at which the learner seeks access to an alternative object or activity. Both blank (Form 10.3a) and filled-in (Form 10.3b) versions are provided on the acompanying CD-ROM.

Step 4: Develop Intervention Strategies

Refer to Chapter 5 for a discussion of choosing intervention strategies. Reinforcement must involve both negative reinforcement (i.e., removing/terminating the nonpreferred object/activity) and positive reinforcement (i.e., providing the desired object/activity).

Step 5: Implement Intervention and Monitor Performance

See the blank (Form 10.4a) and filled-in (Form 10.4b) versions of Form 10.4 on the accompanying CD-ROM.

Step 6: Build Tolerance for Delay

Tolerating a delay in reinforcement means waiting, in the absence of challenging behavior, for the removal of the nonpreferred object or activity and receipt of the desired alternative. For example, when increasing Scott's tolerance for engaging in a nonpreferred reading activity and delaying receipt of the computer, the preferred alternative, his interventionist told Scott, just prior to his request for an alternative, "Read for 1 minute and then you can ask for computer." Once Scott read for 1 minute and requested the computer, he gained access to the computer. The interventionist increased the delay over time so that Scott read for 30 minutes before requesting an alternative.

CASE EXAMPLE

Request for Alternative

Kia, a 14-year-old student with multiple disabilities, used an SGD mounted on her wheelchair to both request and reject food items. Kia liked to eat a variety of salad toppings and sandwiches that she requested from the cafeteria staff during lunch. Sometimes it was difficult for the cafeteria workers to clearly hear what Kia requested in the crowded and noisy cafeteria, resulting in offering Kia something she did not request. When this happened, Kia tried to reach for another item and/or pressed the button on her device that produced the word NO, but would not clarify what she wanted instead (see filled-in Form 10.3b on the accompanying CD-ROM).

To teach requesting an alternative, Kia's device was programmed with a new button that produced the sentence NO THANK YOU, I WANT for Kia to press before touching the button for the item that she had initially requested. The cafeteria staff were recruited to give Kia the wrong food items at least five times during lunch (positive teaching exemplars) but also correctly give Kia the item she requested (negative teaching exemplars). This allowed for a mix of successful requesting opportunities with opportunities to request an alternative. When the cafeteria staff began to put the wrong item on Kia's salad, the interventionist physically prompted touching the buttons for NO THANK YOU, I WANT and then the item that Kia initially requested. The cafeteria worker then immediately gave Kia the requested item. The same intervention procedures were used at home during dinner with her family. Her parents and two siblings prompted Kia's use of the NO THANK YOU, I WANT symbol (see filled-in Form 10.4b on the accompanying CD-ROM).

Rejecting and requesting an alternative allows learners to avoid contact with non-preferred objects or activities altogether. Sometimes, objects or activities become non-preferred when they have been experienced for some time (e.g., dinner conversation, lengthy work period) and simply need to be put aside for a period before reengaging. Communication to escape the object or activity for a brief time (i.e., requesting a break) is appropriate in this case.

REQUESTING A BREAK

Requesting a break involves communication to gain temporary release from an ongoing activity with the expectation of reengaging in that activity. For example, the learner leaves the boring dinner table conversation, returning after a few minutes. In this example, the learner not only removes him- or herself from the boring dinner conversation but also has the opportunity to go into the kitchen and

sneak a bite of dessert. As this illustrates, break requests not only result in negative reinforcement (i.e., removal of the nonpreferred activity) but also positive reinforcement (i.e., access to another object or activity).

Who Might Benefit from Learning to Request a Break?

Break requests are appropriate when it is possible for the learner to leave an activity and then reengage at a later point in time. If the activity is something in which the learner must engage for its entire length (e.g., riding a Ferris wheel), then a break request would not be appropriate. Learners who cannot sustain engagement in an activity for prolonged periods may benefit from breaking up long activities with several shorter periods of activity punctuated by breaks.

What Does the Research Say?
Requesting a Break

An extensive literature effectively demonstrates intervention procedures to teach children and adults to request breaks using sign, graphic systems, microswitches, SGD, and speech to escape from aversive situations (e.g., Carr et al., 1999; Day, Horner, & O'Neill, 1994; Durand, 1993; Mildon, Moore, & Dixon, 2004; Northup et al., 1994). Teaching break requests replaces challenging behavior in much of this literature.

Following a functional analysis confirming escape as the function of participants' challenging behavior, Lalli, Casey, and Kates (1995) taught three participants (ages 10, 13, and 15 years) to request a break from work tasks. The mode was tailored to each participant: one was taught to hand over a card with the word *break,* another to say "no," and the third to shake her head "no." The interventionist presented a work demand and said, "If you do not want to work now, say, 'No,'" (or the way the learner was being taught to express "no") along with physical or modeling prompts. Once the participant indicated "no," the interventionist provided praise and a brief break from the task. Independent requests for breaks gradually increased while rates of challenging behavior decreased during intervention. The interventionist presented a demand and stated

(continued)

the criterion for earning a break (e.g., completing a specific task step) during tolerance building to increase work time. If the participant requested a break prior to completing work, then the interventionist said, "Good saying 'no,' but you have to do [task step] then you can ask for a break," and provided the level of assistance necessary for the participant to complete the task. Rates of challenging behavior remained low even when participants were required to do more to obtain a break.

Using Evidence-Based Strategies to Teach a Break Request

Requesting a break is a viable intervention when the interventionist can allow the learner to briefly disengage from an activity with the expectation of the learner reengaging in the activity. Although there is a limited literature addressing teaching this skill, there are interventionist-directed activities that tend to be commonly applied in instances where requesting a break has been successfully taught.

Steps for teaching a break request

Step 1: Identify situations.
Step 2: Identify the communicative alternative.
Step 3: Identify the point at which to prompt a break request.
Step 4: Develop intervention strategies.
Step 5: Implement intervention, and monitor performance.
Step 6: Build tolerance for delay.

Step 1: Identify Situations

Observe the learner to identify all situations in which he or she engages for some time before attempting to gain access to a break. Appropriate activities in which to teach break requests are those in which a break request can be honored and a request to leave is required. Negative teaching examples include activities the learner prefers; activities the learner could or should simply reject outright without engagement for some time (e.g., going outside in a thunderstorm); activities that do not require a request to leave, rather the learner could just leave (e.g., watching television); and activities

in which a break request cannot and/or will not be honored (e.g., during a required medical procedure).

Step 2: Identify the Communicative Alternative

A break request is typically a general request such as touching a graphic symbol of BREAK, signing BREAK, or verbalizing "break."

Step 3: Identify the Critical Point at Which to Prompt a Break Request

- Observe the learner engaging in the activity across several days.

- Measure the point at which the learner attempts to escape the situation (e.g., as indicated by getting out of the chair) by

  The length of time the learner engages in the activity prior to attempting to escape (e.g., number of minutes the learner sits appropriately at the dinner table)

  The number of discrete tasks/steps the learner completes before engaging in escape motivated behavior (e.g., number of steps in the sequence to make a peanut butter and jelly sandwich)

- Identify the shortest amount of time or the fewest steps across opportunities.

- Prompt a break request prior to the shortest time or fewest steps—the critical point.

Step 4: Develop Intervention Strategies

Provide frequent reinforcement for the learner's engagement in a nonpreferred activity. Consider occasionally using release from the activity (but without the learner's request for a break) as reinforcement for engaging in the nonpreferred activity. This provides the learner with frequent access to highly valued reinforcers for appropriate behaviors (engaging with the activity and requesting a break).

Reinforcement will necessarily involve the termination of the activity (i.e., negative reinforcement) when the learner requests a break. Breaks from an activity often also involve positive reinforcement such as access to other objects or activities (e.g., magazines, toys). Examine what the learner currently gains access to, or seeks to access, while es-

Use a performance monitoring form such as Form 10.5 or Form 10.6. Blank forms (Forms 10.5a and 10.6a) as well as filled-in samples (Forms 10.5b and 10.6b) are provided on the accompanying CD-ROM to record the point at which the learner desires to escape the nonpreferred object or activity.

caping in order to identify potential positive reinforcers to use during intervention. It may be appropriate to identify a specific space for the learner to easily (and with minimal disruption) gain access to other reinforcers while on a break (e.g., a corner of the classroom, a different room in the house).

Consider the following to decrease the likelihood of challenging behavior when asking a learner to return from a break to a nonpreferred activity.

- The reinforcer should ideally be completely consumed during the break time (e.g., provide only a small number of potato chips) or naturally dissipate over the course of the break time (e.g., taking a walk through the school building that ends at the door to the classroom coinciding with the end of the break). This provides a natural cue that the break is over, and may decrease a struggle over removing the positive reinforcers at the end of a break.

- Present antecedent strategies when telling the learner it is time to end the break and return to the activity in order to increase the likelihood of returning to the nonpreferred activity in the absence of challenging behavior.

  Use a **high-probability request sequence** by asking the learner to engage in several easy and/or preferred activities to which the learner has a high probability of responding, presenting reinforcement for each, and then asking the learner to engage in the more difficult or nonpreferred activity to which the learner has a low probability of appropriately responding (the request to return from a break, in this case). For example, after taking a brief dessert break, but before asking

his son to clean up dinner (nonpreferred), the father asked him to tell his sister it was time to clean up dinner, turn off the light in the dining room, and turn on the light in the kitchen. The father provided reinforcement as the learner appropriately responded to each of these requests. Then, he presented the first dinner clean up demand (e.g., "Put the dishes in the dishwasher").

  Offer **choices** by presenting the learner with controlled options about a task. Increasing the learner's control over a less preferred task/activity (i.e., returning to task after a break) can increase the learner's appropriate compliance with that request. For example, following a brief dessert break, the father asked his son whether he would like to put the dishes in the dishwasher or wipe the counters.

  Use a **preferred item as a distractor** by pairing a preferred object or activity with a nonpreferred object or activity. For example, when returning to dinner clean up after a brief break, the father suggested they turn on their favorite evening game show to watch (preferred) while cleaning up.

- In addition to antecedent strategies, specifically reinforce returning from a break. Consider a reinforcer that is only available for returning to the nonpreferred activity from a break without challenging behavior.

Step 5: Implement Intervention and Monitor Performance

Use a form such as Form 10.7 on the accompanying CD-ROM to implement intervention and monitor performance.

Step 6: Build Tolerance for Delay

Once the learner acquires communication to request a break, he or she is likely to use it repeatedly so that he or she soon requests another break after returning to a nonpreferred activity from a break. Although it is terrific that the learner appropriately requests breaks, it is often important for learners to engage with nonpreferred activities for longer periods of time to allow for instruction of a variety of skills. Therefore, tolerance building is important. Tolerating a delay in reinforcement means waiting, in the absence of challenging behavior, before leaving the nonpreferred activity. For example, Julie learned to activate a symbol on her SGD to receive a break from household chores. To increase chore completion and delay breaks, Julie's mother said, "Let's just finish this one task," (e.g., folding a shirt, vacuuming a room) when Julie requested a break. Julie took the break she had requested after she completed that one task. As Julie successfully completed one task, Julie's mother asked her to complete more chores before receiving a break.

Challenging behavior may occur between the break request and receipt of reinforcement (i.e., release from the activity) during tolerance building. If this happens, require the learner to remain in the activity for a brief additional time with no challenging behavior, and then provide the break. Afterward, consider whether the delay was increased too much too quickly (e.g., increasing from one task to five before receiving reinforcement), and decrease the delay period with subsequent increases in smaller increments.

CASE EXAMPLE

Teaching a Break Request

Sam, a kindergarten student diagnosed with autism, often yelled and attempted to rip materials when completing worksheets but readily engaged with and completed other academic activities (e.g., quiet reading). Functional assessment data revealed Sam's behavior served to provide him escape from completing the worksheet. Baseline data showed he generally completed the first two problems prior to engaging in challenging behavior. (See filled-in Form 10.5b on the accompanying CD-ROM.)

Sam was taught to request a break from completing a worksheet by forming the sign for BREAK because he primarily used sign language to communicate (see the intervention planning form in Figure 10.5; Form 6.1 is a blank

version and is included on the accompanying CD-ROM). Sam's interventionists decided that one-to-one sessions with more opportunities would be conducted in the back of the classroom because it would be difficult to provide Sam with enough opportunities to practice requesting a break during regular classroom activities. Sam's teacher or paraprofessional sat with Sam at a table and presented a worksheet. After completing one question, the interventionist said "break" while modeling the sign. Once Sam produced the sign, she removed the worksheet, placed a token on Sam's token board (a reinforcement system already in place for Sam), and Sam enjoyed a break with selected books at the table for 1–2 minutes. Following the break, she put the worksheet back on the table in front of Sam. Because Sam's interventionists were concerned that he might engage in challenging behavior when asked to continue to complete the worksheet following a break, his interventionist delivered a "bonus token" when Sam began the worksheet again without engaging in challenging behavior. Intervention began during regular classroom worksheet activities only once Sam requested a break without any prompts.

Once Sam completed one problem and requested a break without challenging behavior during regular classroom worksheet activities, the interventionist began tolerance building so that Sam would complete more worksheet problems and participate in an increasing number of learning opportunities. At this point, when Sam completed one question and signed for a break, the interventionist told Sam, "First, do one more," and pointed to the next question on the worksheet. He received a break and a token once he completed the next question in the absence of challenging behavior. The interventionist gradually increased the number of questions that Sam needed to complete before receiving a break (1 question at a time up to a total of 10 questions, [the usual length of the worksheets Sam's teacher assigned]). Sam's performance is shown in Figure 10.6 (Form 10.7 is a blank version and is included on the accompanying CD-ROM) and summarized in Figure 10.7. Figure 10.8 shows Sam's successful transitions returning from a break.

Learner's name: Sam   Start date: 1/29

Setting (circle one):   HOME   (SCHOOL)   COMMUNITY   WORK

Communication skill/function: Requesting a break during worksheet tasks

Opportunities

When: While completing worksheets   Where: In the classroom

Minimum opportunities per day/session: 5 opportunities per day during intervention

Context for instruction: Repeated opportunities to learn to request a break provided within one-to-one sessions. Subsequent opportunities will occur within ongoing classroom activities.

Set up: Interventionist says, "Do your work."

Materials: Worksheets, pencils, tokens and token board, books to gain access to while taking a break

Target Behavior

Mode: Manual sign

Augmentative and alternative communication system features: None

Vocabulary: Sign for BREAK

Instructional Strategies

Skill sequence/steps: 1) Present a worksheet and say, "Do your work"; 2) after Sam completes one problem, prompt him to sign BREAK; 3) remove the worksheet and provide Sam with a few books for a 1- to 2-minute break.

Prompts: Model the sign for BREAK and say, "Break." Fade to just a model.

Consequences

Correct response: Provide praise, remove the worksheet, and place a token on Sam's token board followed by a 1- to 2-minute break (when Sam can look at books at the table).

Incorrect response (no response or error response): Immediately increase the prompt level.

Prompt fading: Use most-to-least prompt fading: Fade the verbal praise and model to just a model. Then, fade the model when Sam signs BREAK in the absence of challenging behavior at the designated prompt level—80% of the opportunities across 2 days.

Generalization: Once Sam is signing BREAK independently during one-to-one sessions, implement intervention when worksheets are completed during regular classroom activities. Following mastery in one-to-one sessions and regular classroom activities, gradually increase the amount of work (1 question at a time up to 10 total questions) required before Sam takes a break.

Maintenance: Monitor Sam's performance at least weekly.

Criterion for Mastery

Sam will independently request a break on 80% of the opportunities across 2 days in the absence of challenging behavior.

Performance Monitoring

Document Sam's performance on each opportunity.

Figure 10.5. Intervention Planning Form for teaching Sam to request a break. (*Note:* This is a filled-in version of Form 6.1, Intervention Planning Form. A blank, printable version appears on the accompanying CD-ROM.)

Learner's name: _Sam_   Interventionist: _Gloria_

Activity: _Completing worksheets_   Setting: _Classroom_

Circle one: Baseline   (Intervention)   Maintenance   Generalization

Target response: _Requesting a break_

Instructions: Record the date, the number of tasks/steps the learner should complete before requesting a break (the critical point), and the learner's performance of the response (e.g., a plus [+] for an independent response, a *P* for a prompted response, and a minus [–] for an incorrect response). Calculate percent correct performance. Record whether the learner engaged in challenging behavior during the task and/or at the end of the break (e.g., by making a checkmark in the appropriate space). Record any relevant notes about the learner's performance.

| | | | | | | | | Challenging behavior | | |
Date	Critical point	Performance					Percent	During task	End break	Notes
2/11	1	+	+	+	+	+	100	✓	✓	Full prompt
2/12	1	+	+	+	+	+	100			
2/13	1	+	+	+	+	+	100			
2/14	1	+	+	+	+	+	100			Partial prompt
2/15	1	+	+	+	+	+	100			
2/18	1	+	+	−	+	+	80			Independent
2/19	1	+	+	+	+	+	100			
2/20	1	+	+	+	−	+	80			
2/21	1	+	+	+	+	+	100			
2/22	2	+	+	+	+	+	100			Begin tolerance building
2/25	2	+	+	+	+	+	100			
2/26	3	+	+	+	+	+	100			
2/27	3	+	+	+	+	+	100			

Figure 10.6. Sam's performance during intervention teaching a break request. (*Note:* This is a filled-in version of Form 10.7, Performance Monitoring Form for Break Requests. A blank, printable version appears on the accompanying CD-ROM.)

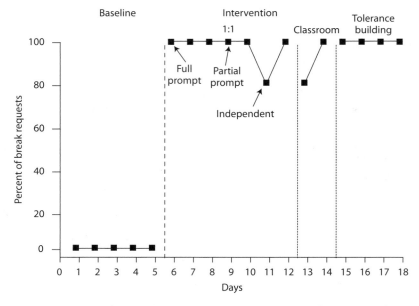

Figure 10.7. Sam's performance during baseline and intervention teaching him to request a break to escape completion of worksheets.

Sometimes nonpreferred activities are difficult for a learner to complete independently in these situations. A break is apt in these situations only to postpone escape, rather than improve the individual's competence. Requesting assistance is more appropriate when escape behavior is linked to the difficulty of the task or activity.

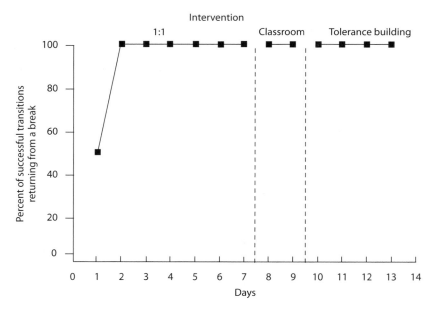

Figure 10.8. Percentage of successful transitions from a break back to a worksheet task (i.e., Sam did not engage in challenging behavior).

REQUESTING ASSISTANCE

A request for assistance can not only result in help, but also allow the learner to escape or avoid difficult and nonpreferred activities. For example, behavior to escape or avoid cleaning up after dinner may be related to difficulty washing the dishes (e.g., adjusting the water temperature, holding the dish and sponge simultaneously). Assistance with washing the dishes would decrease the aversiveness of the task and result in more rapid completion.

Requesting assistance is appropriate when the learner seeks to obtain an object or activity (he or she cannot independently obtain) as well as when he or she is motivated to escape or avoid an object or activity because of difficulty. Requesting assistance taught in the context of access to objects/activities will not necessarily generalize to requesting assistance in the context of escaping/avoiding tasks/activities (Reichle, 1991; Reichle, Drager, & Davis, 2002; Reichle & McComas, 2004); therefore, both situations should be a part of intervention.

Requesting assistance may be particularly appropriate in situations in which it is

> Requesting assistance to obtain an object or activity is discussed in Chapter 9.

undesirable or not possible to reinforce a rejection or break request. Following a rejection, the rejected activity remains incomplete altogether and, following a break request, the activity remains incomplete while the learner receives a break. In contrast, once the learner requests assistance, the activity is immediately completed with assistance, ensuring activity completion and providing specific prompting to teach the learner the requisite task skills. As a result, the learner is likely to become more proficient at the activity that initially caused difficulty, so the need for assistance should decrease. Thus, over time, a given activity should move from a positive teaching example (one for which the learner needs and should request assistance) to a negative teaching exemplar (one for which the learner has now acquired skills

to complete and should not need or request assistance; Reichle et al., 2005).

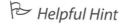 *Helpful Hint*

Even if the learner requests assistance to obtain objects or activities, those responses may not generalize to requesting assistance when presented with a difficult or aversive task/activity and vice versa (Reichle, 1991; Reichle et al., 2002). Therefore, both situations warrant instruction.

Who Might Benefit from Learning to Request Assistance to Escape or Avoid?

Learners who do not have the requisite skills for the task or become easily frustrated by some aspect of the task may benefit from learning to request assistance. If challenging behavior is escape or attention motivated in the presence of difficult activities, then a request for assistance may be particularly appropriate because the resulting reinforcement involves both escape from the difficult task as well as attention in the form of assistance.

What Does the Research Say?
Requesting Assistance

Carr and Durand (1985) taught 3 of 4 children (ages 13–14 years) with developmental disabilities to request assistance using an appropriate vocalization, specifically saying, "I don't understand" (a relevant response that corresponded to the function of the challenging behavior). When the student made an error while working on the difficult task, the interventionist indicated the error and then said, "Do you have any questions? Say, 'I don't understand.'" When the child imitated correctly, the interventionist said, "Okay, I'll show you," and proceeded to indicate the correct response. Participants were also taught an irrelevant response (asking, "Am I doing good work?") that did not match the function of the challenging behavior and resulted in interventionist praise, but no assistance. Results indicated that challenging behavior decreased only when participants were taught the relevant response—a request for assistance.

Horner and Day's (1991) functional analysis showed a 14-year-old boy engaged in aggressive behavior during

(continued)

difficult tasks; however, aggression decreased when assistance was provided. The participant was taught a low-efficiency request for assistance in which he typed each letter of the phrase HELP PLEASE on an AAC device that printed the message on a small strip of paper. He was also taught a high-efficiency request for assistance in which he pressed one button, which resulted in his AAC device producing the whole phrase, HELP PLEASE. Aggression decreased and requests for assistance increased only when using the high-efficiency response, despite the fact that the participant was able to spell out the request. Results indicated the importance of considering response efficiency when choosing the specific communicative alternative.

Task/activity difficulty is likely to change over time as a result of the learner's receipt of assistance upon request. Positive exemplars (i.e., difficult tasks) should become negative exemplars (i.e., easy tasks) over time. In Reichle et al. (2005), intervention resulted in an initial increase in assistance requests and a corresponding decrease in challenging behavior for the participant. Subsequently, assistance requests decreased as the participant became more proficient (through instruction provided when he requested assistance) at completing the task independently, demonstrating conditional use. In Reichle and McComas (2004), however, additional intervention (increasing reinforcement for independent completion of the work task [as that task became easy]) was necessary to teach the participant to request assistance only in situations in which he was unable to complete the task independently. Monitor learner proficiency with the difficult task and corresponding use of requests for assistance, and provide additional intervention if requests for assistance do not decrease as the learner acquires skills to complete the task in order to ensure the learner's conditional use of requesting assistance (i.e., requesting assistance is only used in the face of difficult tasks).

Using Evidence-Based Strategies to Teach Requests for Assistance

Use the following steps to teach requests for assistance in situations that the learner seeks to escape/avoid.

Step 1: Identify Situations

Identify tasks/activities for which the learner engages in behavior to escape or avoid because of difficulty completing the task (i.e., positive teaching exemplars). This may be indicated through a functional assessment

Steps for teaching a request for assistance

Step 1: Identify situations.
Step 2: Identify the communicative alternative.
Step 3: Identify the critical point at which to prompt a request for assistance.
Step 4: Develop instructional strategies.
Step 5: Implement intervention and monitor performance.
Step 6: Build tolerance for delay.

if challenging behavior is present. To assess whether difficulty relates to the learner's desire to escape or avoid the activity, compare the learner's engagement (and escape/avoidance behaviors):

- During easy and difficult versions of an activity (e.g., worksheets [addition versus mixed addition and subtraction problems], cooking tasks [making sandwiches versus risotto])

- Within the difficult situation when assistance is and is not provided; if task difficulty is the issue, then providing assistance should decrease escape or avoidance behavior

Also, identify negative teaching exemplars; in this case, tasks the learner completes independently. As assistance is provided and the learner acquires task-related skills, tasks that are initially difficult (i.e., those for which teaching a request for assistance is appropriate; positive teaching exemplars) should become easy tasks (i.e., negative teaching exemplars). Thus, over time, the positive and negative teaching exemplars will change and intervention may need to change (discussed in Step 4) if the learner does not spontaneously discriminate when to request assistance based on task difficulty.

> See Chapter 1 for information about response efficiency and conditional use.

Step 2: Identify the Communicative Alternative

Consider first teaching a general request (e.g., "Help") that is applicable in multiple situations, followed by more explicit requests for assistance (e.g., "Help wash," "Help. Need soap."). Consider the learner's existing repertoire, usual rate of acquisition, and the number of different situations in which the learner needs to request assistance in making a final decision whether to teach a general or explicit request first, or both simultaneously. Refer to considerations about choosing to teach general versus explicit rejections, which similarly apply to requests for assistance.

Step 3: Identify the Critical Point at Which to Prompt a Request for Assistance

- Observe the learner engaged in the task/activity across several days.

- Note the point at which the learner requires assistance using either a task analysis (see Form 5.4 on the accompanying CD-ROM) or a performance monitoring form that includes space to record the step in the activity at which the learner requires assistance and/or engages in escape/avoidance behavior.

- Identify the earliest step at which the learner demonstrates difficulty across opportunities.

- Implement intervention, prompting a request for assistance just prior to the earliest step at which the learner demonstrates difficulty or after the learner tries to complete the difficult step on his or her own—the critical point. Waiting to prompt until the learner has attempted the difficult step not only teaches requesting assistance but also attempting independent completion first and encountering difficulty before requesting assistance. Waiting until the learner has tried and failed to complete the step may result in challenging behavior. Prompting after the learner has tried and failed may best be done with steps/tasks that are not associated with significant challenging behavior.

Step 4: Develop Instructional Strategies

See Chapter 5 to choose instructional strategies. Reinforcement must include providing enough assistance to decrease the aversiveness of step in the task.

Step 5: Implement Intervention and Monitor Performance

Monitor changes in the learner's abilities that decrease the difficulty of the task, turning positive exemplars into negative exemplars (see Form 10.8 on the accompanying CD-ROM). Requests for assistance in this situation should decrease, demonstrating conditional use of requests for assistance only in the presence of difficult tasks. Although a task may be easy, conditional use may not be established in the absence of additional intervention. Therefore, if the learner requests assistance during easy tasks, then increase the reinforcement value for independent task completion (over the reinforcement for requesting assistance).

- Identify criteria for reinforcement; that is, the number of learner attempts and/or completions of the task. Allow some leeway initially to request assistance even during easy tasks (e.g., criterion of 3 out of 4 tasks independently completed rather than 4 out of 4). Consider also beginning with criteria focused on attempts, and increase criteria to include independent completion of tasks once the learner is successful.

- See Chapter 5 to identify potential reinforcers.

- Prespecify the reinforcer for attempting and/or completing tasks. That is, when presenting the task, tell the learner, "Try on your own, and we can take an extra break."

- Deliver the reinforcer for meeting the criterion number of attempts and/or completions of the activity(ies).

The learner should no longer request assistance when a task becomes easier. Requesting assistance for an unpleasant task, however, may result in faster task completion and quicker escape, even when the learner can independently complete the task. Carefully consider the necessity of independent task completion and reinforcing requests for assistance. This may be especially important if a learner engages in challenging behavior when faced with completing the task inde-

If the learner is not acquiring task-related skills, then reevaluate the type and level of assistance (see Chapter 5 for information about prompting procedures).

pendently. Continued reinforcement of requests for assistance may be warranted in this case and/or more gradual building of tolerance for waiting for assistance.

Step 6: Build Tolerance for Delay

Tolerance for delay when requesting assistance involves the learner waiting until the delay is over without assistance. For example, in a classroom with one teacher and multiple students, it would likely be difficult for the teacher to continue to provide assistance every time the learner requested. Interventionists in these situations may specifically focus on tolerance for delay in providing assistance. After the learner requests assistance, the interventionist delivers a tolerance cue indicating the delay and even requesting the learner attempt further task completion during the delay (e.g., "First try a few more, and I'll help you in a minute").

CASE EXAMPLE

Request for Assistance

Jennifer, a 28-year-old woman, worked in a mailroom with support from her job coach, Jim. Jennifer appeared unsure of what to do when she faced novel tasks, tensing her fists and pacing around the work area, resulting in minimal task completion. Baseline observations showed she never completed the novel tasks and never asked for help.

Jennifer used a few words but primarily communicated by using a picture symbol system. Intervention involved teaching Jennifer to request assistance by handing her job coach a printed card that said, I DON'T UNDERSTAND. I NEED HELP (see Figure 10.9; Form 6.1 is a blank ver-

sion and is included on the accompanying CD-ROM). Jim presented Jennifer with three novel tasks each day, enough opportunities for Jennifer to practice requesting assistance. Jim immediately prompted Jennifer, using physical guidance, to hand him the card and faded prompts using a time delay. When Jennifer requested assistance, Jim provided praise and additional prompts to help Jennifer complete the task. Figure 10.10 illustrates Jennifer's performance learning to request assistance (Form 10.8 is a blank version and is included on the accompanying CD-ROM). Once Jennifer requested assistance from her job coach, Jim taught her to request assistance from her co-workers. At this point, when Jennifer faced a novel task, Jim ensured a co-worker was nearby and immediately prompted Jennifer to request assistance from the co-worker.

Jim and Jennifer's co-workers faded their assistance with a most-to-least prompt hierarchy. Once Jim was delivering minimal prompts to help Jennifer complete the novel tasks, he briefly delayed the presentation of prompts (e.g., for 3–5 seconds), allowing Jennifer to complete the steps of the task more independently; however, she continued to request assistance. Easy tasks and several new difficult tasks were presented to Jennifer to help her learn to request assistance only when she really needed it (i.e., establish conditional use). Jim reminded Jennifer at the beginning of every work day to request assistance only when she really needed it. In addition, Jim told Jennifer to try an easy task on her own and they could take an extra coffee break (a naturally available consequence at Jennifer's work). Jennifer's performance is shown in Figure 10.10 and graphed in Figure 10.11. As Jim increased the value of reinforcement for independent task completion, he also ensured that Jennifer continued to request assistance when she encountered novel tasks, which was immediately honored. As a result, Jennifer demonstrated conditional use and requested assistance with novel tasks. Requests for assistance decreased as the tasks became easier.

Learner's name: _Jennifer_   Start date: _1/29_

Setting (circle one):   HOME   SCHOOL   COMMUNITY   (WORK)

Communication skill/function: _Jennifer will hand over a card to request assistance during novel work_
tasks.

Opportunities

When: _When presented with a novel task_   Where: _In the mailroom at the jobsite_

Minimum opportunities per day/session: _3 opportunities per day (one per novel task)_

Context for instruction: _Naturally occurring opportunities within Jennifer's job activities_

Set up: _Presentation of difficult task_

Materials: _Card, task materials_

Target Behavior

Mode: _Graphic_

Augmentative and alternative communication system features: _None_

Vocabulary: _Printed words "I don't understand. I need help" on card_

Instructional Strategies

Skill sequence/steps: _When encountering a difficult task, 1) Jim or co-worker prompts Jennifer to_
request assistance and 2) provides enough help to complete the task.

Prompts: _Full physical (hand over hand)_

Consequences

     Correct response: _Provide praise for making the correct response and assistance in complet-_
ing the novel task. Once novel (and difficult) tasks become easy, Jennifer will receive an extra
5-minute break for first trying those tasks on her own.

     Incorrect response (no response or error response): _Immediately prompt._

Prompt fading: _Use time delay: Once Jennifer successfully responds to the physical prompt for_
3 days, introduce a 5-second delay before prompting. Fade task-related prompts using a
most-to-least prompt hierarchy and time delay.

Generalization: _Generalize to co-workers once Jennifer requests assistance independently from_
Jim. Once Jennifer begins to independently complete the steps of a task, if a corresponding
decrease in requests for assistance does not occur, deliver an additional reinforcer of an
extra coffee break if Jennifer independently completes a task without requesting assistance.

Maintenance: _Monitor Jennifer's use of the new skill weekly_

Criterion for Mastery

Jennifer will independently request assistance without engaging in challenging behavior on all
opportunities for 3 consecutive days.

Performance Monitoring

Jim will record Jennifer's requests for assistance after each opportunity.

Figure 10.9. Intervention Planning Form for teaching Jennifer to request assistance. (*Note:* This is a filled-in version of Form 6.1, Intervention Planning Form. A blank, printable version appears on the accompanying CD-ROM.)

Learner's name: __Jennifer__   Interventionist: __Jim__

Activity: __Novel task__   Setting: __Work__

Circle one: Baseline   (Intervention)   Maintenance   Generalization

Target response: __Handing Jim a printed card__

Instructions: Record the date, the difficult task, and the learner's request for assistance (e.g., a plus [+] for an independent response, a *P* for a prompted response, and a minus [–] for an incorrect response) and/or the learner's independent task completion (e.g., a plus [+] for independent task completion, a minus [–] for no task completion). Record any relevant notes about the learner's performance.

Date	Difficult task	Request for assistance	Independent task completion	Notes
2/11	Empty mail bin	+	–	Jim; full prompt
2/11	Stock shelves	+	–	Jim
2/11	Sort bulk packages	+	–	Jim
2/12	Stock shelves	+	–	Jim
2/12	Empty mail bin	+	–	Jim
2/12	Stock shelves	+	–	Jim
2/13	Sort bulk packages	+	–	Jim
2/13	Stock shelves	+	–	Jim
2/13	Empty mail bin	+	–	Jim
2/14	Sort bulk packages	+	–	Jim
2/14	Empty mail bin	+	–	Jim; independent
2/14	Stock shelves	+	–	Jim
2/15	Sort bulk packages	+	–	Jim
2/15	Empty mail bin	+	–	Jim
2/15	Stock shelves	+	–	Jim
2/18	Sort bulk packages	+	–	Jim
2/18	Empty mail bin	+	–	Jim
2/18	Stock shelves	+	–	Jim
2/19	Sort bulk packages	+	–	Jim
2/19	Empty mail bin	+	–	Jim
2/19	Stock shelves	+	–	Jim; mastered with Jim
2/20	Sort bulk packages	+	–	Bob; generalization
2/20	Empty mail bin	+	–	Sara; generalization

Figure 10.10. Jennifer's performance during intervention and generalization with her job coach and co-workers. (*Note:* This is a filled-in version of Form 10.8, Performance Monitoring Form for Requests for Assistance. A blank, printable version appears on the accompanying CD-ROM.)

Date	Difficult task	Request for assistance	Independent task completion	Notes
2/20	Stock shelves	+	−	Claire; generalization
2/21	Sort bulk packages	+	−	Bob; generalization
2/21	Empty mail bin	+	−	Sara; generalization
2/21	Stock shelves	+	−	Claire; generalization
2/22	Sort bulk packages	+	−	Andrew; generalization
2/22	Empty mail bin	+	−	Bob; generalization
2/22	Stock shelves	+	−	Andrew; generalization; mastered in generalization
2/25	Sort bulk packages	−	+	Jim; easy task; begin increased reinforcement
2/25	Empty mail bin	+	−	Jim; easy task
2/25	Count rolls of stamps	+	−	Jim; difficult task
2/25	Stock shelves	+	−	Claire; easy use
2/25	Clean employee lounge	+	−	Claire; difficult task; full prompt needed
2/25	Empty mail bin	−	+	Jim; easy use
2/26	Count rolls of stamps	+	−	Jim; difficult task
2/26	Stock shelves	−	+	Sara; easy task
2/26	Sort bulk packages	+	−	Jim; easy task
2/26	Alphabetize mail slots	+	−	Andrew; difficult task
2/26	Sort bulk packages	−	+	Jim; easy task
2/27	Empty mail bin	−	+	Claire; easy task
2/27	Clean employee lounge	+	−	Andrew; difficult task
2/27	Count rolls of stamps	−	−	Jim; difficult task
2/27	Stock shelves	+	+	Andrew; easy task
2/27	Empty mail bin	−	+	Sara; easy task
2/27	Clean employee lounge	+	−	Andrew; difficult task
2/28	Sort bulk packages	−	+	Jim; easy task
2/28	Alphabetize mail slots	+	−	Sara; difficult task
2/28	Empty mail bin	−	+	Claire: easy task
2/28	Count rolls of coins	+	−	Bob; difficult task
2/28	Stock shelves	−	+	Bob; easy task; mastered

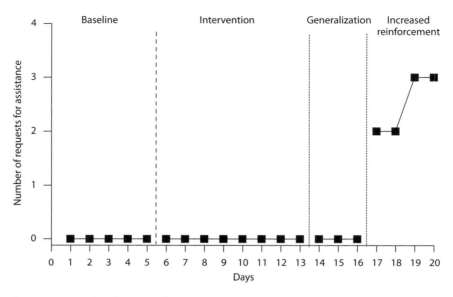

Figure 10.11.   Number of times Jennifer requested assistance.

SUMMARY

Escaping and avoiding objects/activities is an important early developing function of communication. The communicative functions addressed in this chapter allow learners to effectively express their escape-related desires while at the same time creating a mechanism to reduce the aspect of the task that is associated with escape or avoidance. Such communicative responses result in escaping or avoiding nonpreferred objects or activities (as in rejecting and requesting a break) and sometimes can result in gaining access to other needs (as in requesting assistance and requesting an alternative).

REFERENCES

Carpenter, R.L., Mastergeorge, A.M., & Coggins, T.E. (1983). The acquisition of communicative intentions in infants eight to fifteen months of age. *Language and Speech, 26,* 101–116.

Carr, E.G., & Durand, V.M. (1985). Reducing behavior problems through functional communication training. *Journal of Applied Behavior Analysis, 18,* 111–126.

Carr, E.G., Levin, L., McConnachie, G., Carlson, J.I., Kemp, D.C., & Smith, C.E. (1999). Comprehensive multisituational intervention for problem behavior in the community: Long-term maintenance and social validation. *Journal of Positive Behavior Interventions, 1,* 5–25.

Crais, E., Douglas, D.D., & Campbell, C.C. (2004). The intersection of the development of gestures and intentionality. *Journal of Speech, Language, and Hearing Research, 47,* 675–694.

Davis, C.A., Reichle, J.E., & Southard, K.L. (2001). High-probability requests and preferred item as a distractor: Increasing successful transitions in children with behavior problems. *Education and Treatment of Children, 23,* 423–440.

Day, H.M., Horner, R.H., & O'Neill, R.E. (1994). Multiple functions of challenging behaviors: Assessment and intervention. *Journal of Applied Behavior Analysis, 27,* 279–289.

Duker, P.C., Dortmans, A., & Lodder, E. (1993). Establishing the manding function of communicative gestures with individuals with severe/profound mental retardation. *Research in Developmental Disabilities, 14,* 39–49.

Duker, P.C., & Jutten, W. (1997). Establishing gestural yes-no responding with individuals with profound mental retardation. *Education and Training in Mental Retardation and Developmental Disabilities, 32,* 59–67.

Dunlap, G., Kern-Dunlap, L., Clarke, S., & Robbins, F.R. (1991). Functional assessment, curricular revision, and severe behavior problems. *Journal of Applied Behavior Analysis, 24,* 387–397.

Durand, V.M. (1993). Functional communication training using assistive devices: Effects on challenging behavior and affect. *Augmentative and Alternative Communication, 9,* 168–176.

Dyer, K., Dunlap, G., & Winterling, V. (1990). Effects of choice making on the serious problem behaviors of students with severe handicaps. *Journal of Applied Behavior Analysis, 23,* 515–524.

Horner, R.H., & Day, H.M. (1991). The effects of response efficiency on functionally equivalent competing behaviors. *Journal of Applied Behavior Analysis, 24,* 719–732.

Lalli, J.S., Casey, S., & Kates, K. (1995). Reducing escape behavior and increasing task completion with functional communication training, extinction, and response chaining. *Journal of Applied Behavior Analysis, 28,* 261–268.

Mildon, R.L., Moore, D.W., & Dixon, R.S. (2004). Combining noncontingent escape and functional communication training as a treatment for negatively reinforced disruptive behavior. *Journal of Positive Behavior Interventions, 2,* 92–102.

Northup, J., Wacker, D.P., Berg, W.K., Kelly, L., Sasso, G., & DeRaad, A. (1994). The treatment of severe behavior problems in school settings using a technical assistance model. *Journal of Applied Behavior Analysis, 27,* 33–47.

Reichle, J. (1991). Describing initial communicative intents. In J. Reichle, J. York, & J. Sigafoos (Eds.), *Implementing augmentative and alternative communication: Strategies for learners with severe disabilities* (pp. 71–88). Baltimore: Paul H. Brookes Publishing Co.

Reichle, J., Drager, K., & Davis, C. (2002). Using requests for assistance to obtain desired items and to gain release from nonpreferred activities: Implications for assessment and intervention. *Education and Treatment of Children, 25,* 47–66.

Reichle, J., Dropik, P., Alden-Anderson, B., & Haley, T. (2008). Teaching a young child with autism to request conditionally: A preliminary study. *American Journal of Speech and Language Pathology, 17,* 231–240.

Reichle, J., & McComas, J. (2004). Conditional use of a request for assistance. *Disability and Rehabilitation, 26,* 1255–1262.

Reichle, J., McComas, J., Dahl, M., Solberg, G., Pierce, S., & Smith, D. (2005). Teaching an individual with severe intellectual delay to request assistance conditionally. *Educational Psychology, 25,* 275–286.

Romaniuk, C., Miltenberger, R., Conyers, C., Jenner, N., Jurgens, M., & Ringenberg, C. (2002). The influence of activity choice on problem behaviors maintained by escape versus attention. *Journal of Applied Behavior Analysis, 35,* 349–362.

Sigafoos, J., Drasgow, E., Reichle, J., O'Reilly, M., Green, V.A., & Tait, K. (2004). Tutorial: Teaching communicative rejecting to children with severe disabilities. *American Journal of Speech-Language Pathology, 13,* 31–42.

Sigafoos, J., O'Reilly, M.F., Drasgow, E., & Reichle, J. (2002). Strategies to achieve socially acceptable escape and avoidance. In D. Beukelman & J. Reichle (Series Eds.) & J. Reichle, D.R. Beukelman, & J.C. Light (Vol. Eds.), *AAC series: Exemplary practices for beginning communicators: Implications for AAC* (pp. 157–186). Baltimore: Paul H. Brookes Publishing Co.

Sigafoos, J., & Reichle, J. (1991). Establishing an initial repertoire of rejecting. In J. Reichle, J. York, & J. Sigafoos (Eds.), *Implementing augmentative and alternative communication: Strategies for learners with severe disabilities* (pp. 115–132). Baltimore: Paul H. Brookes Publishing Co.

Sigafoos, J., & Roberts-Pennell, J. (1999). Wrong item format: A promising intervention for teaching socially appropriate forms of rejecting to children with developmental disabilities? *Augmentative and Alternative Communication, 15,* 135–140.

Steege, M.W., Wacker, D.P., Cigrand, K.C., Berg, W.K., Novak, C.G., Reimers, T.M., et al. (1990). Use of negative reinforcement in the treatment of self-injurious behavior. *Journal of Applied Behavior Analysis, 23,* 459–467.

Yamamoto, J., & Mochizuki, A. (1988). Acquisition and functional analysis of manding with autistic students. *Journal of Applied Behavior Analysis, 21,* 57–64.

Obtaining and Maintaining Communicative Interactions

Kathleen M. Feeley and Emily A. Jones

▷ CHAPTER OVERVIEW

An individual's ability to establish and maintain communicative interactions facilitates relationships among family members, classmates, co-workers, and others in the community. Communicative disorders negatively affect this process, however, particularly with respect to gaining access to vocabulary and related symbols, motivation to interact socially, rate of message production, and comprehension skills (Reichle, 1997). This chapter begins with an overview of the social-communicative characteristics of learners with severe disabilities (see Chapter 2) then proceeds by discussing initiating, maintaining (including repairing communication breakdowns), and terminating interactions. Procedures and case studies for several interventions to support interactions are presented as well as summaries of research related to teaching these communicative skills to individuals with severe disabilities. Finally, the importance of involving natural social-communication partners in intervention is discussed.

▷ CHAPTER OBJECTIVES

After studying this chapter, readers will be able to

- Identify the social-communicative characteristics of learners with severe disabilities, including those who use AAC systems
- Identify skills necessary to initiate, maintain, and terminate interactions and identify and describe corresponding interventions
- Define communicative breakdowns and repairs and describe how typical learners and those with disabilities respond in the presence of communicative breakdowns
- Identify and describe interventions that address communicative breakdowns
- Describe the importance of natural communicative partners in intervention and identify strategies that can enhance their successful implementation of interventions

▷ KEY TERMS

- commenting
- communication to obtain attention
- communicative breakdown
- conversation books
- initiate social interaction
- learned helplessness

- maintain social interaction
- modifications
- nonobligatory utterance
- obligatory utterance
- partner-focused question
- Picture Exchange Communication System

- reciprocal question
- redirections
- repair behavior
- request for clarification
- response–recode
- terminate an interaction

WHAT IS KNOWN ABOUT THE COMMUNICATIVE INTERACTIONS OF INDIVIDUALS WITH SEVERE DEVELOPMENTAL DISABILITIES?

Delays in communicative behavior are prevalent during the earliest stages of development among children with developmental disabilities, including delays in babbling and vocal and verbal imitation, as well as impairments in a range of communicative functions. As a result, interactions may be affected. For example, the extent to which mothers respond to their children has been found to increase as children's mental age increases (Brooks-Gunn & Lewis, 1984). Also, the extent of caregiver directiveness in interactions may be higher with children with disabilities (Hanzlik & Stevenson, 1986; Light, Collier, & Parnes, 1985). Also, topics of conversation between caregivers and children with and without disabilities differ. Specifically, Ferm, Ahlsén, and Björck-Åkesson (2005) found conversation topics between a typical child and a caregiver included past and future experiences not related to the immediate situation, which differed from conversation between a cognitively typical child with severe communication impairments and a caregiver that were limited to immediate situations. Thus, communicative impairments at the earliest stages of development affect interactions, even those between child and caregiver.

Elementary-age children with severe disabilities using augmentative and alternative communication (AAC) systems are challenged by their tendency for passivity and limited types of interactions. Passivity may possibly result from a history of communicative attempts going unacknowledged. For example, Houghton, Bronicki, and Guess (1987) found that educators responded to only 6% of the communicative acts of students with severe disabilities within unstructured settings. Individuals with severe communicative disorders are at particular risk for **learned helplessness** (Seligman, 1975), a phenomena evident when an individual

stops responding, believing his or her response will have no effect on the environment. This phenomena is avoidable by ensuring others are responsive to the learner's communicative attempts.

Passivity in some learners with motor impairments may be related to the amount of effort required to formulate a message that may be so great they opt out of communicative exchanges (Light et al., 1985). This passivity has been noted within interactions with caregivers as well as peers. Children with severe disabilities also make few social initiations and few positive responses to peer initiations (Beckman & Lieber, 1992). Wilkinson and Romski (1995) noted an increased likelihood of responding to direct questions ("What do you want?") versus comments (e.g., "You're doing well"), as well as increased interaction with same-gender peers in male adolescent AAC users with severe cognitive disabilities. The increased likelihood of learners with severe disabilities responding to direct questions may result in an increase in their use by communicative partners, limiting many learners to responding only to direct questions or instructions (Clarke & Kirton, 2003).

The social-communicative interactions of adults with severe disabilities have revealed that employees with significant communication needs tend to interact more with job coaches than with typically developing co-workers (Storey, Rhodes, Sandow, Loewinger, & Petherbridge, 1991). Individuals with severe disabilities showed similar rates of work-related interactions with co-workers as typically developing peers, but lower rates of non–task-related interactions (e.g., joking, social conversation) (Chadsey-Rusch, Gonzalez, Tines, & Johnson, 1989).

The social-communicative interactions of learners with severe disabilities are greatly affected by their communicative impairments from early stages of development through adulthood. Their role in communicative exchanges is quite different from their communicative partner's, as is the content of the conversation. Several strategies can enhance communicative interactions among individuals with severe disabilities and their partners, however.

Strategies for Supporting Social Interaction

Supporting learners in social interactions not only enhances communication skills but also increases access to inclusive settings/opportunities, increasing learners' quality of life and that of their family members (Carter & Pesko, 2008). Social interaction can be supported by ensuring

- The learner's communication system contains vocabulary that will enhance interactions with familiar and unfamiliar partners
- Caregivers understand the importance of refraining from anticipating and providing for the learner's wants/needs in the absence of communicative responses, thus preparing the learner to interact with others who may not be so accommodating (e.g., unfamiliar partners)
- Communicative partners expand their communicative utterances beyond yes/no questions, a pattern that can discourage conversational initiation
- Frequent opportunities for interaction with unfamiliar individuals

The following sections introduce interventions to address initiation, maintenance (including repairing communication breakdowns), and termination of communicative interactions. They also discuss recommendations for the inclusion of family, peers, and co-workers within intervention to support access to a range of opportunities across a range of situations.

TEACHING LEARNERS TO INITIATE SOCIAL INTERACTIONS

Several factors may influence an individual's propensity to **initiate social interactions**, including the following:

- Familiarity with a communicative partner may increase initiations.
- A learner's disability, specifically, an autism spectrum disorder (ASD), may be associated with a decreased propensity to initiate interactions.
- The lack of a conventional means of initiating communication may result in the learner's attempts going unnoticed, and he or she may stop initiating interactions over time.
- Other learners may rely on challenging behavior to initiate an interaction, particularly if an unconventional means is not successful.
- Communicative partners may "preempt" a learner's communicative attempts, resulting in a lack of attempts to initiate, as reinforcement is consistently delivered in the absence of any effort, another factor that can lead to learned helplessness (Basil, 1992).

Teaching Communication to Obtain Attention

Teaching a request for attention benefits individuals who have appropriate but difficult to interpret means of acquiring attention and individuals who use socially marginal/unacceptable forms (e.g., noises, aggression). It is also beneficial as it can facilitate further social interaction.

Steps to teach communication to obtain attention

Step 1: Identify opportunities when the AAC user is likely to desire attention.

Step 2: Identify when to prompt a request for attention.

Step 3: Identify the communicative behavior.

Step 4: Develop instructional strategies to teach a request for attention.

Step 5: Implement intervention and monitor effectiveness.

Step 6: Build tolerance for delay of reinforcement.

Using Evidence-Based Strategies to Teach Communication to Obtain Attention

Requesting attention is often overlooked as an important social-communicative function to teach to rudimentary communicators. Below is an outline of actions that the interventionist should consider if he or she plans on implementing an AAC system to teach a learner to request attention (**communication to obtain attention**).

Step 1: Identify Opportunities When the AAC User Is Likely to Desire Attention

Identify events that result in an increased desire to interact (e.g., at school with a group of students). Also, identify when it is not appropriate (i.e., negative teaching opportuni-

ties) to request attention (e.g., while doing independent work).

Step 2: Identify When to Prompt a Request for Attention

Some learners may desire attention as soon as they enter a situation; others may not immediately desire attention (e.g., may work up to 2 hours before desiring attention). This can be measured in the amount of time that passes, the number of steps completed, or result from a specific step in a task (e.g., in which assistance is needed). Figure 11.1 contains a performance monitoring form used with Sadie to identify the point at which she should be prompted to request attention. (Form 11.1 is a blank version and is included on the accompanying CD-ROM). As is illus-

---

Learner's name: _Sadie_

Environment observed: _Independent seat work_

Instructions: Fill in the learner's name and the environment in which observations took place. Record the date and the start time of the activity. Note the point in the activity in which the learner indicates a desire for attention under Point at Which Attention-Getting Response Occurred (in terms of time, number of tasks, or specific event), and then note the attention-getting response in the next column. Note the interventionist's initials, and document other information that may be relevant (e.g., if the task was preferred, to whom the attention-getting response was directed).

Date	Activity start time	Point at which attention-getting response occurred (time, number of tasks, or specific event)	Attention-getting response	Interventionist's initials	Notes
4/21	10:00	10:08	Left seat	MK	
4/21	12:40	12:55	Left seat	MK	Approached teacher
4/21	2:00	2:10	Used materials inappropriately	TR	
4/22	10:00	10:15	Pushed materials off desk	TR	
4/22	12:40	12:50	Left seat	MK	Approached teacher
4/22	2:10	2:25	Used materials inappropriately	TR	

Figure 11.1.   Sample performance monitoring form for recording the point at which a learner desires attention. (*Note:* This is a filled-in version of Form 11.1, Performance Monitoring Form for Recording the Point at Which a Learner Desires Attention. A blank, printable version appears on the accompanying CD-ROM.)

trated, during independent seat work, the shortest amount of time Sadie participates, before seeking attention, was 8 minutes before engaging in attention motivated behavior.

Step 3: Identify the Communicative Behavior

Some communicative means require the learner to first gain a communicative partner's attention. For example, signing or selecting a symbol on a low-tech system will be ineffective if the partner is not looking at the AAC user. Consider teaching a learner to tap a partner's shoulder as well as the actual message used to request attention (SPEND TIME WITH ME).

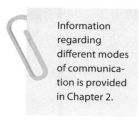

Information regarding different modes of communication is provided in Chapter 2.

Step 4: Develop Instructional Strategies to Teach a Request for Attention

Refer to range of instructional strategies presented in Chapter 5. Make sure to prompt the AAC user to emit the attention-getting response just prior to the point he or she is likely to desire attention (identified in Step 2).

Step 5: Implement Intervention and Monitor Effectiveness

Learner performance should be recorded as intervention is implemented (see Form 11.2 on the accompanying CD-ROM).

Step 6: Build Tolerance for Delay of Reinforcement

A learner may repeatedly request attention once it is acquired. Attention may not be delivered immediately or following every request in some situations; thus, consider teaching the learner to wait for attention.

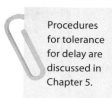

Procedures for tolerance for delay are discussed in Chapter 5.

CASE STUDY

Teaching a Request for Attention and Tolerance for Delay of Reinforcement

Sadie, a girl with Down syndrome, engaged in challenging behavior (leaving her seat and using materials inappropriately) during independent class activities. A functional assessment determined that the behavior was attention motivated. Sadie's interventionists decided to teach her an attention-getting communicative act (i.e., raising her hand) and then to request attention by selecting the symbol CHECK MY WORK in her communication book.

Observation indicated that Sadie worked for at least 8 minutes before desiring attention. Therefore, just prior to 8 minutes, the classroom assistant went to Sadie and said, "If you want Ms. Smith's attention, raise your hand." As soon as Ms. Smith saw Sadie's hand raised, she approached saying, "Yes, Sadie?" Sadie was then prompted to select her CHECK MY WORK symbol. Ms. Smith immediately provided high-quality attention while checking her work.

A tolerance for delay program was implemented because Sadie began to use the requests for attention too often. Initially, when Sadie raised her hand, the teacher would say, "I'll be right there," (tolerance cue) and then go immediately to her. Across opportunities, her teacher waited longer periods of time (e.g., 2 minutes, 4 minutes) between the tolerance cue and going to Sadie.

▷ Helpful Hint

Picture Exchange Communication System

The **Picture Exchange Communication System** (PECS; Bondy & Frost, 1994) is a package intervention in which the learner selects symbols kept in a notebook and sequences them on a sentence strip that he or she then hands to his or her partner in a communicative exchange. The PECS teaches learners to obtain a listener's attention prior to offering a graphic symbol (Bondy & Frost, 1994; Carr & Felce, 2007; Ganz & Simpson, 2004).

What Does the Research Say?

Requesting Attention

Kaczmarek, Evans, and Stever (1995) examined preparatory behaviors in 16 children (3–6 years old) with moderate to severe developmental delays within self-contained classrooms. Two strategies were used to obtain listener attention—delivery of the message itself (occurring more often) or an explicit request for attention before delivering the message. The communicative partner was already in close proximity in most instances, possibly due to the high staff ratio, and, thus, the children rarely needed to establish listener proximity by explicitly requesting attention.

Lancioni et al. (2008) taught three children with severe disabilities to request access to social contact. The children were first taught to select microswitches to gain access to environmental stimuli and then to use a speech-generating device (SGD) to request social contact from a caregiver. Textual prompts (i.e., written words) have also been used to teach children with disabilities, particularly children with autism, to initiate interactions with adults (Krantz & McClannahan, 1998) and peers (Krantz & McClannahan, 1993). Although used to enhance verbalizations, the same strategies can be applied to prompt AAC users to initiate interactions.

Challenging behavior in individuals with severe disabilities was replaced with communicative alternatives, including attention-getting responses (e.g., AM I DOING GOOD WORK?), in Carr and Durand's seminal work (Carr & Durand, 1985; Durand & Carr, 1991). A number of other researchers have demonstrated the effectiveness of requests for attention in replacing challenging behaviors (see Conroy, Dunlap, Clark, & Alter, 2005, and Durand & Merges, 2001).

Introducing One's AAC System to an Unfamiliar Communicative Partner

Because many prospective communicative partners will not have had any experience interacting with an individual who uses an AAC system, it is important to put them at ease by providing a brief explanation of how the system works.

Why Teach Learners to Introduce Their AAC System?

Ensuring partners understand how an AAC user communicates is critical for communication success. Something such as a card with instructions about the AAC device is easy to create and even transport, with significant potential for improving interactions between the learner and unfamiliar partners (Light & Binger, 1998).

What Does the Research Say?

Introducing One's AAC System

Doss et al. (1991) compared the effectiveness/efficiency of various devices with unfamiliar partners (ordering at a fast-food restaurant). In the first experiment, an individual who was acting as an AAC user provided a card stating she did not speak and would use a device to order food. In the second experiment, the card provided explicit instructions about how the individual used the device (e.g., instructions to wait for the AAC user to push the buttons and then listen to the message). Because the focus of these experiments was not on these cards per se, it is not clear what effect the cards alone produced in terms of efficiency and effectiveness, but some findings are suggestive of their usefulness. The more explicit cards may have affected the interactions regarding whether the listener directed requests for clarification to the AAC user or person accompanying the learner. All requests for clarification in the second experiment were directed at the AAC user.

Using Evidence-Based Strategies to Teach a Learner to Introduce His or Her AAC System

The following evidence-based strategies help ensure that interventionists are using instructional procedures that have a history of success. These procedures also provide a list of component parts making it potentially easier for the interventionist to implement procedures with fidelity.

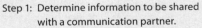

Steps to teach a learner to introduce his or her AAC system

Step 1: Determine information to be shared with a communication partner.
Step 2: Create a display for the introductory message.
Step 3: Develop a strategy for teaching the individual to share the information.
Step 4: Implement intervention and monitor learner performance.

Step 1: Determine Information to Be Shared with a Communication Partner

Consider if the system is the sole mode of communication versus supplemental to speech (i.e., paired with speech or only when clarification is required). Also, consider steps for using the device (e.g., wait for speech output). Then, develop a message with an introduction (i.e., a greeting and learner's name) and information regarding how the learner uses his or her system. A message for a learner using electronic scanning may be HI. I'M JASON. MY DEVICE WILL SCAN THROUGH SEVERAL MESSAGES, SO IT MIGHT TAKE A WHILE FOR ME TO RESPOND. Other learners may indicate how to respond if breakdowns occur (e.g., the message of a learner using an SGD with a dynamic display might be IF YOU CAN'T UNDERSTAND MY SPEECH OUTPUT, THEN LOOK AT MY SYMBOLS).

Step 2: Create a Display for the Introductory Message

When creating a display for the introductory message, consider something easily portable. The message should be in a readable font style and size so that it can be clearly read by the listener. Also, consider creating multiple copies in case one is lost or not retrieved from a listener.

Step 3: Develop a Strategy for Teaching the Individual to Share the Information

Teach the learner to share the message (e.g., hand the card with instructions about the AAC device) with novel listeners at the beginning of an interaction. Teach the learner to discriminate between those with whom the introductory message is necessary (i.e., unfamiliar partners) and those with whom it is not (i.e., familiar partners) to ensure conditional use.

Step 4: Implement Intervention and Monitor Learner Performance

Some learners may benefit from practicing with someone familiar pretending to be a novel partner. For others and those who began instruction in more controlled con-

texts, instruction should take place with unfamiliar partners enabling them to learn to share information while the interventionist monitors if unfamiliar partners understand the information.

The information provided in this section reflects evidence-based practices for teaching AAC users to initiate social interactions. Learners must be able to maintain interactions once they begin, however.

TEACHING LEARNERS TO MAINTAIN INTERACTIONS

Maintaining interactions can be difficult for AAC users (Calculator, 1988; Davis, Reichle, Southard, & Johnston, 1998; Farrier, Yorkston, Marriner, & Beukelman, 1985).

- Partners may not readily recognize a learner's communicative attempts and/or preempt the learner's opportunity to communicate, preventing the learner from engaging in communicative exchanges.

- Partners may inadvertently structure conversation (e.g., ask only yes/no questions), placing the learner in the position of only responding to limited partner initiations.

- The learner may not recognize when it is his or her "turn" to communicate.

- Some learners may not be motivated to **maintain social interactions** and purposefully opt out of communicative exchanges.

- The learner may lack the vocabulary or conversation skills necessary to maintain a conversation.

Learners must recognize their turn in conversation and be versed in contributing to conversations (e.g., initiating topics, asking and answering questions, **commenting**, responding to comments of others) as well as repairing communicative breakdowns.

↳ Helpful Hint

Tips for communication partners to support maintaining a conversation follow.

- Clearly indicate the learner's turn in conversation (e.g., exaggerated pause, expectant look).

- Give the learner time to recognize his or her turn and then additional time to produce a message.

- Use questions, particularly those related to the learner's preceding utterance (Yoder, Davies, & Bishop, 1994). Do not rely on them, however.

- Choose a topic of conversation consistent with learner interests.

- Use additional reinforcers to increase the reinforcing value of maintaining interactions.

- Use antecedent strategies such as high-probability requests, in which a series of obligatory questions (more salient cues to respond) are asked prior to a nonobligatory exchange (less salient), increasing the likelihood the learner will respond (Davis et al., 1998).

Why Teach Learners to Maintain Conversations?

Learners who maintain conversations are likely to be more successful and more independent in interacting with a variety of partners. Maintaining interactions allows for participation in a greater number of learning opportunities, enhances social relationships, and may result in the learner playing a more active role in interactions.

☞ Helpful Hint

Teach AAC users to use "carrier" phrases at the end of a message, which indicate they have more to say. The message AND can be programmed into an SGD to be selected after a message (e.g., I HAD FUN AND), informing the partner he or she has more to communicate. Learners with low-tech systems can be taught to select a symbol or gesture (e.g., put up index finger) to indicate they are not finished taking their turn.

Using Conversation Books to Enhance Communicative Exchanges

Conversation books provide visual prompts to engage in commenting and question ask-

ing (discussed shortly) and help clarify the learner's communication for the partner.

Using Evidence-Based Strategies to Teach Conversation Book Use

The evidence on using conversation books is limited. However, that which is available tends to have common procedures that are reflected in the steps described next.

Steps to teach conversation book use

Step 1: Identify topics about which the learner is likely to communicate.

Step 2: Identify appropriate symbols.

Step 3: Determine a means for displaying symbols and organize how they will be displayed.

Step 4: Teach communicative partners the structure for interaction in the presence of the conversation book.

Step 5: Develop instructional strategies.

Step 6: Implement intervention, and monitor effectiveness.

Step 7: Change symbols to maintain learner and partner interest.

Step 1: Identify Topics About Which the Learner Is Likely to Communicate

It is important to ensure that the learner has topics available that are apt to be of interest to both him or her and the communicative partner. Furthermore, it is important that the list of topics be regularly updated so that they do not become stale. We have found that it works particularly well when participants have a common theme of interest (e.g., football). In the case of football, new information can be infused from text or pictures in the newspaper, which keeps the material new while still building the general theme into a routine of topics that the learner can use.

Step 2: Identify Appropriate Symbols

Choose symbols the learner discriminates and that are appealing (to learner and partner).

Step 3: Determine a Means for Displaying Symbols and Organize How They Will Be Displayed

Consider displays other than a "book" (e.g., a flat display affixed to wheelchair tray, a key ring) as well as technological applications (e.g., personal digital assistant, cell phone, digital camera). Symbols can be organized within the display by environment, by special event (holiday, birthday), or chronologically (e.g., last week's event, this week's event) (Hunt, Alwell, & Goetz, 1991; Shane & Weiss-Kapp, 2007).

Step 4: Teach Communicative Partners the Structure for Interaction in the Presence of the Conversation Book

Communication partners can be provided explicit information regarding why the AAC user has a conversation book and how he or she will use it. Partners can also be taught specific interaction strategies (Hunt et al., 1991)—how to ask questions, wait for the AAC user to respond and make a new comment/question using his or her book, and converse about the symbols the learner referenced.

Step 5: Develop Instructional Strategies

Refer to the instructional strategies presented in Chapter 5 to develop prompting, reinforcement, and error correction procedures.

Step 6: Implement Intervention and Monitor Effectiveness

The frequency with which the learner uses the book to initiate can be measured, as well as the number of conversational turns and/or number of topics raised within an interaction. Figure 11.2 contains a performance

---

Learner's name: __William__

Correct response: __Use of conversation book to initiate and maintain interaction with peers__

Type of prompt: __Visual: cards with SAY HELLO and BOOK symbols__

Level of prompt: F: full prompt   P: partial prompt   I: independent (no prompt)

Instructions: Fill in the learner's name, describe the correct response, and identify the type of prompt that will be used (verbal, gestural, physical, visual) during instruction. For each opportunity, circle *Y* if the learner performed the communicative response or *N* if he or she did not. Identify the communicative partner as well as the level of prompt that was required. Topics of conversation can be recorded under Topics, and the number of conversational turns can be recorded in the last column.

Date	Performed communicative response	Communicative partner	Prompt level	Topics	Number of conversational turns
9/10	Y (N)	Jared	F (P) I	Soccer, movie	3
9/10	Y (N)	Melanie	(F) P I	Soccer, lunch	3
9/10	(Y) N	Sasha	(F) P I	Soccer, movie	5
9/13	Y (N)	Jared	(F) P I	Football game, soccer	6
9/13	(Y) N	Sasha	(F) P I	Art club	6
9/14	(Y) N	Sasha	F (P) I	Football game	5
9/14	(Y) N	Peter	F (P) I	Football game, soccer, lunch	6

Figure 11.2.   Performance Monitoring Form for recording conversation book use for William. (*Note:* This is a filled-in version of Form 11.3, Monitor Learner Progress During Conversational Exchange. A blank, printable version appears on the accompanying CD-ROM.)

monitoring form that was used for William, whose intervention is described in the following case study. (Form 11.3 is a blank version and is included on the accompanying CD-ROM.)

CASE STUDY

Conversation Book Use

William, a 13-year-old boy with autism, used an SGD with line-drawn symbols. Although proficient at answering questions using his SGD, William did not use his system to initiate and engage in conversations. His interventionists developed a conversation book containing photographs of his favorite activities (e.g., soccer, movies, the school football team) placed in sheet protectors and stored on a key ring affixed to his SGD. His speech-language pathologist gathered William's peers and explained how William used his SGD and that he was being taught to use his conversation book to initiate and maintain interactions.

A teaching assistant used a stimulus prompt (i.e., a symbol illustrating, SAY HELLO) to prompt William to approach his peers when he was in close proximity to them during homeroom, in the cafeteria, and during down time in classes. Once he initiated interaction with his peers, the teaching assistant used another visual prompt (i.e., BOOK symbol) to prompt him to use his conversation book. William's peers, both motivated and having been taught how to interact with him, naturally participated in conversational exchanges with William.

Step 7: Change Symbols to Maintain Learner and Partner Interest

Some symbols may remain in the conversation book indefinitely (e.g., favorite musician), whereas others (e.g., holiday photograph) should be rotated to maintain learner and partner interest.

Conversation books can be utilized in conjunction with the interventions described next to address conversation skills. Specifi-cally, they can be used as a means of prompting question asking, commenting, and repairing communication breakdowns.

What Does the Research Say?

Conversation Books

Hunt, Alwell, and Goetz (1988) used a conversation book to address turntaking in high school students with severe disabilities. Learners and their communicative partners were taught a conversation structure requiring them to respond to a question or comment and then cue the partner to communicate. The target students learned to initiate and maintain conversations and generalized skills to a variety of settings with peers without disabilities. Hunt et al. (1991) used similar procedures with elementary-age students with severe disabilities, demonstrating improvements in conversational turntaking. Performance with untrained peers was poorer than with trained peers, however. Training of untrained peers did result in enhanced performance. Hughes et al. (2002) conducted a similar study and demonstrated generalized performance with untrained peers.

Storey and Provost (1996) taught two adults with severe disabilities to use a conversation book within a supported employment setting to initiate a conversation and suggest a topic, expand on and initiate a new topic, and close the conversation. The authors implemented instruction within 5-minute sessions prior to break/lunch/arrival for 2 weeks, resulting in an increase in interactions between participants and typical employees.

Taking Conversational Turns

Several skills are involved in maintaining conversations, most notably, the ability to answer and ask questions as well as comment. A person posing a question during a conversation likely looks in the learner's direction and pauses, providing the learner not only with a clear cue to respond, but also with an obligatory turn (i.e., he or she is obliged to respond). The absence of a response will surely result in a communication breakdown. A less salient indication of a turn is a partner's **nonobligatory utterances.** For example, a comment (e.g., "It's nice outside") does not mandate a response; thus, learners may fail to recognize the opportunity to communicate or, in some cases, choose not to respond. AAC users are less likely to maintain the conversation (Light et al., 1985) when a partner's message is nonobligatory. Unfortunately, continued lack of responding can lead to a termination of the interaction.

Obligatory utterances (i.e., questions) lead to more responses on the part of some learners with severe disabilities because they recognize their turn within an exchange. It is critical for AAC users to learn to respond to obligatory utterances, particularly those that are highly predictable. For example, many adults ask children waiting in line at the store with their parents, "What's your name?" "How old are you?" or "What school do you go to?" Learners can benefit from being taught specific responses to commonly asked questions to address the maintenance of conversation within predictable situations.

Helpful Hint

Identify commonly asked questions when teaching question answering and then

- Consider using discrete trial instruction (see Chapter 6) as a means of providing multiple opportunities to practice answering questions.

- Identify prompting, reinforcement, and error correction procedures.

- Practice the questions and responses within a conversation.

For example, 18-year-old Sam's mother reported that peers often asked questions (e.g., "What's your favorite video?" "What sports do you play?") to which he did not respond. His interventionist used discrete trial instruction—a model of the answer was provided following a question, with praise following correct responses. Then, Sam was engaged in conversation using the questions to maintain interactions. Sam demonstrated some responses with peers but required additional prompting for others. Soon, Sam was readily responding to predictable questions from his peers.

Asking Questions

Question asking provides learners with a means of maintaining interactions, enabling them to exert control over the communicative exchange. They may first respond to a partner's communication and then follow with a related question (e.g., partner asks, "Where did you go?" to which the learner responds, "To a movie," adding, "Where did you go?"). This linguistic form is referred to as a **response–recode** or **reciprocal question**; the response is the answer to a question/ statement, and the recode is the subsequent related question/statement. **Partner-focused questions** ask about the conversation partner (e.g., "What are you doing?") and have been associated with better judgments of communicative competence (Light, Corbett, Gullapalli, & Lepowski, 1995, cited in Beukelman & Mirenda, 2005). Question asking can be used to initiate (e.g., "What's your name?"), maintain, or terminate (e.g., "Should we go?") interactions.

What Does the Research Say?
Asking Questions

Charlop and Milstein (1989) used video modeling to prompt scripted conversations (about a preferred toy and abstract topics) consisting of an answer to the interventionist's question followed by the learner asking questions matching the partner's question and topic-related questions. Children viewed video models three times followed by a test in which a complete correct conversation resulted in praise and a food item. Three children with autism (6–7 years old) learned the conversation skills, generalized to similar conversations, and maintained skills at 15 months follow-up. This approach could be adapted to model AAC system use.

O'Keefe and Dattilo (1992) taught response–recode to three adult AAC users with intellectual disabilities. Clinicians engaged learners in a conversation via statements about preferred activities. If the learner responded with a response–recode, then the clinician also responded with a response–recode, providing another opportunity for the learner to respond. If the learner did not emit a response—

(continued)

recode, the clinician provided instructions, then an example. Results revealed that participants demonstrated increases in response–recodes that maintained at 1- and 3-week probes.

Light, Binger, Agate, and Ramsay (1999) used a least-to-most prompt hierarchy (an expectant look, to a gesture, and then a model) to teach partner-focused questions to six participants (10–44 years old) with a variety of disabilities and communication systems. Instruction involved explaining partner-focused questions, modeling, and providing multiple opportunities in both natural environments and during simulation sessions. All participants acquired question asking that generalized to new natural situations and maintained at 2 months.

Using Evidence-Based Strategies to Teach Learners to Ask Questions

Asking questions represents a strategy that can infuse a conversation to keep it going. In addition, it can be an important strategy during instances in which the learner is attempting to repair a message that was misunderstood by a communicative partner. Below are steps that are addressed in successful strategies that teach learners to ask questions.

Step 1: Identify Types of Questions Appropriate for the Learner to Ask

Consider general questions applicable across multiple contexts (e.g., "Anything new?"). Also, consider a range of questions includ-

Steps to teach learners to ask questions

Step 1: Identify types of questions appropriate for the learner to ask.

Step 2: Identify opportunities for the learner to ask questions.

Step 3: Choose appropriate vocabulary and symbols.

Step 4: Develop instructional strategies.

Step 5: Implement the intervention and monitor effectiveness.

ing partner-focused, reciprocal, and different *wh-* questions (sampling what, where, when, who, and how), making sure the questions a learner asks result in the partner providing information the learner will comprehend.

Step 2: Identify Opportunities for the Learner to Ask Questions

Learners can ask questions at multiple points within a conversation. Make sure the learner has adequate practice with questions immediately following a greeting that begins a conversation as well as after the learner responds to a partner's questions (reciprocal). Consider less salient opportunities (e.g., following a comment or a pause in the interaction) as the learner becomes proficient.

Step 3: Choose Appropriate Vocabulary and Symbols

If possible, questions should use vocabulary items and symbols that are already part of the learner's communicative system. This will allow the learner to focus on the question forms rather than on both the new vocabulary and question forms. Also, remember that, for the learner to participate after the question is asked, he or she needs to have vocabulary and symbols in his or her repertoire that are conducive to potential topic continuation once the communicative partner responds.

Step 4: Develop Instructional Strategies

Choice of prompts is important to help maintain natural interactions. Verbal prompts can be intrusive, particularly when there is only one person present during instruction. In contrast, stimulus prompts can be less disruptive. For example, an interventionist may say to the learner, "I had a great weekend." Instead of saying, "Ask me, 'What did you do?'" a written message "What did you do?" or line drawings representing the question can be used. Refer to Chapter 5 for information about choosing prompting, reinforcement, and error correction procedures.

Step 5: Implement the Intervention and Monitor Effectiveness

Use a performance monitoring form, such as Form 11.3 on the accompanying CD-ROM, to monitor learner performance.

CASE STUDY

Asking Questions

James, a 27-year-old man with cerebral palsy, uses an SGD accessed via a head pointer. College students come by to spend time with him each week. James's support staff noticed James was always in the role of "responder"; he did not ask the same questions back and did not initiate interactions with questions.

Staff taught the young men to implement instruction. Commonly asked questions were identified (e.g., "What's up?" "What do you want to watch?"). Symbols and corresponding messages were identified (i.e., WHAT'S UP WITH YOU? WHAT DO YOU WANT TO WATCH?). The visitors were instructed to approach James, ask one or two questions, and follow James's response with a verbal prompt (e.g., "Don't you want to know what I want to watch?") while pointing to the corresponding symbol on James's SGD. Initially, the guests answered the questions and provided high-quality reinforcement (e.g., "That's great, James! I had a great day today"), then they faded their prompts and faded to more natural reinforcement (e.g., simply answering the question).

James's support staff also prompted him to initiate by saying, "James, here comes Tim. Ask him what he wants to watch." More questions were added to James's SGD (e.g., WHAT DO YOU WANT ON YOUR PIZZA? WHAT ARE YOU DOING TOMORROW?) as he became more proficient.

Commenting

Although speakers use a variety of communicative functions (e.g., requesting social niceties), much of conversation maintenance involves commenting (Buzolich, King, & Baroody, 1991). Comments consist of communication referring to or describing an object or event (present or not) (Pasco, Gordon, Howlin, & Charman, 2008) and are often less prominent in the communicative repertoires of individuals with severe disabilities, limiting the scope and length of communicative interactions.

Commenting begins in infancy with early forms referred to as joint attention or protodeclaratives. Joint attention refers to sharing attention on an object/event with another for the purpose of interacting about that object/event. Infants engage in joint attention through eye gaze and gestures, and they incorporate vocalizations, then words, then sentences as they mature.

> Additional information about early communicative functions, including requesting and joint attention, is discussed in Chapter 1.

Similar vocabulary and communication forms (e.g., gestures) are used to request and to engage in joint attention/comment. Although communication forms may have been taught for requesting, many learners will not necessarily generalize across functions to commenting (Glennen & Calculator, 1985; Reichle, York, & Sigafoos, 1991). Also, learners with certain diagnoses may show specific impairments in commenting (e.g., children with autism; Stone, Ousley, Yoder, Hogan, & Hepburn, 1997). Therefore, specifically teaching commenting skills may be necessary.

What Does the Research Say?
Commenting

Buzolich et al. (1991) added comments represented by single icons to the SGDs of three children with cerebral palsy (9–12 years old). The participants simultaneously received intervention within a class setting. A least-to-most prompting hierarchy was used during opportunities for commenting (from an expectant look, to an open-

(continued)

ended question, to a verbal instruction, to a model of commenting using the learner's SGD). A multiple baseline across participants demonstrated commenting increased (with one participant increasing prior to intervention). A later part of Bondy and Frost's (1994) PECS program also involves teaching commenting, such as responding to a partner's question in reference to an object (e.g., holding an item, an interventionist asks, "What do you see?"). The learner is prompted to choose and exchange relevant symbols (I SEE ___).

Grossi, Kimball, and Heward (1994) taught two adults with developmental disabilities to acknowledge co-workers' initiations by having them listen to recordings of co-worker initiations and learner responses prior to the next work shift, with corrective feedback and role playing. Both participants increased verbal acknowledgments at levels equal to their typically developing co-workers and maintained skills at 4- and 8-week observations.

Conversation skills, including commenting, have been addressed in other studies; however, not within the context of maintaining conversation. Buffington, Krantz, McClannahan, and Poulson (1998) taught four children with autism (4–6 years old) to use gestures and speech to engage in a range of conversational skills (e.g., commenting, answering questions, responding to comments). An item was presented with a question, comment, or directive. If the learner did not respond with the corresponding spoken utterance and gesture (e.g., pointing, shaking head), then a model was provided, with correct responses resulting in token reinforcement. Results showed increases in verbal and gestural responses to trained and untrained stimuli. These procedures could be used to address similar skills within the context of conversations.

Research with scripts (written utterances presented during interactions for a learner to read) has focused on conversation skills, including commenting. Several studies demonstrated improvements in scripted utterances (e.g., Charlop-Christy & Kelso, 2003; Ganz & Flores, 2008; Sarakoff, Taylor, & Poulson, 2001), with some even showing improvements in relevant unscripted or novel utterances (though inconsistent across all participants in all studies). Scripts may also help support speech intelligibility (see Chapter 13) and can be adapted for application across AAC systems (see McClannahan & Krantz, 2006).

Learners have been taught to activate a voice-over recording to prompt spoken utterances (comments, directives) while following activity schedules (see Chapter 12; Wichnick, Vener, Keating, & Poulson, 2010; Wichnick,

Vener, Pyrtek, & Poulson, 2010), which increased initiating and responding to peers. Ongoing conversations were not addressed, however; thus, applications involving maintenance of conversations with multiple turns remain to be examined.

Using Evidence-Based Strategies to Teach Commenting

It is important to ensure that the learner is the recipient of intervention procedures to teach a wide range of communicative functions. One of these that, often, has been overlooked during beginning intervention is comments. Although teaching comments may not represent a high instructional priority for some learners, for those who are interested in approaching others and/or showing or sharing information, commenting may be important.

Steps to teach commenting

Step 1: Identify situations and opportunities.
Step 2: Identify the comments.
Step 3: Identify intervention strategies to teach commenting.
Step 4: Implement intervention, and monitor learner performance.

Step 1: Identify Situations and Opportunities

Select topics and communicative partners that are reinforcing, and consider placing novel or interesting items, photographs, or a conversation book in the environment to stimulate conversation.

Consider salient opportunities, including when a partner answers the learner's question, immediately following a partner's comment (e.g., partner says "That red flower is pretty," to which the learner can be taught to respond THAT PURPLE FLOWER IS, TOO), and when there is a "lull" in the conversation but the learner desires the conversation to continue. Also, opportunities to comment are likely to arise during conversations that are relevant to the learner (e.g., a base-ball fan is more likely to comment following a statement about baseball than following a statement about an unfamiliar sport) (Yoder, Davies, & Bishop, 1994). Less salient oppor-tunities can then be addressed, including when the communicative partner has intro-duced an unfamiliar or less preferred topic or emits a general utterance (e.g., "Hmm") that may be difficult for the learner to interpret.

Step 2: Identify the Comments

Provide the learner with vocabulary neces-sary to produce comments relevant to the situations identified in Step 1. Consider teaching general comments first (e.g., "Wow!"), which require less vocabulary than specific comments (e.g., "What a great shirt!"), potentially less instructional time, and may be more readily generalized to novel contexts. Specific vocabulary can be chained (e.g., "Great" "shirt!") once general comments are acquired.

Step 3: Identify Intervention Strategies to Teach Commenting

Commenting has been taught to AAC users with least-to-most prompt fading strategies—progressing from an expectant look to a model—a strategy appropriate for learners with commenting skills in their repertoire who simply do not take advantage of oppor-tunities. For learners for whom commenting is a new skill, presenting a prompt that reli-ably results in a comment (i.e., most-to-least prompt hierarchy) may result in more suc-cess (e.g., Jones, Carr, & Feeley, 2006). Also, consider stimulus prompts that can be less intrusive (flashing a card with correspond-ing symbols). In addition, if the continua-tion of a conversation does not function as a reinforcer, then consider more powerful reinforcers (e.g., toy, food item) (Jones et al., 2006). See Chapter 5 for a discussion of choosing intervention strategies, including prompting, reinforcement, and error correc-tion procedures.

Use the Intervention Planning Form (Form 6.1 on the accompanying CD-ROM) to ensure the procedures used are well documented and increase the likelihood of reliable implementation.

Step 4: Implement Intervention and Monitor Learner Performance

The next step is to implement the instruc-tional strategy and collect data to monitor ef-fectiveness. Use a performance monitoring from such as Form 11.3 on the accompanying CD-ROM to monitor learner performance.

REPAIRING COMMUNICATION BREAKDOWNS

A **communicative breakdown** occurs when either partner does not receive (e.g., see a gesture/symbol, hear a verbalization), does not understand, or misinterprets the mes-sage. Breakdowns, a common occurrence within any conversational exchange, are ex-perienced more often by learners with se-vere disabilities due to several factors (Fey, Warr-Leeper, Webber, & Disher, 1988).

Core challenges, including deficits in language comprehension, failure to moni-tor listeners' comprehension (and thus de-tect breakdowns), the learner's lack of aware-ness of his or her responsibility to indicate a misunderstanding, a limited communica-tive repertoire, insufficient vocabulary, and failure to be assertive within conversational exchanges, contribute to communication breakdowns. Problems with intelligibility by both familiar and unfamiliar communica-tive partners also affect communicative break-downs, as well as a communicative partner's lack of knowledge or confusion regarding how an AAC user communicates. In addi-tion, the pause time between AAC users and speaking adults is considerably longer, lead-ing to confusion regarding when one turn ends and another begins (Buzolich & Wie-mann, 1988).

Many AAC users essentially give up and refrain from persisting with their message after experiencing failure, forgoing opportunities to repair communicative breakdowns. Other learners may engage in challenging behaviors. If their socially acceptable communicative behavior does not result in a response from the listener, then they may rely on challenging behaviors as a repair strategy rather than more socially appropriate forms that would serve the same function (Brady, McLean, McLean, & Johnston, 1995; Meadan, Halle, Watkins, & Chadsey, 2006). A high probability exists that communicative breakdowns will occur in light of these contributing factors (Light et al., 1985).

Once a breakdown occurs, the recipient of the message (speaking partner or AAC user) typically responds in one of three ways (Halle, Brady, & Drasgow, 2004; Meadan et al., 2006).

1. Requests clarification from the speaker, which can take several forms

   • *Nonspecific/neutral*—listener says something general, "What?" "Huh?"

   • *Specific*—the listener clearly indicates what caused the breakdown, sometimes identifying how it could be repaired (e.g., "I didn't hear you. Say it louder").

   • Request for confirmation ("Did you say cookie?"), for repetition ("Can you say that again?"), or for specification ("What type of cookie would you like?")

2. Ignores the message—the listener attends to the speaker, but does not recognize the communicative message and, thus, redirects the conversation to an unrelated topic (i.e., topic shift); acknowledges the utterance without understanding (e.g., nods and smiles with no understanding); or directs his or her attention away the speaker.

3. Responds incorrectly (e.g., the listener delivers a pancake after the speaker asked for juice).

The speaker must first recognize the listener's indication that the breakdown occurred in order to repair communicative break-

downs. In some instances, the speaker may fail to respond to the listener's indication that a breakdown occurred. The speaker may refrain from responding to a **request for clarification** or his or her partner's ignoring the message, or the speaker may respond in a way that does not address it (i.e., topic shift). For the communicative interaction to be successful in many instances, however, the speaker should respond to the listener's indication the breakdown occurred by attempting to repair the communicative exchange by

• Repeating all or part of the message (repetition)

• Revising the message through

   Modifications—changing the message by adding gestures (speaker says, "I want cookie," partner says "What?" speaker points to cookie); by adding words, phrases, or sentences (i.e., "I want a cookie." "What?" "I want a cookie to eat") (Wetherby, Alexander, & Prizant, 1998); by reducing or simplifying ("Let's go to the park to play." "What?" "Park"); or substituting the original utterance with a different word or form of communication ("Woo woo." "What?" "Dog").

   Redirections—the speaker directs his or her communicative behavior to another person in the environment (Wetherby et al., 1998).

If the speaker's repair strategy was successful, then the recipient of the message indicates understanding (e.g., nods his or her head) and the conversation continues. At times, the first repair strategy chosen by the speaker may not result in understanding on the part of the listener, and, thus, the listener may again request clarification ("stacked" requests) or may respond in a different manner (e.g., ignore the message).

As a participant in a communicative exchange, the AAC user may be in the role of the speaker (i.e., delivers a message that caused the communication breakdown) or in the role of the listener (i.e., he or she does not understand the speaker and, thus, should request clarification). Skills such as noticing when a breakdown occurs and responding appropriately, although seemingly simple, can be a tremendous obstacle for individuals with severe communication impairments. The next section describes the development of repair strategies in speakers who are typically developing and those with developmental disabilities who use AAC, followed by procedures and case examples for teaching repair strategies.

What Is Known About Repair Strategies Used by Typical Learners?

Infants as young as 12 months old perform communicative repairs while interacting with caregivers. For example, Golinkoff (1986) found that infants who were 12 months old engaged in preverbal **repair behaviors,** including negotiating episodes, rejecting incorrect interpretation of their signals (e.g., run away, push or throw an object), and creatively repairing failed signals (e.g., repeat, substitute, or add a communicative behavior). As the infants matured, rejection tended to decrease as use of other repair strategies increased, which Golinkoff attributed to the development of more extensive communicative repertoires. Such early behaviors have led researchers to believe repair behaviors are acquired at the same time as language forms.

Alexander (1994) studied typically developing children (8–24 months old) and found most children who used request behavior produced at least one repair behavior when the request was overlooked. Repetition was used by younger children, and other strategies (changing or adding a communicative behavior) increased as language competence improved. Alexander noted children who exhibited repairs also used gestures as a component. Thus, the addition of gestures is often used as a repair strategy at a very young age, and children increase their use of vocalizations and verbalizations to repair at later ages. Thus, by 2 years old, typically

developing children respond when partners indicate a communication breakdown occurred (Anselmi, Tomasello, & Acunzo, 1986; Wilcox & Webster, 1980). They demonstrate consistent responding to neutral or nonspecific requests for clarification (e.g., "What?" "Huh?") (Anselmi et al., 1986; Gallagher, 1981) and demonstrate increases in the use of repair strategies following their own requests versus their own comments (Shatz & O'Reilly, 1990). Differences in repair strategies at this age have also been found based on communicative partner. Children tend to make reductions to original messages with their mothers and elaborate or substitute in the presence of unfamiliar adults (Tomasello, Farrar, & Dines, 1984).

Children's ability to repair communicative breakdowns improves with age. Brinton, Fujiki, Frome Loeb, and Winkler (1986) demonstrated children (2–9 years old) became more proficient at addressing repeated stacked requests for clarification using a wider range of strategies (i.e., adding more information), and they provided background information, defined terms, and talked about the repair strategy by 9 years of age.

In the role of listener, children as young as 2.6 years of age request clarification; however, it appears those requests are often used to fill a communicative turn rather than a true request for clarification (Shatz & O'Reilly, 1990). Also, children are more likely to respond to a broader range of problematic utterances as they mature (Revelle, Wellman, & Karabenick, 1985).

What Is Known About Repair Strategies Used by Learners with Disabilities?

Despite the presence of significant communication impairments, children and adults with a variety of disabilities not only recognize communicative breakdowns but also engage in communicative repairs (McLean, McLean, Brady, & Etter, 1991). There are differences regarding conditions under which they repair, however, as well as the strategies they choose. Coggins and Stoel-Gammon

(1982) found that children with Down syndrome consistently attempted to repair communicative breakdowns by using revisions more often than repetition. In contrast, Calculator and Delaney (1986) found verbal adults and those using communication boards who had developmental disabilities used repetitions most frequently. Although Brinton and Fujiki (1991) noted repair behaviors exhibited by adults with intellectual disabilities in both institutional and community settings, those within community settings demonstrated more sophisticated strategies.

Brady et al. (1995) examined initiation and repair behaviors in adults with severe/profound cognitive disabilities. The experimenter violated an expectation (e.g., preferred item in view but inaccessible) to evoke requesting and commenting. Following the learner's response, one of five communicative breakdowns was presented (attending to something else while ignoring the communicative act, attending to speaker but ignoring the communicative act, a verbal request for repair, a gestural request for repair, and a wrong response). The majority of participants repaired at least half of their communicative acts and several repaired all, with significant differences noted in types of repairs (recasts were used by the most participants, followed by repetitions, and then the addition of at least one communicative act). The highest percentage of repairs occurred in the "ignore attending" condition; the lowest in the "ignore while not attending" condition. Thus, attention appears to be an important factor regarding repair behaviors. Although Brady et al. did not describe differences in repair associated with level of intelligence or language ability, several researchers have examined this relationship.

Early studies reported individuals with more severe cognitive impairments repaired fewer communicative breakdowns than individuals with less severe cognitive impairments (e.g., Longhurst & Berry, 1975). With respect to language skills, Gallagher and Darnton (1978) found revisions of children with language impairments did not become more sophisticated as their language advanced as noted in typically developing children. Brady, Steeples, and Fleming (2005) did not find a relationship between level of prelinguistic development and responses to communication breakdowns in preschoolers with severe expressive language delays. They did find children, however, attempted to repair more requests than comments, given communicative breakdowns within request and comment conditions, regardless of language level.

Several researchers examined repair strategies of individuals with ASDs. Paul and Cohen (1984) found adults with intellectual disabilities and pervasive developmental disorder (PDD) were less likely to revise a response than adults with intellectual disabilities without a PDD. Meadan, Halle, Ostrosky, and DeStefano (2008) found differences in the repair strategies of two boys with autism (2 years old) with their mothers, which was attributable to the mothers' communicative behaviors (e.g., extent to which they interacted with the child and to which they delivered preferred items contingent on communication) as well as environmental variables (i.e., preferred items in sight but out of reach). Alexander, Wetherby, and Prizant (1997) found children with PDD used modification as a repair strategy more often than a comparison group of children with hearing impairments (who used more repetitions). At varying levels of prelinguistic stages, both groups used gestures within their repairs and both displayed more forceful behaviors during repetitions, with children with PDD increasing their volume.

Researchers have also examined the influence of the listener during breakdowns on repair behaviors. Erbas (2005) found nonverbal preschoolers responded more often to a gestural request for repair than they did to a wrong response or when ignored. The obligatory nature of the request for repair may have resulted in a response by the learner. At the same time, a level of assertiveness would be required for a child to persist within the "ignore" and "wrong response" conditions. Repetition was used most frequently, which is consistent with other studies (Alexander et al., 1997; Calculator & Delaney, 1986). In response to the wrong response condition, however, all participants used a different form of communication more than any other repair behaviors. Meadan et al. (2006) found similar results in two learners with autism (2 and 3 years old) within requesting situations. Most repair behaviors were emitted during requests for clarification, followed by wrong response, and the least when ignored. Also, responses were related to the activity (one learner responded more with food-related activities; the other responded more often in the presence of a preferred toy).

The research discussed to this point focused on learners' responses when their communication results in a breakdown. Equally important, but examined less, is performance of learners in the listener role. Lee, Kamhi, and Nelson (1983) observed 15 preschoolers with language impairments interacting with typical peers. The children with language impairments responded to an average of 9% of the unintelligible utterances with a request for clarification, with only two producing more than one request for clarification. In contrast, typically developing children produced requests for clarification to 59% of the unintelligible utterances, and 13 of the 15 produced more than two requests for clarification.

What Is Known About Repair Strategies Used by AAC Users?

Few researchers have systematically examined performance of AAC users with severe disabilities during communicative breakdowns. Calculator and Delaney (1986) examined use of repair strategies in individuals with disabilities and found that all participants responded to requests for clarification with little difference between those who spoke and those who used AAC. Participants with developmental disabilities utilized rep-

etition in attempting to repair breakdowns, however, rather than using revision as demonstrated by typical counterparts. Light et al. (1985) found children use repair skills discriminately across contexts. Having observed eight children (less than 6 years old) who used Blissymbols on an SGD, only two requested clarification from their parent during a free play activity. All eight, however, requested clarification in response to a clinician purposefully mumbling a statement. The authors noted that parents facilitated their children's communication, thus decreasing communicative breakdowns. All eight children responded to the opportunities provided in a structured context with a clinician purposefully responding with, "I don't understand."

Many learners with severe disabilities have the ability to repair communicative breakdowns, a skill that becomes more sophisticated as a child's communicative repertoire expands. For others, however, it warrants specific instruction.

Important Skills for Repairing Communication Breakdowns

Some learners with severe disabilities recognize when a communicative breakdown occurs, choose a repair strategy, and successfully have their needs met (Brady et al., 1995; McLean et al., 1991). Researchers have identified skills important for repairing communication breakdowns after examining proficient communicators.

Communicative Intentionality

Bates (1976) described communicative intentionality as prior to emitting a communicative behavior—the learner is aware of its effect on the other person(s). Learners progress from using unintentional behaviors (i.e., perlocutionary) to intentional behaviors (i.e., illocutionary); it is believed that repair behaviors emerge in the same manner (Wetherby et al., 1998).

Persistence

An AAC user must demonstrate persistence during communicative breakdowns for the exchange to be successful (Shatz, 1983). Persistence for some learners may take a form not readily interpretable (e.g., the learner may become agitated or emit an idiosyncratic behavior when clarification is requested) (Reichle, Halle, & Drasgow, 1998). These attempts may be missed by communicative partners and ultimately extinguished, or they may be interpreted as "challenging," with intervention in place to extinguish them.

☞ Helpful Hint

Interventionists and family members can make efforts to withhold assistance, leaving natural consequences for communication breakdowns in place to ensure opportunities to practice persistence and repair strategies. To illustrate, when Owen went to a restaurant with his siblings, they anticipate communicative breakdowns, and, thus, one of his siblings immediately ordered Owen's meal. This prevents Owen from having an opportunity to practice ordering and to persist if a breakdown occurs. Owen's siblings were instructed to let him order independently and to leave him on his own to repair a communicative breakdown when the wait staff requested clarification. His preference for restaurant food resulted in Owen quickly learning repair strategies (pointing to photographs on the children's menu and/or slowly recreating the message). Owen is now proficient at ordering his own meals.

Perspective Taking

Taking another's perspective involves understanding the needs of the listener—a sophisticated skill particularly impaired in some learners with severe disabilities, such as those with autism spectrum disorders (Baron-Cohen, Tager-Flusberg, & Cohen, 1997). Taking a listener's perspective helps learners determine how best to repair breakdowns. For example, if given a nonspecific request for clarification ("What?"), the speaker must decide if the listener did not hear or did not understand the message and then decide to repeat the message at an increased volume (in its entirety or in part), add information, or use a different form of communication. Abbeduto and Short-Meyerson (2002) noted this decision is based on the learner's cognizance of the history he or she has with the communicative partner.

A Repertoire of Effective Communicative Forms

Communicative breakdowns will be easier to repair if learners are equipped with an expansive repertoire (i.e., a response class) of effective communicative forms (Brady & Halle, 2002). A response class is a set of behaviors all serving the same function (e.g., gazing, gesturing, vocalizing, or pointing to a photograph may all produce the outcome—delivery of a food item). A learner thus chooses from the response class based on the situation and can change the response form when a breakdown occurs.

What Does the Research Say?
Teaching Repair Behaviors

Few studies have examined interventions to address repair strategies in AAC users with severe disabilities. Duker, Dortmans, and Lodder (1993) taught five individuals with severe disabilities to repeat manual signs as a repair strategy during requests. Although the skill was acquired and would suffice if the partner did not notice the sign the first time, the learner would still lack an effective repair strategy if the sign was not understood. Teaching an alternate form of communication was addressed by Sigafoos et al. (2004), who taught two young adults with severe disabilities to activate an SGD (a switch that activated a recorded message I WANT MORE) to request food items. The communicative form of reaching was immediately reinforced (item delivered) on some occasions. A 10-second delay followed the communicative behavior on other occasions, and the learner was prompted to select the SGD. Both participants learned to use the SGD to repair breakdowns.

(continued)

Weiner (2005) investigated the effect of teaching peers to request repair from elementary-age classmates with severe disabilities (two had Down syndrome and one had autism). Each participant was assigned three different typically developing peers (a peer trained in delivering requests for repair, an informed peer [instructed to request repair but not taught strategies], and an uninformed peer). A multiple baseline across students indicated peers were not likely to make requests for repairs until trained, and, once trained, their requests for and reinforcement of repair behaviors of the learners with disabilities resulted in increased repair behavior and an increase in conversational turns within interactions.

Steps to teach learners to use repair strategies

Step 1: Assess how the AAC user responds to indications of a communicative breakdown.

Step 2: Identify the needs of the AAC user.

Step 3: Teach the learner repair strategies.

Step 4: Implement intervention and monitor learner performance.

Using Evidence-Based Strategies to Teach Learners to Use Repair Strategies

The following steps teach the AAC user to recognize and respond to a partner's indication of a lack of understanding.

Step 1: Assess How the AAC User Responds to Indications of a Communicative Breakdown

Communicative partners indicate a breakdown in a range of ways; thus, it is important to assess the learner's performance in the presence of a variety of partner responses. This allows for identifying situations requiring instruction of repair strategies as well as for identifying breakdowns a learner experiences on a regular basis (e.g., a learner who signs relatively quickly may not be understood by many communicative partners).

The partners' responses should be noted, and the learner should be taught specific strategies to repair (e.g., slowing down sign production) following the specific partner responses (e.g., "Slow down, please").

Conduct observations during both natural and structured interactions. Observe the learner communicating with a variety of familiar and unfamiliar partners during natural interactions, documenting his or her responses and how each partner indicates a lack of understanding. Attend to explicit verbal requests for clarification (e.g., "Where do you want to eat?") as well as gestures (e.g., hand to one's ear) and facial expressions (e.g., quizzical look). Figures 11.3 and 11.4 illustrate data collected during naturalistic observations of communication breakdowns.

Structured observations can be used because the natural environment may not yield the full range of potential responses from communicative partners. Figure 11.5 (Form 11.4 is a complete blank version and is included on the accompanying CD-ROM)

Partner utterance	Learner utterance
"What did you have for lunch?"	Selects the symbol SANDWICH on communication board
"Huh?"	Selects the symbol TASTES GOOD
"But, what did you have for lunch?"	Again selects the symbol TASTES GOOD
"I still don't know what you had for lunch."	[No response]

Figure 11.3. Example of an augmentative and alternative communication user failing to repair a communicative breakdown.

Partner utterance	Learner utterance
"What did you have for lunch?"	Selects the symbol SANDWICH on the communication board
"Can you show me again?"	Selects the symbol SANDWICH on the communication board
"That's what I had."	

Figure 11.4.   Example of a successful repair of a communicative breakdown.

shows a form for documenting learner performance in the presence of a range of partner responses to communicative breakdowns.

Step 2: Identify the Needs of the AAC User

It is important to determine if the learner is not responding because he or she did not recognize the breakdown or because he or she lacks the necessary vocabulary or response forms to repair the communicative breakdown. Possible outcomes include:

- The learner recognizes the partner's response to a breakdown and appropriately repairs it.
- The learner does not recognize the partner's response and does not engage in repair responses.

- The learner recognizes the partner's response but fails to respond or does so inappropriately (e.g., the learner becomes frustrated and cries in response to the partner saying, "What?").
- The learner recognizes and responds to some but not all of the partner's responses.

Step 3: Teach the Learner Repair Strategies

Instruction can proceed based on performance during the assessment process. Interventions can be designed to address specific needs of the AAC user using the range of instructional strategies provided in Chapter 5. Table 11.1 consists of three likely scenarios of learner performance in the presence of

Learner's name: _Juanita_   Date: _5/2_

Communicative partner: _Mark_

Responses to communicative breakdowns	Examples	Describe learner performance
Explicit request for clarification—identifying the cause of the communication breakdown	"Show me the symbol again. I didn't see what you selected." "Show me that sign again. I didn't see you."	Learner selects the symbol again.
Explicit request for clarification—without identifying the cause of the communicative breakdown	"Show me the symbol again." "Show me that sign again."	Learner selects the symbol again.
General request for clarification	"What?" "Huh?"	No response from learner.

Figure 11.5.   Range of learner responses to communicative breakdowns. (*Note:* This is a filled-in version of Form 11.4, Monitor Learner Progress During a Structured Observation. A blank, printable version appears on the accompanying CD-ROM.)

Table 11.1. Likely scenarios of learner performance during communicative breakdowns and corresponding intervention procedures

AAC user does not respond to any requests for clarification	AAC user responds to some but not the full range of requests for clarification	AAC user can benefit from expansion of his or her repertoire of repair strategies	
Begin instruction with a salient request for clarification (e.g., "I didn't understand. Say it again.").	If a learner is responding to some requests for clarification (e.g., an explicit request), then pair that request with a less explicit request.	Having several ways to communicate the same message is vital once the learner is able to recognize a breakdown. Consider the following example.	
• The interventionist initiates interaction (e.g., "What did you do last night?").	• If the learner responds to "Say it again," then pair it with a less salient request for clarification, "Say it again. What?"	Partner:	"I had a great weekend."
• After the learner responds, the interventionist explicitly requests clarification (e.g., "I didn't understand. Say it again.").		Learner:	Signs I WENT DANCING.
		Partner:	Quizzical facial expression.
• The learner is prompted to either repeat the response or use an alternative form of communication.	• If the learner does not recognize facial gestures, then pair the more explicit request "Say it again" with a quizzical expression.	Learner:	Signs I WENT DANCING.
		Partner:	Continues quizzical expression.
• The interventionist immediately provides reinforcement.	• Gradually fade the more explicit verbal statement.	Learner:	Points to graphic symbol DANCE
Requests can be paired with less salient forms once the learner is consistently responding to explicit requests (see next scenario).	Some learners will have repair strategies in their repertoire and can readily repair the interaction once they are taught to recognize a breakdown. Others may require specific instruction in using repair strategies (see next scenario).	Partner:	"That's great. It's fun to go dancing."
		Expanding this AAC user's response classes enables her to communicate messages in different manners (e.g., gesture, point to a graphic symbol, verbal approximation).	

Key: AAC, augmentative and alternative communication.

communicative breakdowns and corresponding intervention procedures.

Step 4: Implement Intervention and Monitor Learner Performance

The learner's progress should be monitored within both the intervention setting and during natural interactions with a variety of communicative partners (see Figure 11.6; Form 11.5 is a blank version and is included on the accompanying CD-ROM).

Using Evidence-Based Strategies to Teach Learners to Request Clarification from Communicative Partners

AAC users will fail to understand a message at times and should, in turn, request clarification.

Steps to teach learners to request clarification from communicative partners

Step 1: Observe the learner engaged in conversation with several partners.

Step 2: Identify one or more requests for clarification to be taught.

Step 3: Teach the learner to respond to misunderstood messages by requesting clarification.

Step 4: Monitor learner performance.

Step 1: Observe the Learner Engaged in Conversation with Several Partners

Observe the AAC user to determine if he or she indicates that a message is not understood. Consider contrived opportunities such as purposefully emitting unintelligible utterances (garbled/inaudible), then wait for

Learner's name: __Nayla__

Repair behavior being addressed: __Repeat selection of line-drawn symbols on communication board.__

Type of prompt: __Gestural and visual prompt: Interventionist points to communication board and__

__holds up symbol for "slow down."__

Level of prompt: F: full prompt   P: partial prompt   I: independent (no prompt)

Instructions: Fill in the learner's name, identify the repair behavior being addressed, and describe the type of prompt that will be used (verbal, gestural, physical, visual) during instruction. Noting the date of observation, record messages that were misunderstood and how the communicative partner responded. Note the repair strategy used by the learner, and circle the level of prompt utilized. In the last column, circle *Y* if the breakdown was successfully repaired or *N* if the communicative partner continued to experience difficulty understanding the learner.

Date	Misunderstood message	Partner response to breakdown	Repair strategy	Prompt level	Was breakdown repaired?
3/11	Selection of symbols I, WANT, and BAGEL	"What? I didn't see what you wanted."	Repeat message, maintaining contact with the symbols for a longer amount of time.	Ⓕ P I	Ⓨ N
3/11	Selection of symbols I, GOING, and MOVIES	"Where are you going, Nayla? I didn't see it."	Repeat message, maintaining contact with the symbols for a longer amount of time.	Ⓕ P I	Ⓨ N
3/12	Selection of symbols THIS IS and FUN	"What did you say, Nayla?"	Repeat message, maintaining contact with the symbols for a longer amount of time.	F Ⓟ I	Ⓨ N

Figure 11.6. Sample form for monitoring learner progress during communicative breakdowns (augmentative and alternative communication user in the role of speaker). (*Note:* This is a filled-in version of Form 11.5, Monitor Learner Progress During Communicative Breakdowns [Augmentative and Alternative Communication User in the Role of Speaker]. A blank, printable version appears on the accompanying CD-ROM.)

the learner to respond. The left-hand column of Table 11.2 lists a variety of communicative breakdowns used to sample learner performance.

Step 2: Identify One or More Requests for Clarification to Be Taught

A request for clarification may take several forms (see the right-hand column of Table 11.2). Learners with limited verbal repertoires can be taught to say "Huh?" or raise a hand to their ear (i.e., general requests). The WHAT? symbol can be provided for

graphic mode users, as well as symbols for explicit requests for clarification (e.g., I DON'T UNDERSTAND).

Step 3: Teach the Learner to Respond to Misunderstood Messages by Requesting Clarification

Instruction can proceed once a request for clarification response has been identified.

- The interventionist can purposefully emit messages that are unintelligible.
- Prompt the learner to produce a request for clarification.

Table 11.2.   List of potential communicative breakdowns and sample responses

Communicative breakdown	Sample learner responses
The message is not loud enough.	*General response* Select the symbol WHAT? Raise hand to ear. *Explicit response* Select the symbol SAY IT LOUDER.
The message is unintelligible due to environmental noise/event.	*General response* Sign WHAT? Raise hand to ear. *Explicit response* Sign SAY THAT AGAIN.
The message is too complex.	*General response* Select the message WHAT? *Explicit response* Select the message I DON'T UNDERSTAND.

- Repeat or modify the message after the learner requests clarification.
- If the repetition of the message alone is not reinforcing, then consider using reinforcement unrelated to the specific utterance (e.g., verbal praise). For example,

Interventionist:	"Let's make (interventionist mumbles the word)?"
Learner:	Looks confused.
Interventionist:	Points to the learner's symbol for WHAT?
Learner:	Selects the WHAT? symbol.
Interventionist:	"Great question! I said, 'Let's make pancakes?'"

Step 4: Monitor Learner Performance

Progress should be monitored within the intervention setting and during natural interactions with a variety of communicative partners to ensure performance is generalized (see Figure 11.7; Form 11.6 is a blank version and is included on the accompanying CD-ROM).

TERMINATING INTERACTIONS

One or both partners take initiative to **terminate an interaction** at some point, possibly by commenting, "I have to go." Interactions may be terminated due to environmental variables (e.g., end of break, the need to attend to something else) and, although both participants may wish to continue the interaction, it may be necessary to terminate the interaction due to environmental events (e.g., the recess bell rings, which signals children to return to their classroom). Alternatively, a partner may desire to terminate a conversation due to loss of interest or anticipation of it heading in a direction he or she would rather avoid (e.g., a reprimand, the topic of household chores).

Many learners with severe disabilities lack an appropriate means of terminating interactions. Some engage in challenging behaviors, whereas others fail to engage in any type of response to indicate the termination of an interaction.

Using Evidence-Based Strategies to Terminate Conversational Exchanges

If a learner is to engage in conversations, it is important that he or she not only be able to initiate and maintain them but also to terminate them appropriately (e.g., not walking away; not saying, "I'm done," abruptly). We have found the following steps useful in establishing a socially acceptable method of terminating a communicative exchange.

Learner's name: __Marcel__

Repair behavior being addressed: __Select the graphic symbol I DON'T UNDERSTAND on speech-generating__
__device (SGD)__

Type of prompt: __Gestural: Interventionist points to symbol on SGD__

Level of prompt: F: full prompt   P: partial prompt   I: independent (no prompt)

Instructions: Fill in the learner's name, identify the repair behavior being addressed, and describe the type of prompt that will be used (verbal, gestural, physical, visual) during instruction. Note the date of observation, identify the communicative partner, and record his or her misunderstood message. Note the repair strategy used by the learner to indicate the message was misunderstood, and circle the level of prompt utilized. In the last column, circle *Y* if the communicative partner understood the learner's request for repair and, in turn, responded so that the learner understood the message. Circle *N* if the learner's request did not result in a successful communicative exchange.

Date	Communicative partner	Partner's misunderstood message	Repair strategy	Prompt level	Was breakdown repaired?
4/8	Classroom teacher	"Do you want to finish your work here, go with Ms. Web, or go with the other students?"	Select the symbol I DON'T UNDERSTAND on SGD.	(F) P I	(Y) N
4/9	Hall monitor	"Are you going to the assembly or your classroom?"	Select the symbol I DON'T UNDERSTAND on SGD.	(F) P I	(Y) N
4/10	Art teacher	"Marcel, I saw your artwork in the superintendent's office."	Select the symbol I DON'T UNDERSTAND on SGD.	(F) P I	Y (N)
4/10	Classroom teacher	"You can put your things away now or go with your group and put them away later."	Select the symbol I DON'T UNDERSTAND on SGD.	F P (I)	(Y) N

Figure 11.7. Sample form for monitoring learner progress during communicative breakdowns (augmentative and alternative communication user in the role of listener). (*Note:* This is a filled-in version of Form 11.6, Monitor Learner Progress During Communicative Breakdowns [Augmentative and Alternative Communication User in the Role of Listener]. A blank, printable version appears on the accompanying CD-ROM.)

Steps to teach learners to terminate conversational exchanges

Step 1: Identify situations and opportunities.
Step 2: Identify responses to be used to terminate an interaction.
Step 3: Identify intervention strategies.
Step 4: Implement intervention and monitor learner performance.

Step 1: Identify Situations and Opportunities

A range of opportunities should be considered when identifying situations and opportunities to terminate a conversation. Begin with those that are salient—a specific event (e.g., bell rings to indicate change in school periods); a cue that can be easily incorporated (e.g., setting a watch or cell phone to ring/vibrate in 15 minutes, indicating the need to terminate the conversation.); or a nonpreferred interaction appropriate for the learner to terminate. Consider teaching in the presence of less salient opportunities (a communicative partner looking at his or her watch, contributing less and less to the conversation, or when a preferred activity becomes less interesting) once a leaner terminates more salient interactions.

Step 2: Identify Responses to Be Used to Terminate an Interaction

Identify an appropriate response the learner can use to terminate an interaction. Consider symbols representing the messages EXCUSE ME or GOT TO GO or the sign for I'M DONE.

Step 3: Identify Intervention Strategies

Prompt the learner to emit the response to terminate the conversation following a clear environmental cue. Role-play to create opportunities to teach a learner to respond to less salient cues (e.g., act out how a communicative partner may act when desiring to end a conversation—check watch, look over one's shoulder, gather belongings). Less salient cues can initially be paired with more salient cues to which the learner already appropriately responds.

Step 4: Implement Intervention and Monitor Learner Performance

A performance monitoring form such as Form 11.3. on the accompanying CD-ROM can be used to monitor performance across both instructional and generalization settings.

Use the intervention planning form (Form 6.1 on the accompanying CD-ROM) to ensure the procedures used are well documented and increase the likelihood of reliable implementation.

INVOLVING COMMUNICATIVE PARTNERS IN INSTRUCTION OF SOCIAL-COMMUNICATION SKILLS

The mere placement of individuals with disabilities in settings alongside typical peers does not automatically result in social interaction or improved social-communicative skills. Instead, training of natural communicative partners (e.g., peers, interventionists) within those settings is critical and can have a tremendous effect on learners. Parent implementation of interventions within home and community settings (Bruno & Dribbon, 1998; Girolametto, 1988) and peer participation in interventions within school settings (Carter & Maxwell, 1998; Goldstein & Ferrell, 1987) has positively affected the social-communicative skills of children with developmental disabilities. Staff and peers within residential settings and staff and co-workers within places of employment have been taught to deliver systematic instruction improving social-communicative interactions (Light, 1989; McNaughton & Light, 1989). The following recommendations should be considered as natural communication partners are involved in instruction.

- A range of individuals, including interventionists (e.g., related services personnel, job coach), peers (e.g., classmates, co-workers), and support personnel (e.g., lunch monitors, coaches), should provide support to AAC users.

- Consider selecting "high-status" peers. Sasso and Rude (1987) demonstrated that more social initiations were made by untrained peers when high-status peers interacted with children with severe disabilities than when "low-status" peers were instructed to do so.

- Some support personnel will be naturally attuned to the needs of the AAC user and others might require individualized training to address their specific strengths and weaknesses.

- Ensure procedures provided to support personnel are not burdensome; it is essential to identify procedures that are palatable to support personnel (Carter & Pesko, 2008).

- Develop ways to monitor support personnel's use of strategies (e.g., Finn & Sturmey, 2009; Ward-Horner & Sturmey, 2008).

Empowering peers, parents, teachers, and other interventionists with strategies to support social-communicative interactions is particularly important for learners using AAC. It not only increases the number of teaching opportunities, but also results in instruction taking place in natural environments in which the learner is likely to communicate.

SUMMARY

In addition to communicative impairments (e.g., cognitive challenges, limited opportunities), several factors related to severe disabilities can have an effect on social interactions with both familiar and unfamiliar partners. Individually designed interventions can be used to teach a variety of conversational skills, including initiating, maintaining (including signaling and repairing of communicative breakdowns), and terminating interactions. Such strategies have the potential to improve the communicative skills of learners with developmental disabilities, thus increasing the likelihood of successful social-communicative interactions.

REFERENCES

Abbeduto, L., & Short-Meyerson, K. (2002). Linguistic influences on social interaction. In S.F. Warren & M.E. Fey (Series Eds.) & H. Goldstein, L.A. Kaczmarek, & K.M. English (Vol. Eds.), *Communication and language intervention series: Promoting social communication: Children with developmental disabilities from birth to adolescence* (pp. 27–54). Baltimore: Paul H. Brookes Publishing Co.

Alexander, D. (1994). *The emergence of repair strategies in chronologically and developmentally young children.* Unpublished dissertation, Florida State University, Tallahassee.

Alexander, D., Wetherby, A., & Prizant, B. (1997). The emergence of repair strategies in infants and toddlers. *Seminars in Speech and Language, 18,* 197–212.

Anselmi, D., Tomasello, M., & Acunzo, M. (1986). Young children's responses to neutral and specific contingent queries. *Journal of Child Language, 13,* 135–144.

Baron-Cohen, S., Tager-Flusberg, H., & Cohen, D.J. (1997). *Understanding other minds: Perspectives from autism.* Oxford, England: Oxford University Press.

Basil, C. (1992). Social interaction and learned helplessness in severely disabled children. *AAC:*

Augmentative and Alternative Communication, 8, 188–199.

Bates, E. (1976). *Language and context: The acquisition of pragmatics.* San Diego: Academic Press.

Beckman, P.J., & Lieber, J. (1992). Parent–child social relationships and peer social competence of preschool children with disabilities. In S.L. Odom, S.R. McConnell, & M.A. McEvoy (Eds.), *Social competence of young children with disabilities: Risk, disability, and intervention* (pp. 65–92). Baltimore: Paul H. Brookes Publishing Co.

Beukelman, D.R., & Mirenda, P. (2005). *Augmentative and alternative communication: Supporting children and adults with complex communication needs* (3rd ed.). Baltimore: Paul H. Brookes Publishing Co.

Bondy, A.S., & Frost, L.A. (1994). The Picture Exchange Communication System. *Focus on Autistic Behavior, 9,* 1–19.

Brady, N.C., & Halle, J.W. (2002). Breakdowns and repairs in conversations between beginning AAC users and their partners. In D. Beukelman & J. Reichle (Series Eds.) & J. Reichle, D.R. Beukelman, & J.C. Light (Vol. Eds.), *AAC series: Exemplary practices for beginning communicators: Implications for AAC* (pp. 323–351). Baltimore: Paul H. Brookes Publishing Co.

Brady, N.C., McLean, J.W., McLean, L.K., & Johnston, S. (1995). Initiation and repair of intentional communication acts by adults with severe to profound cognitive disabilities. *Journal of Speech and Hearing Research, 38,* 1334–1348.

Brady, N.C., Steeples, T., & Fleming, K. (2005). Effects of prelinguistic communication levels on initiation and repair of communication in children with disabilities. *Journal of Speech, Language, and Hearing Research, 48,* 1098–1113.

Brinton, B., & Fujiki, M. (1991). Responses to requests for conversational repair by adults with mental retardation. *Journal of Speech and Hearing Research, 34,* 1087–1095.

Brinton, B., Fujiki, M., Frome Loeb, D., & Winkler, E. (1986). Development of conversational repair strategies in response to requests for clarification. *Journal of Speech and Hearing Research, 29,* 75–81.

Brooks-Gunn, J., & Lewis, M. (1984). Maternal responsivity in interactions with handicapped infants. *Child Development, 55,* 782–793.

Bruno, J., & Dribbon, M. (1998). Outcomes in AAC: Evaluating the effectiveness of a parent training program. *Augmentative and Alternative Communication, 14,* 59–70.

Buffington, D.M., Krantz, P.J., McClannahan, L.E., & Poulson, C.L. (1998). Procedures for teaching appropriate gestural communication skills to children with autism. *Journal of Autism and Developmental Disorders, 28,* 535–545.

Buzolich, M.J., King, J.S., & Baroody, S.M. (1991). Acquisition of the commenting function among system users. *Augmentative and Alternative Communication, 7,* 88–99.

Buzolich, M., & Wiemann, J.M. (1988). Turn taking in atypical conversations: The case of the speaker/augmented-communicator dyad. *Journal of Speech and Hearing Research, 31,* 3–18.

Calculator, S.N. (1988). Promoting the acquisition and generalization of conversational skills by individuals with severe disabilities. *Augmentative and Alternative Communication, 4,* 94–103.

Calculator, S., & Delaney, D. (1986). Comparison of nonspeaking and speaking mentally retarded adults' clarification strategies. *Journal of Speech and Hearing Disorders, 51,* 252–259.

Carr, E.G., & Durand, V.M. (1985). Reducing behavior problems through functional communication training. *Journal of Applied Behavior Analysis, 18,* 111–126.

Carr, D., & Felce, J. (2007). The effects of PECS teaching to phase III on the communicative interactions between children with autism and their teachers. *Journal of Autism and Developmental Disabilities, 37,* 724–737.

Carter, E.W., & Pesko, M.J. (2008). Social validity of peer interaction intervention strategies in high school classrooms: Effectiveness, feasibility, and actual use. *Exceptionality, 16,* 156–173.

Carter, M., & Maxwell, K. (1998). Promoting interaction with children using augmentative communication through a peer-directed intervention. *International Journal of Disability, Development, and Education, 45,* 75–96.

Chadsey-Rusch, J., Gonzalez, P., Tines, J., & Johnson, J.R. (1989). Social ecology in the workplace: Contextual variables affecting social interactions of employees with and without mental retardation. *American Journal on Mental Retardation, 94,* 141–151.

Charlop, M.H., & Milstein, J.P. (1989). Teaching autistic children conversational speech using video modeling. *Journal of Applied Behavior Analysis, 22,* 275–285.

Charlop-Christy, M., & Kelso, S.E. (2003). Teaching children with autism conversational speech using a cue card/written script program. *Education and Treatment of Children, 26,* 108–127.

Clarke, M.T., & Kirton, A. (2003). Patterns of interaction between children with physical disabilities using augmentative and alternative communication systems and their peers. *Child Language Teaching and Therapy, 19,* 135–151.

Coggins, T.E., & Stoel-Gammon, C. (1982). Clarification strategies used by four Down's syndrome children for maintaining normal conversational behaviors. *Education and Training of the Mentally Retarded, 17,* 65–67.

Conroy, M.A., Dunlap, G., Clark, S., & Alter, P.J. (2005). A descriptive analysis of proactive behavior intervention research with young children with challenging behaviors. *Topics in Early Childhood Special Education, 25,* 157–166.

Davis, C.A., Reichle, J., & Southard, K., & Johnston, S. (1998). Teaching children with severe disabilities to utilize nonobligatory conversational opportunities: An application of high-probably requests. *Journal of The Association for Persons with Severe Handicaps, 23,* 57–68.

Doss, L.S., Locke, P.A., Johnston, S.S., Reichle, J., Sigafoos, J., Charpentier, P.J., et al. (1991). Initial comparison of the efficiency of a variety of AAC systems for ordering meals in fast food restaurants. *Augmentative and Alternative Communication, 7,* 256–265.

Duker, P.C., Dortmans, A., & Lodder, E. (1993). Establishing the manding function of communicative gestures with individuals with severe/profound mental retardation. *Research in Developmental Disabilities, 14,* 39–49.

Durand, V.M., & Carr, E. (1991). Functional communication training to reduce challenging behavior: Maintenance and application in new settings. *Journal of Applied Behavior Analysis, 24,* 251–264.

Durand, V.M., & Carr, E. (1992). An analysis of maintenance following functional communication training. *Journal of Applied Behavior Analysis, 25,* 777–795.

Durand, V.M., & Merges, E. (2001). Functional communication training: A contemporary behavior analytic intervention for problem behaviors. *Focus on Autism and Other Developmental Disabilities, 16,* 110–119.

Erbas, D. (2005). Response to communication breakdowns by nonverbal children with developmental disabilities. *Education and Training in Developmental Disabilities, 40*(2), 145–157.

Farrier, L.D., Yorkston, K.M., Marriner, N.A., & Beukelman, D.R. (1985). Conversational control in nonimpaired speakers using an augmentative communication system. *Augmentative and Alternative Communication, 1,* 65–73.

Ferm, U., Ahlsén, E., & Björck-Åkesson, E. (2005). Conversational topics between a child with complex communication needs and her caregiver at mealtime. *Augmentative and Alternative Communication, 21,* 19–40.

Fey, M.C., Warr-Leeper, G., Webber, S.A., & Disher, L.M. (1988). Repairing children's repairs: Evaluation and facilitation of children's clarification requests and responses. *Topics in Language Disorders, 8,* 63–84.

Finn, L.L., & Sturmey, P. (2009). The effect of peer-to-peer training on staff interactions with adults with dual diagnoses. *Research in Developmental Disabilities, 22,* 179–186.

Gallagher, T. (1981). Contingent query sentences with adult-child discourse. *Journal of Child Language, 8,* 51–62.

Gallagher, T., & Darnton, B.A. (1978). Conversational aspects of speech of language-disordered children: Revision behaviors. *Journal of Speech and Hearing Research, 21,* 118–135.

Ganz, J.B., & Flores, M.M. (2008). Effects of the use of visual strategies in play groups for children with autism spectrum disorders and their peers. *Journal of Autism and Developmental Disabilities, 38,* 926–940.

Ganz, J.B., & Simpson, R.L. (2004). Effects on communicative requesting and speech development of the Picture Exchange Communication System in children with characteristics of autism. *Journal of Autism and Developmental Disabilities, 34,* 395–409.

Girolametto, L.E. (1988). Improving the social-conversational skills of developmentally delayed children: An intervention study. *Journal of Speech and Hearing Disorders, 53,* 156–167.

Glennen, S.L., & Calculator, S.N. (1985). Training functional communication board use: A pragmatic approach. *Augmentative and Alternative Communication, 1,* 134–142.

Goldstein, H., & Ferrell, D.R. (1987). Augmenting communicative interaction between handicapped and nonhandicapped preschool children. *Journal of Speech and Hearing Disorders, 52,* 200–211.

Golinkoff, R.M. (1986). "I beg your pardon?": The preverbal negotiation of failed messages. *Journal of Child Language, 13,* 455–476.

Grossi, T.A., Kimball, J.W., & Heward, W.L. (1994). What did you say?: Using review of tape-recorded interactions to increase social acknowledgments by trainees in a community-based vocational program. *Research in Developmental Disabilities, 15,* 457–472.

Halle, J., Brady, N.C., & Drasgow, E. (2004). Enhancing socially adaptive communicative repairs of beginning communicators. *American Journal of Speech-Language Pathology, 13,* 43–54.

Hanzlik, J., & Stevenson, M. (1986). Mother–infant interaction in families with infants who are mentally retarded, mentally retarded with cerebral palsy or nonretarded. *American Journal of Mentally Deficiency, 90,* 513–520.

Houghton, J., Bronicki, G.J., & Guess, D. (1987). Opportunities to express preferences and make choices among students with severe disabilities in classroom settings. *Journal of The Association for Persons with Severe Handicaps, 12,* 18–27.

Hughes, C., Rung, L., Wehmeyer, M.L., Agran, M., & Copeland, S.R. (2002). Self-prompted communication book use to increase social interaction among high school students. *Journal of The Association for Persons with Severe Handicaps, 25,* 153–166.

Hunt, P., Alwell, M., & Goetz, L. (1988). Acquisition of conversation skills and the reduction of inappropriate social interaction behaviors. *Journal of The Association for Persons with Severe Handicaps, 13,* 20–27.

Hunt, P., Alwell, M., & Goetz, L. (1991). Interacting with peers through conversation turntaking with a communication book adaptation. *Augmentative and Alternative Communication, 7,* 117–126.

Jones, E., Carr, E., & Feeley, K. (2006). Multiple effects of joint attention intervention for children with autism. *Behavior Modification, 30,* 782–834.

Kaczmarek, L.A., Evans, B.C., & Stever, N.M. (1995). Initiating expressive communication: An analysis of the listener preparatory behaviors of preschoolers with developmental disabilities in center-based programs. *Journal of The Association for Persons with Severe Handicaps, 20,* 66–79.

Krantz, P.J., & McClannahan, L.E. (1993). Teaching children with autism to initiate to peers: Effects of a script-fading procedure. *Journal of Applied Behavior Analysis, 26,* 121–132.

Krantz, P.J., & McClannahan, L.E. (1998). Social interaction skills for children with autism: A script-fading procedure for beginning readers. *Journal of Applied Behavior Analysis, 31,* 191–202.

Lancioni, G.E., O'Reilly, M.F., Singh, N.N., Sigafoos, J., Oliva, D., & Severini, L. (2008). Three persons with multiple disabilities accessing environmental stimuli and asking for social contact through microswitch and VOCA technology. *Journal of Intellectual Disability Research, 52,* 327–336.

Lee, R., Kamhi, A., & Nelson, L. (1983, November). *Communicative sensitivity in language-impaired children.* Paper presented at the meeting of the American Speech-Language-Hearing Association, Cincinnati, OH.

Light, J. (1989). Toward a definition of communicative competence for individuals using augmentative and alternative communication devices. *Augmentative and Alternative Communication, 5,* 137–144.

Light, J.C., & Binger, C. (1998). *Building communicative competence with individuals who use augmentative and alternative communication.* Baltimore: Paul H. Brookes Publishing Co.

Light, J.C., Binger, C., Agate, T.L., & Ramsay, K.N. (1999). Teaching partner-focused questions to individuals who use augmentative and alternative communication to enhance their communicative competence. *Journal of Speech, Language, and Hearing Research, 42,* 241–255.

Light, J., Collier, B., & Parnes, P. (1985). Communicative interaction between young nonspeaking physically disabled children and their primary caregivers: Part l: Discourse patterns. *Augmentative and Alternative Communication, 1,* 74–83.

Light, J., Corbett, M.B., Gullapalli, G., & Lepkowski, S. (1995, December). *The effect of other orientation on the communicative competence of students who use AAC.* Poster presented at the annual convention of the American Speech-Language-Hearing Association, Orlando, FL.

Longhurst, T.M., & Berry, G.W. (1975). Communication in retarded adolescents: Response to listener feedback. *American Journal of Mental Deficiency, 80,* 158–164.

McClannahan, L.E., & Krantz, P.J. (2006). *Teaching conversation to children with autism: Scripts and script fading.* Bethesda, MD: Woodbine House.

McLean, J.E., McLean, L.K., Brady, N.C., & Etter, R. (1991). Communication profiles of two types of gesture using nonverbal persons with severe to profound mental retardation. *Journal of Speech and Hearing Research, 34,* 294–308.

McNaughton, D., & Light, J. (1989). Teaching facilitators to support the communication skills of an adult with severe cognitive disabilities: A case study. *Augmentative and Alternative Communication, 5,* 35–41.

Meadan, H., Halle, J., Ostrosky, M.M., & DeStefano, L. (2008). Communicative behavior in the natural environment: Case studies of two young children with autism and limited expressive language. *Focus on Autism and Other Developmental Disabilities, 23,* 37–48.

Meadan, H., Halle, J.W., Watkins, R.V., & Chadsey, J.G. (2006). Examining communication repairs of two young children with autism spectrum disorder: The influence of the environment. *American Journal of Speech-Language Pathology, 15,* 57–71.

O'Keefe, B.M., & Dattilo, J. (1992). Teaching the response-recode form to adults with mental retardation using AAC systems. *Augmentative and Alternative Communication, 8,* 224–233.

Pasco, G., Gordon, R.K., Howlin, P., & Charman, T. (2008). The Classroom Observation Schedule to Measure Intentional Communication (COSMIC): An observational measure of the intentional communication of children with autism in an unstructured classroom setting. *Journal of Autism and Developmental Disabilities, 38,* 1807–1818.

Paul, R., & Cohen, D. (1984). Responses to contingent queries in adults with mental retardation and pervasive developmental disorders. *Applied Psycholinguistics, 5,* 349–357.

Reichle, J. (1997). Communication intervention with persons who have severe disabilities. *Journal of Special Education, 31,* 110–134.

Reichle, J., Halle, J.W., & Drasgow, E. (1998). Implementing augmentative communication systems. In S.F. Warren & M.E. Fey (Series Eds.) & A. Wetherby, S.F. Warren, & J. Reichle (Vol. Eds.), *Communication and language intervention series: Vol. 7. Transitions in prelinguistic communication* (pp. 417–436). Baltimore: Paul H. Brookes Publishing Co.

Reichle, J., York, J., & Sigafoos, J. (1991). *Implementing augmentative and alternative communication: Strategies for learners with severe disabilities* (pp. 115–132). Baltimore: Paul H. Brookes Publishing Co.

Revelle, G.L., Wellman, H.M., & Karabenick, J.D. (1985). Comprehension monitoring in preschool children. *Child Development, 56,* 654–663.

Sarakoff, R.A., Taylor, B.A., & Poulson, C.L. (2001). Teaching children with autism to engage in conversational exchanges: Script fading with embedded textual stimuli. *Journal of Applied Behavior Analysis, 34,* 81–84.

Sasso, G.M., & Rude, H.A. (1987). Unprogrammed effects of training high-status peers to interact with severely handicapped children. *Journal of Applied Behavior Analysis, 20,* 35–44.

Seligman, M.E.P. (1975). *Helplessness: On depression, development, and death.* San Francisco: Freeman.

Shane, H.C., & Weiss-Kapp, S. (2007). *Visual language in autism.* San Diego: Plural Publishing.

Shatz, M. (1983). Communication. In J. Flavell & E.M. Markman (Eds.), *Handbook of child psychology* (pp. 841–889). New York: Wiley.

Shatz, M., & O'Reilly, A.W. (1990). Conversational or communicative skill? A reassessment of two-year-olds' behavior in miscommunication episodes. *Journal of Child Language, 17,* 131–146.

Stone, W.L., Ousley, O.Y., Yoder, P.J., Hogan, K.L. & Hepburn, S.L. (1997). Nonverbal communication in two-and three-year-old children with autism. *Journal of Autism and Developmental Disorders, 27,* 677–696.

Storey, K., & Provost, O. (1996). The effect of communication skills instruction on the integration of workers with severe disabilities in supported employment settings. *Education and Training in Mental Retardation, 31,* 123–141.

Storey, K., Rhodes, L., Sandow, D., Loewinger, H., & Petherbridge, R. (1991). Direct observations of social interactions in a supported employment setting. *Education and Training in Mental Retardation, 26,* 53–63.

Tomasello, M., Farrar, M., & Dines, H. (1984). Children's speech revisions for a familiar and an unfamiliar adult. *Journal of Speech and Hearing Research, 27,* 359–363.

Ward-Horner, J.C., & Sturmey, P. (2008). The effects of general-case training and behavioral skills training on the generalization of parents' use of discrete-trial teaching, child correct responses, and child maladaptive behavior. *Behavioral Interventions, 23,* 271–284.

Weiner, J.S. (2005). Peer-mediated conversational repair in students with moderate and severe disabilities. *Research and Practice for Persons with Severe Disabilities, 30,* 26–37.

Wetherby, A.M., Alexander, D.G., & Prizant, B.M. (1998). The ontogeny and role of repair strategies. In S.F. Warren & M.E. Fey (Series Eds.) & A. Wetherby, S.F. Warren, & J. Reichle (Vol. Eds.), *Communication and language intervention series: Vol. 7. Transitions in prelinguistic communication* (pp. 135–161). Baltimore: Paul H. Brookes Publishing Co.

Wichnick, A.M., Vener, S.M., Keating, C., & Poulson, C.L. (2010). The effect of a script-fading procedure on unscripted social initiations and novel utterances among young children with autism. *Research in Autism Spectrum Disorders, 4,* 51–64.

Wichnick, A.M., Vener, S.M., Pyrtek, M., & Poulson, C.L. (2010). The effect of a script-fading procedure on responses to peer initiations among young children with autism. *Research in Autism Spectrum Disorders, 4,* 290–299.

Wilkinson, K.M., & Romski, M.A. (1995). Responsiveness of male adolescents with mental retardation to input from nondisabled peers: The summoning power of comments, questions, and directive prompts. *Journal of Speech and Hearing Research, 38,* 1045–1053.

Wilcox, J.M., & Webster, E.J. (1980). Early discourse behavior: An analysis of children's responses to listener feedback. *Child Development, 51,* 1120–1125.

Yoder, P.J., Davies, B., & Bishop, K. (1994). Reciprocal sequential relations in conversations between parents and children with developmental delays. *Journal of Early Intervention, 18,* 362–379.

Yoder, P.J., Davies, B., Bishop, K., & Munson, L. (1994). Effect of adult continuing *wh*-questions on conversational participation in children with developmental disabilities. *Journal of Speech and Hearing Research, 37,* 193–204.

Using AAC to Support Language Comprehension

12

Emily A. Jones and Meredith Bailey-Orr

Speech comprehension plays a silent yet critical role in the language development process (Sevcik & Romski, 2002, p. 258).

▷ CHAPTER OVERVIEW

The majority of this book focuses on the use of augmentative and alternative communication (AAC) to provide the learner with a means of conveying information. AAC is also an important tool to enhance the learner's role as a listener. The role of listener requires **comprehension;** that is, understanding the communicative behavior produced by a partner. Providing additional input to spoken information presented to learners may not only improve comprehension but also productive communication.

▷ CHAPTER OBJECTIVES

After studying this chapter, readers will be able to

- Describe the importance of comprehension
- Describe, develop, and implement augmented input using the learner's AAC system
- Develop and implement visual supports to enhance comprehension and adaptive functioning

▷ KEY TERMS

- ▶ aided language stimulation
- ▶ augmenting input
- ▶ choice boards
- ▶ comprehension
- ▶ contingency maps

- ▶ message board
- ▶ picture recipes
- ▶ rule cards
- ▶ shopping lists
- ▶ simultaneous communication

- ▶ System for Augmenting Language (SAL)
- ▶ to-do and reminder lists
- ▶ visual schedules
- ▶ visual stories
- ▶ visual supports

WHY USE AAC TO SUPPORT COMPREHENSION?

The ability to comprehend spoken language represents a critical skill. In school settings, comprehending language makes it much easier to learn one's daily routine. It also makes it possible to easily learn of changes in the regular routine. Understanding sequences of actions that may be required to complete an activity (e.g., steps to microwave one's favorite meal) is also easier when one comprehends spoken language.

Why Is Comprehension Important?

Comprehension begins to emerge in the first year of life and rapidly increases in typically developing children (Miller, Chapman,

Branston, & Reichle, 1980). Comprehension of spoken language often precedes production and may facilitate the development of speech (Fenson et al., 1994; Hirsh-Pasek & Golinkoff, 1991). Speaking children tend to comprehend and produce the words most frequently spoken to them (Huttenlocher, Haight, Bryk, Seltzer, & Lyons, 1991). This is not an exact relationship, however, with some words produced that are not comprehended. Language comprehension alone is not likely to result in productive use, and learners with significant disabilities are not likely to generalize from comprehension to productive use without intervention (e.g., Romski & Sevcik, 1991).

The relationship between comprehension and production may be more complex in other modes and across modes. Comprehension of a symbol is assessed by showing the learner a graphic symbol (the sample), and the learner responds by selecting the corresponding object (choices); production of a symbol is assessed by showing the learner the object (sample), and the learner responds by selecting the graphic symbol (choices). Matching symmetry is the ability to match referents regardless of whether they are used as the sample or a choice. Some learners with severe disabilities do not show matching symmetry so that teaching one relationship does not guarantee the other (see Chapter 8). Drager et al. (2006) found symbol comprehension emerged before productive use; but productive use began before the learner demonstrated mastery of comprehension for that symbol. Harris and Reichle (2004) found comprehension and production of graphic symbols emerged simultaneously for some learners.

Productive use of graphic symbols also influences comprehension of speech for those symbols (Brady, 2000), facilitating acquisition across modes. Speech comprehension also influences acquisition of AAC (comprehension and production). Romski and Sevcik (1996)

The effect of augmented input on production is discussed in Chapter 2.

found that learners showing speech comprehension prior to intervention showed a pattern of simultaneous acquisition of comprehension and production of symbols with a speech-generating device (SGD), but those with little to no speech comprehension at the start showed comprehension first, followed by productive use of an SGD. Similarly, Clarke, Remington, and Light (1986, 1988) found speech comprehension influenced sign production acquisition.

Many learners with developmental disabilities show significant delays in comprehension (Beukelman & Mirenda, 2005; Wood, Lasker, Siegel-Causey, Beukelman, & Ball, 1998). Coexisting sensory (e.g., hearing impairments) or auditory processing impairments (difficulty recognizing, interpreting, and remembering auditory information, especially speech sounds and discriminating sounds in words; Lincoln, Dickstein, Courchesne, Elmasian, & Tallal, 1992) may negatively affect comprehension (Grandin, 1995; Quill, 1995; Schopler, Mesibov, & Hearsey, 1995). Memory difficulties may also negatively affect language comprehension. Learners with Down syndrome show specific impairments in auditory short-term memory (Byrne, Buckley, MacDonald, & Bird, 1995; Jarrold, Baddeley, & Phillips, 2002) that may affect comprehension and production of language (Fidler, 2005). Speech is a transient production, placing significant processing as well as memory demands on a learner. Sign is also somewhat transient, requiring significant recall memory requirements (Mirenda, 2003) and may be more difficult than graphic symbols for learners with memory difficulties.

USING AAC TO SUPPORT COMPREHENSION

Poor comprehension can influence a learner's ability to understand messages (conveyed through speech), affect participation in activities that require considerable spoken direction, and lead to challenging behavior. Using AAC to augment input and provide visual supports can help learners comprehend spoken information and begin to make associations between speech, AAC symbols, and referents, building the foundation of comprehension on which eventual expressive use of the AAC system may be based (Wood et al., 1998).

AUGMENTING INPUT

AAC users are not necessarily exposed to partner use of the AAC user's primary mode of communication. In a way, that more closely resembles the language learning experience of typically developing children learning speech. **Augmenting input,** also referred to as **aided language stimulation,** involves providing exposure to communication through partner use of the learner's AAC system. Augmenting input provides a model of how and where the AAC system can be used during communicative exchanges, demonstrates the effect that mode of communication can have in interactions, and destigmatizes its use (Romski & Sevcik, 1996). Augmenting input maps (i.e., pairs) spoken words, symbols, and their referents in the environment to help learners associate each of those elements. Augmenting input can be done with different modes of communication. Augmenting input in graphic communication involves the partner pointing to key graphic symbols corresponding to his or her spoken words.

ment their spoken messages. Interventionists also took advantage of naturally occurring opportunities for the child to use the communication display, initially to make requests using eye gaze (i.e., looking at her partner, a symbol, and again at her partner). The child acquired the use of eye gaze to communicate and even used 2- to 3-word spoken utterances during 7 months of intervention.

Examinations of augmented input alone (without prompting use of the communication system) with a graphic display reveal improvements in both learner comprehension and production of symbols (e.g., Bruno & Trembath, 2006; Cafiero, 2001; Drager et al., 2006; Heller, Alberto, & Romski, 1995). Harris and Reichle (2004) used augmented input with 3 preschool children (ages 3–5 years) with moderate cognitive disabilities who each spoke less than 30 words, but showed some preexisting speech comprehension. The experimenter provided augmented input during scripted classroom routines by pointing to a referent in the environment and then pointing to its corresponding Picture Communication Symbols (PCSs; Mayer-Johnson, 1992) while saying the name of referent. Unlike Goossens' (1989), experimenters did not prompt participants to use the picture symbols for production. All three participants acquired the target symbols (both receptively [when asked to show an object while pointing to the symbol] and expressively [when asked to identify the symbol corresponding to the object]) with some evidence of faster rate of acquisition as successive symbols were targeted for intervention.

What Does the Research Say?

Aided Language Stimulation

Goossens' (1989) implemented aided language stimulation involving augmented input with picture symbol communication boards with a 6-year-old girl with severe spastic-athetoid cerebral palsy and estimated developmental level of 16–20 months. She knew 5 Korean and 10 English words. Clinicians and her parents spoke in simple phrases and simultaneously pointed to corresponding symbols on her communication display during functional (e.g., dressing, eating) and age-appropriate (e.g., doll and toy play) activities. Communication displays created by activity included a vest worn by the communication partner, an eye gaze display, and a frame on the child's wheelchair. Displays contained an array of graphics reflecting different parts of speech and vocabulary for partners to use to aug-

In augmented input with an SGD, the partner speaks a word and the device produces the word after the partner selects the symbol. Romski and Sevcik (1993a) suggested the speech output of the device may specifically aid in developing comprehension. Schlosser, Belfiore, Nigam, Blischak, and Hetzroni (1995) compared the presence versus absence of speech from an SGD during receptive symbol instruction. The interventionist modeled use of the SGD simultaneous with his or her instruction (e.g., "Point to ___"). The interventionist's use of the SGD also produced speech output from the SGD only in the

See Chapter 2 for a discussion of the effect of SGD on speech production.

condition with the speech output turned on. Comprehension of symbols was only acquired by one of the participants when speech output was operational. The other two adults with severe to profound intellectual disabilities acquired symbol comprehension when speech output was on or off, but more efficiently, with fewer errors, when speech output was operational. Blischak (1999), Brady (2000), and Sigafoos, Didden, and O'Reilly (2003) found improved speech comprehension and production associated with an SGD.

What Does the Research Say?

System for Augmenting Language

Romski and Sevcik's (1996) **System for Augmenting Language (SAL)** involves augmented input using an SGD with visual graphic symbols, intervention within natural interactions encouraging but not requiring learner use of the SGD, and ongoing resources and feedback. Romski and Sevcik examined SAL with 13 males (ages 6–20 years) with moderate to severe intellectual disabilities who showed little to no functional speech (less than 10 word approximations). Partners learned to operate the device, viewed videotapes of others providing augmented input, and helped choose graphic symbol vocabulary in three 1-hour sessions. SAL began with one symbol on the SGD during mealtime at school or home. The SGD contained 13 social regulative symbols (e.g., THANK YOU, HELP) after 6 months and 35–44 symbols by the end of the second year. Participants used it for a range of functions (e.g., requesting, answering questions) (Romski & Sevcik, 1996). Participants showed two outcome patterns: Four participants showed a beginner pattern of slow acquisition of 20–30 single symbols for which comprehension emerged before production. Nine participants showed an advanced pattern of rapid and simultaneous acquisition of comprehension and production of symbols. The advanced group also showed speech comprehension prior to the study. Communication generalized across settings (i.e., home or school) and adults (i.e., parents and teachers) (Romski, Sevcik, Robinson, & Bakeman, 1994) and, for some participants, interactions with peers (Romski, Sevcik, & Wilkinson, 1994). Some also began to show related skills including symbol combinations in both production and comprehension that were not directly taught (Wilkinson, Romski, & Sevcik, 1994), recognition of written words (which were printed above the symbols) (Romski & Sevcik, 1993b), increased intelligible speech (Romski & Sevcik, 1993b),

and, when assessed 5 years later, fast mapping abilities (i.e., the ability to learn a new word with little exposure) (Romski, Sevcik, Robinson, Mervis, & Bertrand, 1995). Only one of the advanced achievers did not fast map; it may be that speech comprehension also indicates fast mapping ability and this was one way learners acquired AAC and speech.

Sevcik and colleagues extended SAL to preschoolers (Sevcik & Romski, 2005; Sevcik, Romski, & Adamson, 2004). In Sevcik and Romski (2005), 10 children (26–41 months old) with severe developmental delays and less than 10 spoken words participated in 12 months of SAL with similar results as Romski and Sevcik (1996).

Another method of augmenting input in the gestural mode, termed **simultaneous communication** or total communication, involves the partner simultaneously speaking and signing their communication.

Augmenting input is based on the premise that spoken language input in typically developing children provides a model for children's developing language abilities, both comprehension and production. Augmenting input provides that model using multiple modes of communication. If done prior to or in the early stages of learning an AAC system, then the learner begins to take part in the communicative process within an alternative mode of communication prior to actually taking on the role of speaker in that mode (Sevcik et al., 2004). Doing so should help build a foundation of comprehension skills and may result in a more typical language development path, decreasing other associated negative outcomes (e.g., challenging behavior, poor social development) (Romski & Sevcik, 1996; Sevcik et al., 2004).

The referents and spoken words are repeatedly paired when augmenting input. The corresponding elements of the referent, speech, and symbol should become equivalent through a process of stimulus equivalence, resulting in the establishment of the speech–referent relation (i.e., speech comprehension) (Remington & Clarke, 1993). The learner's existing speech comprehension also influences acquisition. As the spoken word is paired with the graphic symbol or sign, the relation between the graphic symbol or sign and corresponding referent is easily established for learners with existing speech comprehension (i.e., who have already established the relation between the spoken word and referent). In the absence of speech comprehension, despite the pairing of speech with graphic/sign in augmented input, the learner must rely on visual stimuli to establish the relation between the symbol and corresponding referent. Once that is established, the relation between the referent and speech may emerge.

What Does the Research Say?
Simultaneous Communication

Simultaneous/total communication is an effective way to teach sign comprehension and production to learners with developmental disabilities (e.g., Barrera, Lobato-Barrera, & Sulzer-Azaroff, 1980; Carr & Dores, 1981) and speech comprehension (e.g., Carr & Dores, 1981) and production (e.g., Kouri, 1988, 1989) for some learners. Carr and Dores taught receptive signs to six children with autism (6–11 years old). When the interventionist touched an object and said its name while also signing the label, he or she prompted the learner to touch the object. Two participants who showed poor verbal imitation skills acquired sign comprehension but not speech comprehension. The other four participants who had better verbal imitation skills acquired both speech and sign comprehension.

Several studies found that simultaneous/total communication is more effective than instruction using sign or speech alone (e.g., Barrera et al., 1980), but others found no differences (e.g., Remington & Clarke, 1983). Outcomes may differ depending on existing learner abilities. Layton (1988) found that learners with good verbal imitation skills benefitted from simultaneous communication, speech only, or sign only, but those with poor verbal imitation skills did the worst when presented with speech-only instruction. The four participants who acquired both speech and sign comprehension in Carr and Dores's (1981) study showed better verbal imitation skills.

Existing speech comprehension abilities are associated with faster sign acquisition with simultaneous/total communication than instruction with sign alone (Clarke et al., 1986, 1988) and may relate to overselectivity observed by Carr, Binkoff, Kologinsky, and Eddy (1978). After teaching expressive signing using a simultaneous communication approach, three of four children were primarily responding to the visual stimuli (i.e., referent), whereas only one child showed signing in the presence of either the referent or speech alone.

Who Might Benefit From Augmented Input?

It makes sense that most learners would benefit from receiving language input within the mode they are learning to use for production, but existing skill repertoires including speech comprehension, fast mapping abilities, and verbal imitation abilities may influence the effectiveness of augmenting input. Augmented input has resulted in positive outcomes for learners without these skills in their repertoire (e.g., Carr et al., 1978; Romski & Sevcik, 1996) and, in fact, may be particularly beneficial (Drager et al., 2006). Augmenting input may also result in decreases in challenging behavior (Peterson, Bondy, Vincent, & Finnegan, 1995).

Augmenting Input

Even though there has been limited implementation of augmented input, the existing evidence base is promising and suggests certain key steps that may be associated with a more desirable outcome. These steps are addressed below.

Steps for implementing augmented input

Step 1: Identify necessary vocabulary.
Step 2: Train partners.
Step 3: Use the AAC system during interactions with the learner.

Step 1: Identify Necessary Vocabulary

Choose the initial vocabulary supporting augmented input after identifying an AAC system for a learner, taking into consideration learner characteristics and needs (described in Chapter 2). Goossens' (1989) displays with a large vocabulary of graphic symbols for individual activities allowed partners to provide input across a variety of communicative functions related to ongoing activities (e.g., commenting, requesting, delivering instructions). Romski and Sevcik (1996) limited the initial display to only one symbol, however, because of the difficulty some learners have acquiring the association between symbols and referents. It may be that learners who show some existing skills that facilitate acquisition of AAC and speech (e.g., verbal imitation, speech comprehension) may respond better to starting with a larger vocabulary array.

Step 2: Train Partners

Train partners (e.g., parents, teachers, siblings) to use the AAC system that the learner is or will be using. If learners are using an SGD, then partners need basic information about the device and its programming. Partners must also learn how to communicate using the AAC system. Training may involve didactic instruction, modeling the use of the AAC system to provide augmented input, and practice with feedback.

Step 3: Use the AAC System During Interactions with the Learner

- Goossens' (1989) suggested partners specifically speak in shorter phrases, use a slower rate, and pause regularly when augmenting input.

- Pair spoken utterances with use of the AAC system for the key words/phrases in the communication exchange. Sevcik, Romski, Watkins, and Deffebach (1995) found partners most often used one symbol and augmented the last word in an utterance.

- Make the presentation of the graphic or signed communication salient for the AAC user. Produce gestures in clear view of the learner (e.g., close enough so learner can easily see the signs). Select graphic symbols in the same way as the learner's (e.g., direct selection with finger). Use additional means (e.g., pointing with a small squeaker in the palm, handheld stick, or light pointer) to help attract the learner's attention. If using tactile symbols for a learner with visual

impairments, then assist the learner in feeling the relevant symbol(s). Use the learner's own materials (e.g., device, book) to augment input with a graphic system, making sure they are in plain view and close enough the learner can see the selections easily. A teacher might more easily use his or her own communication display (e.g., a poster board of relevant symbols positioned on an easel in the front of the group) with a group of students (e.g., during a science lesson).

- Specifically highlight the referent (Drager et al., 2006; Harris & Reichle, 2004); consider pointing at the referent or showing or moving the object (e.g., shaking a toy, picking it up).

CASE STUDY

Augmented Input

Malcolm, a 4-year, 1-month-old boy with Down syndrome, showed delays in comprehension and production of language. All of his spoken words were highly unintelligible and many could not even be understood by familiar communication partners. An SGD was added to his individualized education program due to his age and degree of unintelligibility. Introducing the SGD to Malcolm included the interventionists providing augmented input.

Playing board games in his preschool classroom with his teacher and peers was one of the situations in which interventionists first introduced the SGD. The content of the SGD included colors, comments, and turn-taking phrases (e.g., IT'S YOUR TURN. IT'S MY TURN.). Intervention procedures are described in detail in the intervention planning form in Figure 12.1 (Form 6.1 is a blank version and is included on the accompanying CD-ROM). Intervention involved providing augmented input as well as specific prompts to assist Malcolm in productive use of his SGD. To illustrate, when the interventionist took her turn, she picked a card, spoke the label of the color card picked, and depressed the correct symbol on the SGD. When Malcolm took his turn, he picked a card, and the interventionist also spoke the label of the color and then used gestures to prompt

Learner's name: _Malcolm_   Start date: _1/3_

Setting (circle one):   HOME   (SCHOOL)   COMMUNITY   WORK

Communication skill/function: _Color identification_

Opportunities

When: _During tabletop activity time_   Where: _In classroom_

Minimum opportunities per day/session: _10 opportunities per day_

Context for instruction: _Instruction embedded within an activity_

Set up: _Playing a board game_

Materials: _Speech-generating device (SGD), board game_

Target Behavior

Mode: _Graphic, verbal_

Augmentative and alternative communication system features: _Direct selection of pictures on SGD_

Vocabulary: _Red, yellow, blue, green, your turn, my turn, I have, you have_

Instructional Strategies

Skill sequence/steps: _1) Pick a game to play; 2) the teacher provides augmented input during his or her turn by picking a card, labeling the color, and depressing the correct membrane on the SGD; 3) Malcolm takes a turn and picks a card, then the teacher prompts him to depress the corresponding symbol display._

Prompts: _Gesture to the correct color symbol._

Consequences

     Correct response: _Continue game uninterrupted and provide verbal praise._

     Incorrect response (no response or error response): _Stop the game, and model the use of the SGD following no response or an incorrect response. Use hand-over-hand assistance to select and depress the correct color symbol, and say the color name._

Prompt fading: _Use a time delay—begin by immediately prompting the correct response, and fade by delaying the prompt 5 seconds._

Generalization: _Examine generalization with peers and then across contexts: during game play at home, during coloring activities during occupational therapy, and during a bean bag toss game in physical therapy._

Maintenance: _Record performance one time per week to ensure the skill is maintained._

Criterion for Mastery

Malcolm will show 80% correct selection of targeted colors across 2 days and two partners. Use Performance Monitoring Form.

Figure 12.1. Intervention Planning Form to address colors. (*Note:* This is a filled-in version of Form 6.1, Intervention Planning Form. A blank, printable version appears on the accompanying CD-ROM.)

Learner's name: __Malcolm__   Activity: __Board game__

Instructions: Fill in each goal for the activity indicated above. In the Set up column, describe what the interventionist should do within the activity to provide the learner with an opportunity to practice that goal. Fill in the date of an observation, and record the learner's performance on that goal. For example, record a plus (+) if the learner demonstrated the correct response for that goal and a minus (–) if he or she did not demonstrate a correct response or demonstrated no response. Additional information about learner performance may include whether the interventionist presented a prompt (e.g., record a *P* for that step) or the learner did not respond at all for that step (e.g., record an *NR* for no response).

Goal	Set up	Performance
Labeling colors	When Malcolm picks a color card on his turn in the game, prompt him to press corresponding color symbol button.	Date: _1/10_ Interventionist's initials: _BP_ P | P | P | P | P | P | P | + | P | P | Date: _1/12_ Interventionist's initials: _SJ_ P | P | P | P | P | P | P | P | + | P | Date: _1/14_ Interventionist's initials: _BP_ P | P | + | + | P | + | + | + | P | + |

Goal	Set up	Performance
Identifying whose turn it is	At the beginning of Malcolm's turn, prompt him to press the MY TURN symbol button. At the completion of Malcolm's turn, prompt him to press the YOUR TURN symbol button.	Date: _1/10_ Interventionist's initials: _BP_ P | P | P | P | P | P | P | P | P | P | Date: _1/12_ Interventionist's initials: _SJ_ P | P | P | P | + | P | P | P | P | P | Date: _1/14_ Interventionist's initials: _BP_ P | P | + | P | + | + | + | P | P | + |

Figure 12.2.   Performance Monitoring Form for communication goals within games for Malcolm. (*Note:* This is a filled-in version of Form 6.4, Performance Monitoring Form for Instruction Embedded within an Activity. A blank, printable version appears on the accompanying CD-ROM.)

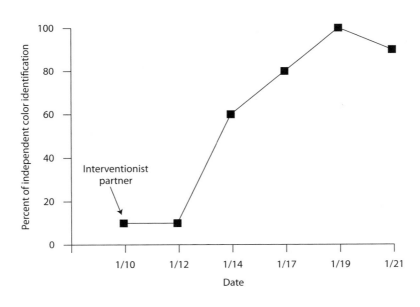

Figure 12.3.   Malcolm's color identification performance during games.

Malcolm to depress the corresponding color symbol on the SGD. Malcolm quickly progressed to independently depressing the color symbol and even using a word approximation for the colors. A portion of Malcolm's progress was recorded in detail on the performance monitoring form in Figure 12.2 (Form 6.4 is a blank version and is included on the accompanying CD-ROM) and illustrated graphically in Figure 12.3.

Efforts to generalize Malcolm's emerging color identification skills with peers will begin with one peer (Joseph) performing the same actions as the interventionist and then additional peers as Malcolm is successful. The interventionist will observe from another table as the children become proficient in using the device during the game. Additional vocabulary buttons will be added so that Malcolm can identify the agent of the action (e.g., I HAVE GREEN. YOU HAVE BLUE.) and create a sentence.

Augmenting input involves partner use of AAC to support learner comprehension and, ultimately, productive use of an AAC system. The latter half of this chapter focuses on using AAC within a variety of visual supports to specifically enhance learner comprehension.

VISUAL SUPPORTS

Visual supports include aids using photographs, pictures, line drawings, and so forth (see Earles-Vollrath, Cook, & Ganz, 2006; Ganz, 2007; Ganz, Cook, & Earles-Vollrath, 2006; Hodgdon, 1995; Mirenda & Brown, 2009) to enhance understanding of events. instruction. Using visual supports may

- Increase learner comprehension of spoken language as well as task/activity demands and expectations (that are often primarily conveyed through spoken language)
- Decrease challenging behavior by increasing learner understanding of expectations
- Help gain and maintain learner attention to tasks
- Help learners self-regulate

- Decrease the need for interventionist direction and enhance independent functioning

Who Might Benefit from Using Visual Supports?

Learners who show the following might benefit from using visual supports:

- Poor speech comprehension
- Difficulty learning the expectations and rules for certain situations or activities
- Improved performance in structured and predictable environments
- Difficulty remembering to engage in activities or components of an activity
- Reliance on extensive interventionist-delivered prompts to complete activities
- Challenging behavior

VISUAL SCHEDULES

Groups of symbols that inform the learner about activities that will occur during a designated period of time (e.g., a learner's entire day or week, a portion of the day) are called **visual schedules,** also referred to as *picture schedules* or *activity schedules*. Schedule following (i.e., generalized use of schedules in a variety of activities and tasks) across settings is an important part of a learner's skill repertoire. Schedules can be applied in many ways to support independence, active participation, and appropriate behavior in many situations.

Visual schedules should reflect a learner's choices both to engage and not engage in activities, increasing the learner's control over his or her environment (Brown, 1991). A schedule can indicate that something more preferred also is coming when upcoming activities are nonpreferred. If the learner does not want to stop an activity, then a schedule can indicate when he or she can engage in that activity again. Visual schedules increase independent engagement and active participation (rather than waiting for interventionist direction), allowing caregiver proximity to be faded (e.g., Irvine, Erickson,

Singer, & Stahlberg, 1992; MacDuff, Krantz, & McClannahan, 1993; Pierce & Schreibman, 1994). Visual schedules can provide an important component of behavioral support (e.g., Brown, 1991; Dooley, Wilczenski, & Torem, 2001; Dunlap & Fox, 1999; Marshall & Mirenda, 2002).

Visual schedules can depict multiple activities (also referred to as *daily schedules* and *picture or photographic activity schedules*) (e.g., McClannahan & Krantz, 1999) or components of a single activity (also referred to as *within-activity schedules, task organizers*, and *minischedules*) (e.g., Earles-Vollrath et al., 2006; Hogdgon, 1995). A schedule depicting a single activity provides detailed step-by-step information about the individual steps/actions within a task. For example, a within-activity schedule for brushing one's teeth might contain steps for getting the toothpaste and toothbrush, wetting the toothbrush, opening the toothpaste, and so forth. A schedule of multiple activities provides information about a sequence of activities such as the chores one must complete over the weekend or the errands a learner must complete after work.

What Does the Research Say?

Visual Schedules

MacDuff et al. (1993) examined the use of a photographic activity schedule displayed in a three-ring binder with six photographs of leisure and homework activities. Interventionists used graduated guidance delivered from behind the learners to teach picking up the schedule, carrying it to the location, opening the schedule, pointing to the first photograph, obtaining the necessary materials, completing the activity, putting the materials away, turning the page to the next photograph, and so forth. All four participants (9–14 years old) with autism learned to follow the schedule, showing both on-schedule and on-task behavior. Participants demonstrated generalized performance with new activity pictures and the interventionist absent.

Pierce and Schreibman (1994) taught daily living skills (e.g., doing laundry, making lunch, getting dressed) to three children with autism using visual schedules. Schedules consisted of pictures in a photograph book with a

---

smiley face on the last page, indicating the learner's opportunity for reinforcement. Children first learned to discriminate pictures of the steps in a given task (i.e., the interventionist presented three pictures and asked the learner to point to a given picture). The steps for interacting with the schedule were taught sequentially, beginning with just the first step in the task. As the learner independently completed the first step, the second symbol was added, chaining the two steps together, and so forth. Finally, the interventionist gradually increased the amount of time outside the room or his or her distance until he or she was out of the learner's view. Intervention resulted in acquisition of daily living skills, decreases in challenging behavior, and generalization across settings and a new sequence of pictures. In addition, the new tasks presented through visual schedules required considerably fewer intervention sessions for learners to acquire than the initial tasks. Several other studies obtained similar results (e.g., Berg & Wacker, 1989; Robinson-Wilson, 1977).

See McClannahan and Krantz (1999) and Hodgdon (1995) for additional information about creating visual schedules.

Steps for implementing visual schedules

Step 1: Choose tasks/activities and a time period for the schedule.
Step 2: Construct the sequence of activities/ steps in the schedule.
Step 3: Choose materials and vocabulary for the schedule.
Step 4: Create the schedule display.
Step 5: Develop instructional strategies.
Step 6: Implement the schedule, and monitor learner performance.

Step 1: Choose Tasks/Activities and a Time Period for the Schedule

For what time period should a schedule be created?

- Times when independent activity is appropriate, but the learner requires extensive prompting to engage in appropriate behavior

- Times when there are changes in schedule that can be difficult for the learner to comprehend and follow

- Times associated with challenging behavior, particularly related to the lack of predictability of routines and/or understanding of expectations

- Transitions may be difficult for some learners. If transitions are a problem in general, then consider a schedule for the learner's entire day. If only certain transitions are an issue, then a more circumscribed schedule just for those transitions may be helpful. Include symbols for specific learner behaviors during a transition (e.g., obtaining materials, getting in line), rules for transition behavior (e.g., keep your hands to yourself; see additional information on **rule cards** later in this chapter), and reinforcers for appropriate transition behavior. The learner can carry the graphic symbols (or objects) during transitions to the next activity.

- A longer period of time (e.g., a date book) to plan vacations, appointments, and events

For what tasks/activities should a schedule be created?

- Choose relatively brief tasks/activities for the first schedule. The first schedule for a learner may contain only one activity or take an "if . . . then . ." or "first . . . then . . ." format. Removable symbols or a dry erase board allows interventionists to continuously modify brief schedules as new demands are presented to a learner.

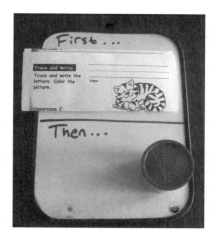

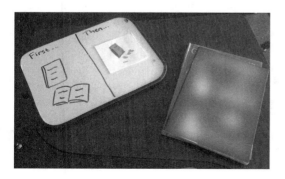

- Choose activities with which the learner is already relatively proficient if

  The learner is new to activity schedules and must learn schedule following

  The goal is the learner's independent engagement

- If developing a daily schedule, then divide up the day into meaningful and obvious units as the activities (e.g., by changes in location, materials, staff).

- Include those activities that are already a required part of the schedule time period (e.g., after-school activities might already include a snack and homework; classroom schedule might already include morning meeting, reading time, art).

- Identify additional activities for the time period such as daily living skills, vocational skills, skills to increase independence, and so forth (e.g., in addition to homework after school, activities could include playing a game and completing one household chore).

- For schedules depicting a single activity, choose activities that can be broken down into smaller steps:

  Novel activities for which the learner is just acquiring the individual steps

  Familiar activities for which the learner needs to master the steps

  Activities the learner should complete more independently

Activities with an object referent that clearly goes with each step/instruction (this makes it easier to develop a visual representation)

Activities that do not occur often (e.g., washing the car, hooking up a computer) may be particularly suited to schedules to support comprehension

- If a learner shows difficulty with an activity in a schedule of multiple activities, then create a single activity schedule for that activity to embed in the schedule for multiple activities.

- Include preferred activities and/or reinforcers on the schedule (Lancioni et al., 2000; Thineson & Bryon, 1981), which encourages the learner to check the schedule. Choose the last activity in the schedule to function as a reinforcer for engagement with all the preceding activities in the schedule.

- Activities should have clear endings (e.g., all the pieces are placed in the puzzle), or identify additional cues to signify the ending so the learner knows when each task is completed:

Flashing the lights and ringing a bell are some cues common in schools.

Providing the learner with his or her own clock to reference for the end of activities (e.g., Dettmer, Simpson, Smith Myles, & Ganz, 2000; Newman et al., 1995).

Teaching the learner to set a timer as part of a particular activity (e.g., McClannahan & Krantz, 1999). For example, the learner retrieves a bin containing a book and timer and sets the timer for 10 minutes before he or she begins reading.

- Graphic symbols can also represent specific learner interactions to practice expressive communication and social skills; for example, seeking out a parent to show him or her the homework just completed or asking a co-worker if he or she is also ready for a break.

- Schedules may also indicate when activities are not available.

☞ *Helpful Hint*

Communicating "No"

Use a NO symbol (e.g., X, Ø) across various types of visual supports to indicate activities, choices, and so forth that are not available or behavior that is inappropriate. Position the NO symbol next to or on top of the picture. Alternatively, turn over, cover up, or remove a graphic symbol to indicate it is not available. Affix the NO symbol to materials and spaces in the environment to indicate the learner is not to touch or gain access to them. Having a visual way to indicate "no" provides a permanent visual representation of the information to increase learner understanding.

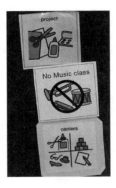

Step 2: Construct the Sequence of Activities/Steps in the Schedule

List and sequence all the activities/steps.

- Note any activities/steps that are fixed in order or time when they must be completed (e.g., the dog must be walked at 4:30 in the afternoon).

- Alternate different types of activities ensuring the same activity does not occur repeatedly (e.g., do not sequence three puzzles or three cleaning chores).

- Alternate preferred and nonpreferred or neutral activities/steps. Use participation in an activity in which the learner readily engages as a consequence following the learner's participation in an activity in which he or she is less likely to engage. This is the Premack principle—engaging in one activity can function as a reinforcer for engaging in another.

- Alternate novel with familiar activities.

- Alternate easier and more difficult activities/steps.
- Vary the sequence of activities/steps across instructional opportunities so the learner engages in generalized schedule following and not a memorized order.
- The schedule may apply to a group of learners (e.g., family calendar on the refrigerator) and/or be individualized for a specific learner (e.g., personal date book).

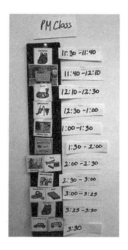

- Schedules are often prepared for the learner, but learners can also sequence their own schedule of activities (e.g., Bevill, Gast, Maguire, & Vail, 2001; Morrison, Sainato, Benchaaban, & Endo, 2002). Anderson, Sherman, Sheldon, and McAdam (1997) taught three adults with intellectual disabilities (21, 22, and 37 years old) in a group home to choose amongst line-drawn pictures and/or photographs of personal care, housekeeping, and recreational activities for a visual schedule of activities for the late afternoon/evening (after returning home from school or work). Participant engagement increased, and the need for interventionist prompting decreased.

☞ Helpful Hint

A **message board** informs the learner or group (e.g., family, class) about activities/tasks to do (not necessarily on a schedule or in a sequence) or even

changes in routine (e.g., substitute teacher, change in lunch menu).

Step 3: Choose Materials and Vocabulary for the Schedule

Practitioners should carefully select materials and vocabulary to create meaningful symbols that will represent components of events that will enhance self regulatory skills.

See Chapter 3 for additional information on selecting vocabulary and types of symbols.

What Vocabulary Will Be Used for Each Activity/Step?

- Choose a single graphic symbol for each activity/step (e.g., photograph containing just the game the learner will play; the label from the cookies the learner will eat to indicate snack time on the schedule).
- Use the same graphic symbol for a given activity/step throughout and across schedules.
- Include symbols for reinforcers.
- Use familiar vocabulary when possible so that instruction can focus on "schedule following" rather than on the meaning of the symbols. If novel symbols are used, then teach symbol discrimination and matching the symbol with the object/activity either while teaching the visual schedule or before introducing the symbols in a schedule.

☞ Helpful Hint

Symbols can be affixed to the object and/or location of materials.

- If the symbol corresponding to the one in the schedule is affixed to the materials required for the step/activity (e.g., on the drawer, cabinet door, container where the materials are located) or at the location of the step/activity (e.g., Dooley et al., 2001), then the learner relies on his or her matching skills to locate the required materials and/or location for an activity/step.

- Affixing symbols to specific objects or locations may also be helpful in conveying possession or personal space (e.g., learner's bedroom). For example, only shelves on which the learner's photograph is affixed are available for the learner to gain access to materials.

- Affix additional symbols (not necessarily those in the schedule) to other locations (e.g., drawers, closets) and materials to assist learners in completing activities (e.g., putting laundry away with drawers labeled for shirts and pants).

What Types of Symbols Will Be Used to Create the Schedule?

Use objects, line drawings, text, photographs, package labels, and so forth to create a schedule. Consider a variety of graphic symbols because it is not necessary to use the same type of symbol for every activity/step throughout the schedule. If the learner comprehends black-and-white line drawings for several of the activities, but would more easily recognize a photograph for others, then use both.

> See Chapter 3 for additional information about considerations in choosing AAC systems.

Step 4: Create the Schedule Display

The type of display that houses a learner's symbols represents a very important feature. The method used to configure the placement of and portability of the symbols may have a direct effect on the efficiency of the overall system.

What Kinds of Displays Can Be Used for a Schedule?

Consider using pages in a three-ring binder, date book, photograph album, chart affixed to a learner's desk, wall display (e.g., bulletin board), magnet board, sequence of boxes on a shelf, or even a plastic bag hung on the wall (allowing an actual object to be used as the symbol). Use durable materials, laminate paper materials, enclose symbols in clear protective sheets or photograph album pages, and use stronger cardboard or poster board on which to mount symbols. Utilize hook and loop tape, magnets, and so forth to allow the sequence of symbols on the schedule to be rearranged. Even if the schedule is relatively fixed (e.g., classroom activities), there will be days when things change (e.g., half day, assembly, substitute paraprofessional). The schedule needs to accommodate such changes as these are probably the most important events to communicate effectively to learners. Regularly rearrange the schedule sequence to ensure generalization of schedule following.

Technology, such as cell phones and computers, can be used to display schedules. Some SGDs come with scheduling software to create visual schedules. Mechling and Gast (1997) used a schedule created with a Digivox using photographs for each step of the task that, when pressed, also provided digitized speech instructions for that step. Four children (10–13 years) with moderate intellectual disabilities learned tasks such as making popcorn and using the dishwasher.

What Does the Research Say?
Creating Computer-Aided Visual Schedules

Computer technology provides a variety of ways of presenting visual schedules that take advantage of digital photographs, video, and sound as well as scanners to scan other pictures, drawings, and so forth. Lancioni et al. (2000) compared a computer-based visual schedule with simple color pictures of each step along with smiley face pictures cuing reinforcement to picture cards in a booklet to teach several tasks (e.g., cleaning, preparing food). The computer schedule was more effective for all six participants (23–47 years old), and it was possible to cluster the steps into a smaller number of groupings during maintenance.

PowerPoint has been used to present computer-aided visual schedules (e.g., Dauphin, Kinney, & Stromer, 2004; Kimball, Kinney, Taylor, & Stromer, 2004; Stromer, Kimball, Kinney, & Taylor, 2006). Dauphin et al. taught a 3-year-old

(continued)

child with autism and attention-deficit/hyperactivity disorder sociodramatic play skills (a play action and verbalization) using a computer-aided visual schedule. The participant already knew how to use the computer mouse and basic computer activity schedules for other tasks (e.g., puzzles, sorting shapes). Computer schedules were presented on a laptop computer with digital photographs, video, text, and sound on PowerPoint slides. The participant used the mouse to click the page turner and the picture, watched the video of a child modeling a script and action with specific materials, obtained the required materials, said the script in the video and completed the action, and put away the materials. Upon completion and return to the computer, advancing to the next page resulted in spoken praise and tokens to later receive a break. The participant acquired all three sociodramatic play actions and verbalizations and also generalized to similar action-verbalization combinations.

Davies, Stock, and Wehmeyer (2002a, 2002b) used palmtop computer technology to develop software that incorporates video and audio signals to teach vocational tasks. Davies et al. (2002b) compared a written scheduling system (written instructions with the designated time indicated) with a palmtop computer, and the palmtop personal computer system was associated with a decreased need for assistance and fewer errors. The computer system was associated with timely completion of scheduled tasks for 11 of 12 adults with developmental disabilities (only 1 participant completed the tasks in a timely fashion with the written schedule). This software and the use of commonly available technology provide natural supports for learners with developmental disabilities in inclusive settings.

Some computer skills (e.g., use of a mouse) may ease the introduction of computer-aided visual schedules. If a learner is new to visual schedules, then a first schedule could be on the computer (especially for a learner with computer experience and/or interest), though instruction could also begin with a regular paper schedule and then transfer to a computer presentation.

> See Rehfeldt, Kinney, Root, and Stromer (2004) for detailed step-by-step instructions for setting up a computer-aided visual schedule in PowerPoint.

How Will the Schedule Be Used and Where Will It Be Located?

Schedules should be easily accessible to the learner and within the location they will be used or near transition points between environments (e.g., on the table by the door to retrieve when leaving the house).

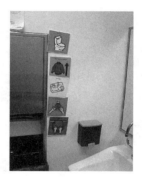

Schedules used across multiple environments should be relatively small and contain storage places for potential symbols, used symbols, and so forth. In some situations, however, storing the symbols in a separate location (e.g., keeping symbols for a schedule for recess at school in the classroom) will likely be less cumbersome and help keep distractions (e.g., extra symbols) to a minimum when initially teaching schedule following. Schedules on cell phones or personal digital assistants (PDAs) are portable and easily blend with the gadgets that are carried around all the time.

How Will the Learner Signify Completion of an Activity/Step?

- Make a mark (e.g., a checkmark) on top of, next to, or below the symbol upon completion.

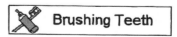

- Remove the symbol and place it in a designated "finished"/"done" area of the schedule display. Alternatively, place the symbol in a separate storage area or hand it to the interventionist.

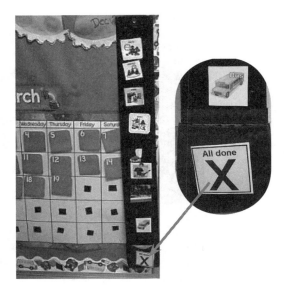

- Turn the page in a book/binder schedule to signify completion of that activity. Copeland and Hughes (2000) found that turning the page at the completion of a step was related to successful completion of the activities.

- Cover the symbol by turning it face down on the schedule display, or place another symbol representing finished (e.g., an *x*) on top of or next to the symbol for the completed activity.

☞ Helpful Hint

Completed schedules can be used as a visual prompt for the learner to share information about his or her day or to request a work check. For example, the learner uses a visual schedule at school that he or she brings home with each completed activity marked with an *x*. This visual then serves as a prompt for him or her to communicate with his or her parents about his or her activities that day.

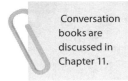

Conversation books are discussed in Chapter 11.

Step 5: Develop Instructional Strategies

- If the vocabulary on the schedule is new to the learner, then teach the learner to discriminate the symbols. Show the learner several (e.g., three) symbols from those on the schedule and ask him or her to point to a specified task/action/object (e.g., point to homework). Learners may also need instruction to match the symbols to the corresponding materials. Present the symbol and ask the learner to choose the corresponding item(s) from an array. Teach discrimination and matching while also teaching schedule following or prior to introducing the schedule.

- Construct a task analysis of how the learner will interact with the schedule (see Form 12.1 on the accompanying CD-ROM). Steps in schedule following might include opening the schedule book, removing the symbol and bringing it to the activity area, obtaining the necessary materials and completing the activity designated on that symbol, bringing the symbol back to the schedule upon completion, placing symbol in "finished" pocket, and locating the next symbol.

- Prepare materials.

- Ensure necessary materials are available and in the correct locations.

- Make sure reinforcers are ready.

- Sequence the symbols on the schedule following the information in Step 2.

  Involve the learner in creating the schedule (e.g., learner chooses the order of leisure activities; learner chooses the last activity in the schedule). Choice of activities increases engagement and on-task behavior (e.g., Bannerman, Sheldon, Sherman, & Harchik, 1990; Dunlap et al., 1994; Watanabe & Sturmey, 2003). At first, teach the learner to place symbols on the schedule as the interventionist identifies them. Then, the learner can make choices of activities when the interventionist presents a few at a time. Over time, the learner may be able to create the entire schedule given all the available options.

- Identify the natural cue to remind the learner to check the schedule (e.g., the bell ringing, the teacher telling everyone to get ready for the next activity). Use additional cues such as a vibrating pager or timer to help increase independent use of the schedule, requiring less interventionist direction.

- Utilize chaining and prompting procedures to teach the learner to complete the schedule.

Schedule following consists of a sequence of learner responses that together form a chain. (See filled-in Form 12.1b, Task Analysis, included on the accompanying CD-ROM. A blank, printable version, Form 12.1a, is also available on the accompanying CD-ROM.) All of the activities/steps and schedule following responses (e.g., turning the page, pointing at the symbol) can be taught simultaneously as in total task presentation (McClannahan & Krantz, 1999). For example, MacDuff et al. (1993) taught all the steps of schedule following simultaneously to four children with autism (9–14 years old).

Forward or backward chaining can also be used. Backward chaining involves teaching the last step in schedule following first; the interventionist completes all the steps, except for the last one—the one targeted for instruction. Once the learner masters the last behavior in the chain, the interventionist teaches the second to last, the third to last, and so forth. Forward chaining involves teaching the chain of schedule-following behaviors in temporal order, beginning with the first behavior in the sequence (the interventionist completes the rest of the steps in the chain). Instruction continues once the learner masters the first behavior, teaching one additional behavior within the chain at a time. Pierce and Schreibman (1994) first taught the picture schedule with the first photograph for a task on page one and a smiley face on page two (to indicate completion and the opportunity to obtain reinforcers). The interventionist provided praise and the learner gained access to reinforcers once the learner opened the book, pointed

to the picture, completed the step illustrated on the first page, and turned to the smiley face page. Interventionists delayed the prompts to allow the learner to respond independently. When the learner independently used the schedule with one picture and the smiley face page, the second picture (step) was added, chaining each picture (step) to the initial one.

> See Chapter 5 about prompting and chaining.

Choice of prompts to direct the learner to follow the schedule and complete the activities must be individualized to focus learner attention on the schedule and activity and so they can be easily faded. Verbal prompts may prove difficult to fade and be disruptive to independent schedule completion. McClannahan and Krantz (1999) suggested using graduated guidance from behind the learner in an effort to facilitate independent completion of the schedule. If physical or modeling prompts are used, then make sure the prompts do not block the learner from the schedule or the activities.

> See prompt fading in Chapter 5 to fade additional cues.

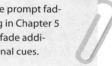

Fade the presence of the interventionist by gradually increasing his or her distance from the learner in order to facilitate independence. The interventionist might also leave intermittently for short periods of time (e.g., 10 seconds), gradually increasing the time absent.

- Reinforce checking and using the schedule as well as completing the activities/steps.

- If the learner makes an error (e.g., not completing the activity, not returning to the schedule after completing an activity), then return to the previous prompting procedure (i.e., the higher prompt level in the hierarchy); introduce a reference to the visual (e.g., using a gestural prompt directed at the picture of the correct activity in the schedule) (Martin,

Mithaug, & Frazier, 1992) for errors such as obtaining the wrong materials; begin that activity/step again; and begin the entire schedule again (McClannahan & Krantz, 1999).

Also consider the effectiveness of the reinforcers.

☞ Helpful Hint

Use visual schedules in conjunction with other self-management strategies such as self-reinforcement when the learner judges his or her completion of the schedule and then gains access to a reinforcer (Berg & Wacker, 1989; Pierce & Schreibman, 1994).

Step 6: Implement the Schedule and Monitor Learner Performance

Schedules must be used consistently and remain available to the learner. Record learner performance for each of the activities/steps of using the schedule and completing the activity(ies) using the task analysis developed in Step 5 (see Form 12.1 on the accompanying CD-ROM) or similar performance monitoring forms such as Figure 12.4 (Form 12.2 is a blank version and is included on the CD-ROM).

CASE STUDY

Multiple Activity Schedule

Samuel, a 4-year, 5-month-old boy diagnosed with Pervasive Developmental Disorder-Not Otherwise Specified (PDD-NOS), was familiar with picture symbols and used them to communicate. Samuel screamed and/or threw himself on the floor when he was taken out of the room by any of his therapists (e.g., occupational therapist, physical therapist, speech-language pathologist [SLP]) or went to computer class. The only transitions outside the classroom with which Samuel did not have difficulty were going to the playground and

music with his class; Samuel's music teacher always played an instrument while walking the class to the music room, and Samuel went with all the other children to the playground for recess. In contrast, Samuel was "pulled out" for speech four times a week, occupational therapy two times a week, and physical therapy one time a week. In addition to probable reinforcers available in music and recess (e.g., peers, music, play), the extra visual cues at transition time may have increased their success.

Samuel's teachers introduced a vertical picture schedule of the events of the day. The picture schedule was posted near his cubby for easy access. The symbols (line drawings and pictures) were printed on laminated photograph paper (with hook and loop tape backing for affixing to and removing from the schedule). Intervention procedures are described in detail on the intervention planning form in Figure 12.5 (Form 6.1 is a blank version and is included on the accompanying CD-ROM). Prior to each transition, Samuel consulted the schedule, removed the picture symbol, took it with him as a transition object, and returned it to the "all done" pocket when he reentered the classroom. The last symbol on the schedule offered Samuel a choice of highly preferred activities (e.g., using playdough, helping his friends make a puzzle) if he did not engage in challenging behavior. If Samuel exhibited challenging behavior during a transition, then the interventionist directed him to return to the schedule, used hand-over-hand guidance to take the picture off the schedule, and escorted him to the next activity. Challenging behavior decreased significantly during transitions to his therapies and to computer class as recorded on the performance monitoring form in Figure 12.4 (Form 12.2 is a blank version and is included on the accompanying CD-ROM) and depicted graphically in Figure 12.6. After approximately 4 weeks, Samuel only consulted the schedule briefly when entering and exiting the classroom.

Learner's name: _Samuel_

Correct response: _Samuel will remove the symbol from his schedule and take it with him to transition without challenging behaviors (e.g., screaming, falling to the floor)._

Instructions: Fill in the prompts to be used (e.g., full prompt: hand over hand; partial prompt: pointing to picture schedule). Record the date and the learner's performance of the response for each observation. Record whether the learner engaged in challenging behavior (e.g., Y for yes, N for no). Record the initials of the interventionist and any notes relevant to learner performance.

F (full prompt): Hand over hand

P (partial prompt): Pointing to picture schedule

I (independent): No prompt

Date	Response	Challenging behavior	Delay in prompt	Initials	Activity	Notes
4/8	F	Yes	0 seconds	LS	Speech	Intervention
4/8	F	Yes	0 seconds	TO	Computer	Intervention
4/9	F	Yes	0 seconds	PK	Occupational therapy	Intervention
4/9	F	No	0 seconds	LS	Speech	Intervention
4/10	F	No	0 seconds	LS	Speech	Intervention
4/10	F	No	0 seconds	PK	Occupational therapy	Intervention
4/11	P	Yes	0 second	LS	Speech	Intervention; sent home after therapy with fever
4/12	P	No	0 seconds	AK	Physical therapy	Intervention
4/15	P	No	0 seconds	LS	Speech	Intervention
4/16	P	No	0 seconds	LS	Speech	Intervention
4/16	P	No	10 seconds	PK	Occupational therapy	Intervention
4/17	P	No	10 seconds	PK	Occupational therapy	Intervention
4/17	I	No	10 seconds	AK	Physical therapy	Intervention
4/17	P	No	10 seconds	LS	Speech	Intervention
4/18	I	No	10 seconds	TO	Computer	Intervention
4/19	I	No	10 seconds	LS	Speech	Intervention

Figure 12.4. Performance Monitoring Form for Samuel's use of an activity schedule for transitions. (*Note:* This is a filled-in version of Form 12.2, Performance Monitoring Form for Use of an Activity Schedule for Transitions. A blank, printable version appears on the accompanying CD-ROM.)

(continued)

Figure 12.4.   *(continued)*

Date	Response	Challenging behavior	Delay in prompt	Initials	Activity	Notes
4/22	I	No	10 seconds	PK	Occupational therapy	Intervention
4/22	I	No	10 seconds	LS	Speech	Intervention
4/23	I	No	10 seconds	AK	Physical therapy	Intervention
4/24	I	No	10 seconds	LS	Speech	Intervention
4/24	I	No	10 seconds	LS	Speech	Intervention
4/25	I	No	10 seconds	LS	Speech	Intervention
4/25	I	No	10 seconds	TO	Computer	Intervention
4/26	I	No	10 seconds	PK	Occupational therapy	Intervention
4/27	P	No	0 seconds	Mom	Home	Generalization; stopped playing computer and came to dinner
4/27	P	No	0 seconds	Mom	Home	Generalization
4/27	P	No	0 seconds	Dad	Home	Generalization; left synagogue with Dad after service
4/28	I	No	10 seconds	Dad	Home	Generalization
4/29	I	No	10 seconds	Dad	Home	Generalization
4/30	I	No	10 seconds	Sister	Home	Generalization; stopped playing computer and drew pictures
4/30	I	No	10 seconds	Sister	Home	Generalization; left library with sister after program's conclusion
5/1	I	No	10 seconds	LS	Speech	Maintenance
5/1	I	No	10 seconds	Dad	Home	Generalization; stopped playing computer and drew pictures

Learner's name: _Samuel_   Start date: _4/1_

Setting (circle one):   HOME   (SCHOOL)   COMMUNITY   WORK

Communication skill/function: _Use of vertical activity schedule_

Opportunities

When: _Throughout the day_   Where: _Classroom and in hallways while making a transition_

Minimum opportunities per day/session: _One opportunity per therapeutic session as well as a weekly computer class resulting in eight opportunities per week_

Context for instruction: _Naturally occurring opportunities to travel from the classroom to therapy or computer room_

Set up: _When the therapist or computer instructor comes into the classroom and indicates it is time to go (e.g., "Samuel, time for occupational therapy")_

Materials: _Vertical picture schedule, pictures, photograph paper, hook-and-loop tape_

Target Behavior

Mode: _Graphic_

Augmentative and alternative communication system features: _Direct selection of line-drawn symbols_

Vocabulary: _Teacher's and therapists' names, occupational therapy, physical therapy, speech, and computer_

Instructional Strategies

Skill sequence/steps: _1) The therapist or teacher calls Samuel's name when it is time for him to make a transition to therapy or computer class; 2) prompt schedule use; 3) provide verbal praise if Samuel responds by taking the picture off the schedule and walking with his teacher or therapist._

Prompts: _Use hand-over-hand assistance faded to a gesture to the correct symbol._

Consequences

   Correct response: _Allow participation in therapies and computer class, and offer verbal praise._

   Incorrect response (no response or error response): _Use hand-over-hand assistance to select the correct symbol following no response or an incorrect response, and escort Samuel to his destination._

Prompt fading: _First fade from most to least (from full prompt [physical guidance] to partial prompt [gesture]). Then, use a time delay—begin by immediately prompting the correct response and fade by delaying the prompt 10 seconds. Fade when Samuel shows correct schedule use on three opportunities across 2 days in the absence of challenging behavior._

Generalization: _Address making a transition at home and in community with family members, using a similar schedule format for difficult home transitions._

Maintenance: _Record performance one time per week to ensure the skill is maintained._

Criterion for Mastery

Samuel will show independent schedule use and the absence of challenging behavior on three opportunities across 2 days.

Performance Monitoring

See Performance Monitoring Form.

Figure 12.5. Intervention Planning Form to address challenging behaviors during transitions. (*Note:* This is a filled-in version of Form 6.1, Intervention Planning Form. A blank, printable version appears on the accompanying CD-ROM.)

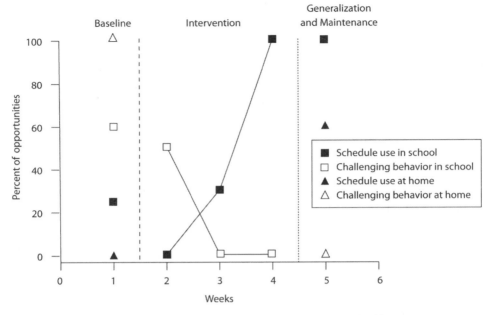

Figure 12.6. Samuel's use of vertical activity schedule during transitions within school and home.

☞ *Helpful Hint*

Within Activity Schedule: Picture Recipe

Picture recipes are one example of a single or within-activity schedule. Use picture recipes to teach cooking and other food-related skills (e.g., cutting, cleaning up), expand a learner's repertoire of foods, and ensure learners eat a variety of healthy foods. Picture recipes can increase the independence of a learner who otherwise requires extensive and intrusive prompting and supervision from an interventionist (e.g., Martin et al., 1992; Taylor, 1987).

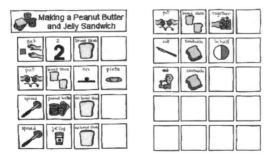

TO-DO AND REMINDER LISTS

Everyone makes **to-do and reminder lists** for weekend chores, daily tasks, shopping,

items to pack for vacation, and so forth. Lists may be traditional paper or use technology. Myles, Ferguson, and Hagiwara (2007) taught a 17-year-old with Asperger syndrome to use a PDA to list his homework assignments (including the subject area, due date, and details of the work). Lists also increase learner independence. A **shopping list** is a group of items that need to be purchased.

What Does the Research Say?

Shopping Lists

Sarber, Halasz, Messmer, Bickett, and Lutzker (1983) taught both menu planning and shopping to an adult with an intellectual disability. A weekly menu chart included slots for each of the four color-coded food groups at each of three meals per day for 7 days and the number of servings from each food group that should be consumed per day. The participant learned to place food cards in the corresponding food group columns on the menu, tally the servings per day, and plan a menu of meals. Using her menu, the participant then located the food cards corresponding to the ones on the menu and checked for food already in her home, creating a final group of needed food items. She

(continued)

placed the food cards in a binder to bring to the store. When the learner located the corresponding items at the store, she used a yellow marker to cover the food card (to indicate it had been put in the cart).

Morse and Schuster (2000) examined a multicomponent intervention including the use of shopping lists to teach shopping skills to elementary students (5–12 years old) with moderate intellectual disabilities. The teacher and each learner created shopping lists using photographs of the aisle signs and corresponding items to purchase, with yellow directional arrows to indicate the order of items (in the students' community shopping store). Teachers immediately prompted use of the shopping list with a model and verbal direction and introduced a 4-second time delay during the first two opportunities. Six children mastered shopping skills, two other children improved, and two did not begin intervention because the school year ended.

Step 1: Choose Symbols for the List

Refer to guidelines about visual schedules in this chapter. Choose familiar symbols, such as from the learner's own AAC system and labels from boxes or cans of shopping items (these are also easily matched to the items in the store). Use different types of symbols depending on their familiarity to the learner.

Consider also affixing symbols to the storage locations for the corresponding items within the learner's kitchen (e.g., cereal box label affixed to the inside of the cabinet door where the cereal is stored). This may help with putting purchased items away after a shopping trip.

- An initial list might contain just a few items.

- Vary the items on the list to ensure the learner continues to check the list and does not simply memorize the items needed.

- Include preferred items so the list is not aversive, but make sure to include less preferred or neutral items so the list can be useful across situations and needs.

- Learners may have a history of using graphic symbols to request highly pre-

Steps for teaching use of shopping lists

Step 1: Choose symbols for the list.
Step 2: Choose a system to store, display, and transport the symbols/list to the store.
Step 3: Identify the steps of developing a shopping list (as well as putting away the purchases).
Step 4: Develop instructional strategies.
Step 5: Use the shopping list and monitor learner performance.

ferred items that are on the list. Once obtained, learners may seek to immediately consume those items. This may result in challenging behavior if they cannot do so. The pragmatic use of the symbol must shift away from just requesting. Consider using tolerance for delay of reinforcement. Once the learner obtains the preferred item (e.g., coffee beans), identify a way to gain access to it appropriately (e.g., get a cup of coffee from an in-store coffee shop). Then, delay gaining access to the cup of coffee from the point of placing coffee beans in the cart.

See Chapter 5 for information about tolerance for delay.

Step 2: Choose a System to Store, Display, and Transport the Symbols/List to the Store

- Consider how the storage system is organized—group symbols by frequently used items placed together in the front, location of items in the stores' aisles, major food groups, and so forth.

- Store symbols in a small box (e.g., recipe box) or binder, ideally, in the kitchen area.

- Use hook and loop tape, magnet boards, or the refrigerator door to display the shopping list as it is created and to easily add and remove symbols. If necessary, transfer the symbols to a more portable device such as a small clipboard, binder, or wallet with a long fold-out section for transport to the store. Consider technology such as PDAs, cell phones, or a handheld SGD on which to create the list. These are easily portable, less cumbersome, and may be less stigmatizing as many people carry electronic gadgets with them in stores.

Step 3: Identify the Steps of Developing a Shopping List (as Well as Putting Away the Purchases)

Complete a task analysis of the steps for developing the shopping list, using the list while shopping, and putting away the groceries. To create the shopping list: 1) prompt the learner to obtain the corresponding symbol and add it to the list as items are used up, 2) schedule times to check for used-up items (e.g., keep used-up items in a designated location, the learner checks for empty containers), or 3) the learner creates a list with his or her symbols after someone else identifies needed items. Depending on how the list is developed, steps might include gaining access to symbol storage location, selecting symbols corresponding to empty products, and affixing symbols to the display device.

The learner will need to create the list when it is time to go shopping (and, if necessary, transfer symbols for transport to the store [e.g., wallet]), which may involve a series of substeps. Shopping also involves a series of steps. Once home, items need to be put away, the symbols from the list returned to their storage location, and the list returned to its display location. This is just a sample of the general steps involved in using a shopping list. The task analysis for each learner will reflect the unique needs of that learner and the specific materials and display involved.

See Chapter 5 for more information about task analysis and tolerance for delay.

Step 4: Develop Instructional Strategies

Assess learner competence with each step by using the task analysis created in Step 3. Use the information in Chapter 5 to choose instructional strategies.

Step 5: Use the Shopping List and Monitor Learner Performance

Monitor performance on a form such as the task analysis created in Step 3.

CASE STUDY

Shopping List

Julie, age 32, is learning to shop for groceries to increase her independence. Actual labels and line drawings of foods Julie ate on a weekly basis were housed in a recipe box next to the shopping list binder in the kitchen cabinet. Each page of the shopping binder as well as the pictures themselves had hook and loop tape for affixing the pictures to the binder. The binder was divided into sections according to the layout of the shopping store. A pocket in the back of the binder was designated to move the picture symbols once the actual items were placed in the shopping cart.

The evening before shopping, the interventionist taught Julie to take the needed symbols out of the recipe box and place them in her binder according to the layout of the store. If any items on the shopping list required a quantity greater than one, then they put that number next to the symbol in her binder as an additional reminder. The initial shopping list was limited to five items and gradually increased as Julie successfully created and used her shopping list.

Julie obtained her own cart and placed the shopping list binder in the front of the cart. Using her list, Julie obtained the item, placed it in her cart, removed the symbol from the list, and placed it in the back pocket, indicating that the item had been obtained. Julie tended to put more of an item in her cart than needed. If this happened, then the interventionist pointed to her book and presented a visual cue (e.g., holding up two fingers) to indicate how many of the same item to put in her cart. Julie independently obtained the necessary food items on her list in the right quantities after approximately 10 weekly shopping trips. Julie continued to require assistance putting the shopping list together in the correct order (according to the store's layout) each week, however.

VISUAL STORIES

Visual stories incorporate graphic symbols such as photographs and line drawings with written text in a book format that describes a situation in detail, focusing on social cues, events, and reactions that might occur and what the learner should do and why. Gray's (2004; Gray & Garand, 1993) Social Stories are one example of visual stories specifically designed to address the difficulties children with autism have in understanding and navigating social situations.

- The visual format may be consistent with many learners' strengths (in visual as opposed to auditory processing), providing a concrete, nontransient visual presentation.

- Visual stories involve repeated exposure to information a learner may not readily glean about specific situations.

- Visual stories provide a structure with rules that works well for learners who rely heavily on rules and routines (e.g., those with autism) (Sansosti & Powell-Smith, 2006).

As a result, visual stories may increase learner understanding of and engagement in appropriate behavior within a situation.

What Does the Research Say?
Visual Stories
Stories have been a component of intervention to decrease challenging behavior (e.g., Kuttler, Myles, & Carlson, 1998;

Reynhout & Carter, 2007) and increase social (Crozier & Tincani, 2007; Sansosti & Powell-Smith, 2006) and play behaviors (Barry & Burlew, 2004). Stories have been used to improve participation in lunchtime at school (Toplis & Hadwin, 2006) and novel situations (Ivey, Heflin, & Alberto, 2004). Barry and Burlew (2004) examined the use of a visual story (i.e., a social story based on Gray's Social Story guidelines) with two children (7 and 8 years old) with autism with little expressive language who required excessive prompting to choose a play activity and play appropriately during free time in their classroom. On a daily basis, just prior to free time, teachers read two stories with simple sentences and photographs of the children to the participants. Teachers continued to provide prompts to help the children choose a play activity and refer back to the story if they did not play appropriately, as well as provide praise for appropriate play. Following the introduction of the two stories, teachers introduced a third story, about sharing and playing with a peer, using a similar format and procedures. Participants' independent choice making and duration of time spent playing appropriately increased (though increases were greater for one participant than the other). The stories remained in the classroom for review each morning, but teachers decreased their prompts during free time.

Gray's (2004; Gray & Garand, 1993) Social Stories were originally described for learners with autism. Much of the research on stories involves children with autism (Ali & Frederickson, 2006), some with overlapping intellectual disability (e.g., Kuttler et al., 1998; Reynhout & Carter, 2007). Most studies show at least modest improvement for participants (Ali & Frederickson, 2006). Maintenance of gains is more inconsistent, and generalization across settings and partners has only recently been examined, with some positive results (Reynhout & Carter, 2007; Sansosti, Powell-Smith, & Kincaid, 2004). Much of the research on visual stories includes other intervention strategies (e.g., reinforcement contingencies), thus, the specific effects of the stories remains to be clearly determined. It also remains to be examined which components of stories (e.g., how and when the learner reviews the story, types of sentences) are necessary for behavior change (Ali & Frederickson, 2006; Sansosti et al., 2004).

The following procedures are partially based on Gray's (2004; Gray & Garand, 1993) Social Stories.

Steps for implementing visual stories

Step 1: Identify the situation about which to
write a story.
Step 2: Draft the story.
Step 3: Choose graphic symbols.
Step 4: Decide how the learner will review the
story.
Step 5: Review the story with the learner.
Step 6: Monitor learner performance in the
target situation.

Step 1: Identify the Situation About Which to Write a Story

Identify situations through consultation with the learner and/or relevant caregivers as well as through a functional behavioral assessment (see Chapter 1). Consider situations:

- In which the learner behaves inappropriately
- In which the learner does not participate at all
- That are completely new to the learner
- That reflect the learner's accomplishments

  For example, when Sam spent the afternoon at a friend's house, his mother created a visual story describing how much fun he had, what he and his friend had played, and how much Sam would enjoy visiting his friend's house again. Gray (2004) suggested 50% of Social Stories should reflect positive social situations.

☞ *Helpful Hint*

Interventionists can develop a visual story for a learner; however, a learner can also help create his or her own visual story, including identifying the situation, filling in parts of the story (e.g., from partially written sentences), and actually creating the entire story.

Step 2: Draft the Story

Write the story with an introduction, body, and conclusion, answering who, what, when, where, how, and why questions about the situation (Gray, 2004).

- Use the present tense.
- Phrase sentences in the positive; that is, what the learner should do, rather than not do, in a situation.
- Highlight relevant cues to help improve the learner's understanding of the situation.
- Use vocabulary within the learner's existing repertoire.
- Ask others who know the learner and situation to provide feedback on a draft of the story.
- Consider style. Repetition and rhyme may be appropriate and more interesting for younger children. A newspaper, pamphlet, or flier format may be more age appropriate and motivating for adolescent and adult learners.

Step 3: Choose Graphic Symbols

Use graphic symbols to augment the written text of the story to support the learner's understanding. Symbols should illustrate key words and/or concepts.

Consider video in conjunction with the story and/or displaying the story on a computer. Hagiwara and Myles (1999) created stories presented on a computer involving text read with synthesized speech and video of the participant's actions related to the story (see Hagiwara & Myles, 1999, for specific procedures for creating a story on the computer). Sansosti and Powell-Smith (2008) utilized a computer-based story presented within an automatically progressing PowerPoint slideshow that also included a video model of appropriate behaviors.

Step 4: Decide How the Learner Will Review the Story

- The learner reads the story him- or herself.
- The learner listens while an interventionist reads the story.
- The learner listens to an audio recording and follows along with the story. This could also be paired with music (espe-

cially if music is motivating to the learner) (Brownell, 2002).

- The learner views and listens to the story on video while following along.
- The learner listens while a peer reads the story. Peers can then prompt the learner within the target situation (e.g., reminding the learner, "Remember your story").

Step 5: Review the Story with the Learner

Review the story prior to the target activity; for example, at the beginning of the day for situations that arise throughout the learner's day (e.g., keeping hands to oneself) or at a specific point in time just before the situation (e.g., just before making a transition to the cafeteria). Place the story in a visible location within that situation (e.g., inside the learner's lunchbox). Learner comprehension should be assessed for at least the first review of the story.

Step 6: Monitor Learner Performance in the Target Situation

As the learner improves his or her participation in the target social situation, fade the visual story by decreasing the frequency with which it is reviewed or rewriting the story with select sentences omitted or partially omitted for the learner to "fill in." Even as the learner is successful, keep the story available to ensure maintenance of behavior change.

If the learner's participation within the target situation does not improve, then examine the content and visuals used in the story for accuracy. Did the learner demonstrate comprehension of the text (when questioned or during role play)? Have reinforcers been delivered contingent on the learner's successful participation in the target situation?

CASE STUDY

Visual Story

Joe is a 14-year-old student diagnosed with autism starting his first year of high school. He attends a general education class with 22 other students. In the first four assemblies of the school year, Joe shouted loudly and then walked out without permission and was sent to the vice principal. Joe had never before encountered such large and noisy assemblies (e.g., sports team pep rally accompanied by the high school band).

Joe's SLP drafted a story with feedback from Joe's parents and teachers to help Joe participate in assemblies. The visual story included information about why students go to assemblies (e.g., "Sometimes we go to an assembly to listen to someone speak."), expected assembly behaviors (e.g., "I will try to stay in my seat."), and things that might happen (e.g., "The band makes loud sounds with their instruments. This is okay.") with corresponding photographs from previous assemblies. Joe was expected to attend an assembly with the rest of his class, stay in his seat, sit quietly while the speaker was talking, and exit the assembly with the rest of his class. The story also included information about the ways he could be involved, such as clapping and cheering when he saw his peers doing the same. Joe's SLP recorded the story and uploaded the sound file onto Joe's iPod. Joe enjoyed the idea of listening to a story on his iPod; he and his parents referred to it as the assembly "podcast."

Joe reviewed the story during the week prior to an upcoming assembly by listening to the story while reading the text and looking at the accompanying photographs. Joe's parents also helped him at home by reviewing the story and asking him questions about the situation and what behaviors were required. Joe's parents faded the use of the text with pictures, just using the iPod prior to school assemblies. Eventually, Joe did not need to listen to the iPod prior to assemblies, his parents just reminded him in the morning that "today is an assembly 'podcast' day."

☞ *Helpful Hint*

Rule cards or rule scripts are more proscriptive directions about behavior that convey information about appropriate behaviors (e.g., "quiet hands," "all done") using graphic symbols (Mirenda, Mac-Gregor, & Kelly-Keough, 2002). Rule cards may depict a specific situation and the expected behaviors. **Contingency maps** are similar to rule cards; however, they also specifically illustrate the contingencies (i.e., antecedents and consequences) related to both the occurrence of problem behavior as well as more appropriate behavior (Brown & Mirenda, 2006). The rule card/contingency map can be referenced for reinforcement for appropriate rule following behavior and, if necessary, prompt more appropriate behavior.

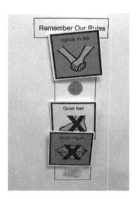

VISUALLY PRESENTED CHOICES

Choices involve selecting an item or activity from an array of options (two or more) that may or may not be explicitly presented. Many learners prefer situations in which they can make choices over situations in which the choices are made for them (Bannerman et al., 1990; von Mizener & Williams, 2009). Increasing choice-making opportunities improves engagement and performance and decreases challenging behavior (e.g., Dunlap et al., 1994; Dyer, Dunlap, & Winterling, 1990; Parsons, Reid, Reynolds, & Bumgarner, 1990; Watanabe & Sturmey, 2003).

Elicited choices are often presented verbally (e.g., the server lists the soups of the day), thus the learner must possess adequate speech comprehension to make a choice. The transient nature of speech means verbally represented choices also make significant memory demands (Beukelman & Mi-

renda, 2005). Self-initiated choices such as choosing a route home also rely on recall memory for the range of options. In contrast, choosing what to eat for dinner from the options in the refrigerator is a more visually based choice with lower memory requirements. Choices that require significant speech comprehension and recall memory may be more difficult than those supported by visual presentations. In fact, the choices learners make when options are only presented verbally may not reflect their true preferences (e.g., Vaughn & Horner, 1995).

Choice boards or choice menus (Hodgdon, 1995) provide a visual representation of the options available to a learner (e.g., a menu in a restaurant) so the options are no longer transient and the process is about recognition rather than recall. Visual choices support independence and may decrease challenging behavior as well as limit the infinite number of options that may be available, but are overwhelming or too numerous to recall; expand the variety of options presented to a learner; increase the likelihood of the learner choosing more varied options (rather than the same thing every time) by limiting and varying the options available; and communicate when an option is not available (the option is not on the board or crossed out).

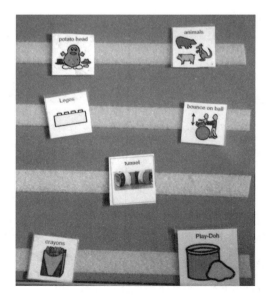

What Does the Research Say?
Choices

Vaughn and Horner (1995) compared verbally presented choices with the combination of visually and verbally presented choices during meals for an adult with autism. Visual choices were presented in three columns representing breakfast, lunch, or snack options. The choice display was always available, but interventionists changed options as they were available. The participant made choices when options were presented verbally, but often then refused (e.g., by throwing) the actual food items once prepared and offered. In contrast, when choice options were presented visually and verbally, the participant not only made a choice, but also increased his acceptance of the food item presented.

Visual presentation of choices is often applied along with other strategies. Dauphin et al. (2004) included a choice board for the learner to create his or her own visual schedule of activities. Barry and Burlew (2004) constructed a visual story about choosing play activities from a choice board.

Steps for implementing visually based choices

Step 1: Identify about what (and when and where) choices can be made.
Step 2: Identify the vocabulary and materials for the choice board.
Step 3: Create the choice board.
Step 4: Introduce the choice board and monitor learner performance.

Visually Based Choices

Use the following steps to create meaningful accessible ways for learners to make choices.

Step 1: Identify About What (and When and Where) Choices Can Be Made

Identify situations in which the learner might not already be making choices, but could and should (e.g., meals, leisure activities, clothing); the learner consistently picks the same option in a situation; some options are occasionally not available (not only would a choice board help to convey the lack of availability, but also alternative options).

Step 2: Identify the Vocabulary and Materials for the Choice Board

Conduct a preference assessment (see Chapter 5) to identify specific items to include on a choice board for a given topic and situation.

Step 3: Create the Choice Board

Begin with a few options on the choice board and gradually increase the number of options presented as the learner successfully makes choices. Presenting preferred options is the most natural choice format (Beukelman & Mirenda, 2005). If a learner consistently chooses and then rejects an option once it is provided, then consider a different format, such as presenting one preferred option with one nonpreferred option or one preferred option with a distractor (e.g., blank card) to first teach choice making.

If a goal is to encourage the learner to increase the variety of items chosen, then cover up or remove the choice once it is made (e.g., the computer is chosen as a leisure activity) to indicate that it is no longer available (until it reappears on the board). A NO symbol is a useful addition to indicate that a choice is not available (e.g., the playground on a rainy day).

Step 4: Introduce the Choice Board and Monitor Learner Performance

Identify the cue for the learner to consult his or her choice board. This could be the teacher's statement that it is free time (for choices of free time activities), a timer sounding, the completion of an activity in a learner's activity schedule (with the next page representing the learner's choices of reinforcers, the next activity). Place the choice board in an easily accessible and visible location near the situation about which choices are being made (e.g., on the refrigerator for food choices, on the wall as a child enters the play room) for self-initiated choice making. Present the choice board within the learner's line of sight along with a verbal offer (e.g., "What do you want?") for elicited choices. This might also be paired with a verbal and visual (e.g., through pointing or showing) review of the available options on the board.

The learner's choice response involves indicating an option (e.g., pointing to the symbol, moving the symbol on the board) and/or acting on an option (e.g., seeing the symbol for trains on the board and proceeding to take out the trains in the play area). Choose prompts to help learners select an option and/or act on it (e.g., prompting the learner from behind may increase independence).

Use natural consequences by providing the item chosen when a learner makes a choice, even if he or she chose "incorrectly" (e.g., chose a known nonpreferred item). Do not try error correction at this point as it may perpetuate the learner's incorrect choosing. Instead, provide natural consequences and then quickly provide another choice opportunity, adding prompts as necessary (Beukelman & Mirenda, 2005). Consider checking the accuracy of the learner's choice. Present the items (or symbols) for a choice. Once the learner selects one, present the other mode (i.e., symbols or items) to confirm the choice. If the learner selects the symbol (or item) that corresponds to the one initially chosen, then this indicates comprehension of the choice. If the learner chooses the other available option, then repeat the comprehension check and use prompting or error correction procedures to assist the learner in making the correct choice.

CASE STUDY

Choices

Sheri, a 7-year-old girl diagnosed with autism, communicated primarily using an SGD. Sheri's teacher was planning to begin game activities in which pairs of students choose a game (e.g., Candyland, Connect Four, Bingo) to play with each other and practice making choices, turn-taking, and counting during game playing. Sheri's teacher created a choice board with photographs of all the available games. She hung the board on the inside of the game closet. Her teacher began by presenting two pictures of available game options on the choice board.

At game time, Sheri and the teacher went to the closet, opened the door, and observed the choice board. Sheri's teacher prompted Sheri to point toward whichever game she wanted to play. The choice board presented limited options but also contained a wide array of potential options, which allowed Sheri's teacher to rotate the game options so each student, including Sheri, played different games. As Sheri independently chose from an array of two options, Sheri's teacher gradually increased the number of games from which to choose. Eventually, Sheri independently opened the closet door, chose a game picture, and gained access to the corresponding game.

SUMMARY

AAC is primarily used to provide an output mode for learners who do not have functional speech. AAC can also be used in the input mode, however, which facilitates comprehension of speech as well as specific situations and demands, helping learners function more independently and successfully.

REFERENCES

Ali, S., & Frederickson, N. (2006). Investigating the evidence base of social stories. *Educational Psychology in Practice, 22,* 355–377.

Anderson, M.D., Sherman, J.A., Sheldon, J.B., & McAdam, D. (1997). Picture activity schedules and engagement of adults with mental retardation in a group home. *Research in Developmental Disabilities, 18,* 231–250.

Bannerman, D.J., Sheldon, J.B., Sherman, J.A., & Harchik, A.E. (1990). Balancing the right to habilitation with the right to personal liberties: The rights of people with developmental disabilities to eat too many doughnuts and take a nap. *Journal of Applied Behavior Analysis, 239,* 79–89.

Barrera, R.D., Lobato-Barrera, D., & Sulzer-Azaroff, B. (1980). A simultaneous treatment comparison of three expressive language training programs with a mute autistic child. *Journal of Autism and Developmental Disabilities, 10,* 21–37.

Barry, L.M., & Burlew, S.B. (2004). Using social stories to teach choice and play skills to children with autism. *Focus on Autism and Other Developmental Disabilities, 19,* 45–51.

Berg, W.K., & Wacker, D.P. (1989). Evaluation of tactile prompts with a student who is deaf, blind, and mentally retarded. *Journal of Applied Behavior Analysis, 22,* 93–99.

Beukelman, D.R., & Mirenda, P. (2005). *Augmentative and alternative communication: Supporting children and adults with complex communication needs* (3rd ed.). Baltimore: Paul H. Brookes Publishing Co.

Bevill, A.R., Gast, D.L., Maguire, A.M., & Vail, C.O. (2001). Increasing engagement of preschoolers with disabilities through correspondence training and picture cues. *Journal of Early Intervention, 24,* 129–145.

Blischak, D.M. (1999). Increases in natural speech production following experience with synthetic speech. *Journal of Special Education Technology, 14,* 44–53.

Brady, N.C. (2000). Improved comprehension of object names following voice output communication aid use: Two case studies. *Augmentative and Alternative Communication, 16,* 197–204.

Brown, F. (1991). Creative daily scheduling: A nonintrusive approach to challenging behaviors in community residences. *Journal of The Association for Persons with Severe Handicaps, 16,* 75–84.

Brown, K.E., & Mirenda, P. (2006). Contingency mapping: Use of a novel visual support strategy as an adjunct to functional equivalence training. *Journal of Positive Behavior Interventions, 8,* 155–164.

Brownell, M.D. (2002). Musically adapted social stories to modify behaviors in students with autism: Four case studies. *Journal of Music Therapy, 39,* 117–144.

Bruno, J., & Trembath, D. (2006). Use of aided language stimulation to improve syntactic performance during a weeklong intervention program. *Augmentative and Alternative Communication, 22,* 300–313.

Byrne, A., Buckley, S., MacDonald, J., & Bird, G. (1995). Investigating the literacy, language, and memory skills of children with Down's syndrome. *Down Syndrome: Research and Practice, 3,* 53–58.

Cafiero, J.M. (2001). The effect of an augmentative communication intervention on the communication, behavior, and academic program of an adolescent with autism. *Focus on Autism and Other Developmental Disabilities, 16,* 179–189.

Carr, E.G., Binkoff, J.A., Kologinsky, E., & Eddy, M. (1978). Acquisition of sign language by autistic children: I: Expressive labeling. *Journal of Applied Behavior Analysis, 11,* 489–501.

Carr, E.G., & Dores, P.A. (1981). Patterns of language acquisition following simultaneous communication with autistic children. *Analysis and Intervention in Developmental Disabilities, 1,* 347–361.

Clarke, S., Remington, B., & Light, P. (1986). An evaluation of the relationship between receptive speech skills and expressive signing. *Journal of Applied Behavior Analysis, 19,* 231–239.

Clarke, S., Remington, B., & Light, P. (1988). The role of referential speech in sign learning by mentally retarded children: A comparison of total communication and sign-alone training. *Journal of Applied Behavior Analysis, 21,* 419–426.

Copeland, S.R., & Hughes, C. (2000). Acquisition of a picture prompt strategy to increase independent performance. *Education and Training in Mental Retardation and Developmental Disabilities, 35,* 294–305.

Crozier, S., & Tincani, M. (2007). Effects of social stories on prosocial behavior of preschool children with autism spectrum disorders. *Journal of Autism and Developmental Disabilities, 37,* 1803–1814.

Dauphin, M., Kinney, E.M., & Stromer, R. (2004). Using video-enhanced activity schedules and matrix training to teach sociodramatic play to a child with autism. *Journal of Positive Behavior Interventions, 6,* 238–250.

Davies, D.K., Stock, S.E., & Wehmeyer, M.L. (2002a). Enhancing independent task performance for individuals with mental retardation through the use of a handheld self-directed visual and audio prompting system. *Education and Training in Mental Retardation and Developmental Disabilities, 37,* 209–218.

Davies, D.K., Stock, S.E., & Wehmeyer, M.L. (2002b). Enhancing independent time-management skills of individuals with mental retardation using a palmtop personal computer. *Mental Retardation, 40,* 358–365.

Dettmer, S., Simpson, R.L., Smith Myles, B., & Ganz, J.B. (2000). The use of visual supports to facilitate transitions of students with autism. *Focus on Autism and Other Developmental Disabilities, 15,* 163–169.

Dooley, P., Wilczenski, F.L., & Torem, C. (2001). Using an activity schedule to smooth school transitions. *Journal of Positive Behavior Interventions, 3,* 57–61.

Drager, K.D.R., Postal, V.J., Carrolus, L., Castellano, M., Gagliano, C., & Glynn, J. (2006). The effect of aided language modeling on symbol comprehension and production in two preschoolers with autism. *American Journal of Speech-Language Pathology, 15,* 112–125.

Dunlap, G., DePerczel, M., Clarke, S., Wilson, D., Wright, S., White, R., & Gomez, A. (1994). Choice making to promote adaptive behavior for students with emotional and behavioral challenges. *Journal of Applied Behavior Analysis, 279,* 505–518.

Dunlap, G., & Fox, L. (1999). A demonstration of behavioral support for young children with autism. *Journal of Positive Behavior Interventions, 1,* 77–87.

Dyer, K., Dunlap, G., & Winterling, V. (1990). Effects of choice making on the serious problem behaviors of students with severe handicaps. *Journal of Applied Behavior Analysis, 239,* 515–524.

Earles-Vollrath, T.L., Cook, K.T., & Ganz, J.B. (2006). *PRO-ED series on autism spectrum disorders: How to develop and implement visual supports.* Austin, TX: PRO-ED.

Fenson, L., Dale, P.S., Reznick, J.S., Bates, E., Thal, D.J., & Pethick, S.J. (1994). Variability in early communicative development. *Monographs of the Society for Research in Child Development, 59* (5, Serial No. 242).

Fidler, D.J. (2005). The emerging Down syndrome behavioral phenotype in early childhood: Implications for practice. *Infants and Young Children, 18,* 86–103.

Ganz, J.B. (2007). Classroom structuring methods and strategies for children and youth with autism spectrum disorders. *Exceptionality, 15,* 249–260.

Ganz, J.B., Cook, K.T., & Earles-Vollrath, T.L. (2006). *PRO-ED series on autism spectrum disorders: How to write and implement social scripts.* Austin, TX: PRO-ED.

Goossens', C. (1989). Aided communication intervention before assessment: A case study of a child with cerebral palsy. *Augmentative and Alternative Communication, 5,* 14–26.

Grandin, T. (1995). The learning style of people with autism: An autobiography. In K.A. Quill (Ed.), *Teaching children with autism: Strategies to enhance communication and socialization* (pp. 33–52). New York: Delmar Publishers.

Gray, C. (2004). Social Stories 10.0: The new defining criteria and guidelines. *Jenison Autism Journal: Creative Ideas in Practice, 15,* 2–21.

Gray, C., & Garand, J.D. (1993). Social stories: Improve responses of students with autism with accurate social information. *Focus on Autistic Behavior, 8,* 1–10.

Hagiwara, T., & Myles, B.S. (1999). A multimedia social story intervention: Teaching skills to children with autism. *Focus on Autism and Other Developmental Disabilities, 14,* 82–95.

Harris, M.D., & Reichle, J. (2004). The impact of aided language stimulation on symbol com-

prehension and production in children with moderate cognitive disabilities. *American Journal of Speech-Language Pathology, 13,* 155–167.

Heller, K.W., Alberto, P.A., & Romski, M.A. (1995). Effect of object and movement cues on receptive communication by preschool children with mental retardation. *American Journal on Mental Retardation, 99,* 510–521.

Hirsh-Pasek, K., & Golinkoff, R.M. (1991). Language comprehension: A new look at some old themes. In N.A. Krasnegor, D.M. Rumbaugh, R.L. Schiefelbusch, & M. Studdert-Kennedy (Eds.), *Biological and behavioral determinants of language development* (pp. 301–320). Mahwah, NJ: Lawrence Erlbaum Associates.

Hodgdon, L.A. (1995). *Visual strategies for improving communication: Vol. 1: Practical supports for school and home.* Troy, MI: Quirk Roberts Publishing.

Huttenlocher, J., Haight, W., Bryk, A., Seltzer, M., & Lyons, T. (1991). Early vocabulary growth: Relation to language input and gender. *Developmental Psychology, 27,* 1236–1248.

Irvine, A.B., Erickson, A.M., Singer, G.H.S., & Stahlberg, D. (1992). A coordinated program to transfer self-management skills from school to home. *Education and Training in Mental Retardation, 27,* 241–254.

Ivey, M.L., Heflin, L.J., & Alberto, P. (2004). The use of social stories to promote independent behaviors in novel events for children with PDD-NOS. *Focus on Autism and Other Developmental Disabilities, 19,* 164–176.

Jarrold, C., Baddeley, A.D., & Phillips, C.E. (2002). Verbal short-term memory in Down syndrome: A problem of memory, audition, or speech? *Journal of Speech, Language, and Hearing Research, 45,* 531–544.

Kimball, J.W., Kinney, E.M., Taylor, B.A., & Stromer, R. (2004). Video enhanced activity schedules for children with autism: A promising package for teaching social skills. *Education and Treatment of Children, 27,* 280–298.

Kouri, T.A. (1988). Effects of simultaneous communication in a child-directed treatment approach with preschoolers with severe disabilities. *Augmentative and Alternative Communication, 4,* 222–232.

Kouri, T. (1989). How manual sign acquisition relates to the development of spoken language: A case study. *Language, Speech, and Hearing Services in Schools, 20,* 50–62.

Kuttler, S., Myles, B.S., & Carlson, J.K. (1998). The use of social stories to reduce precursors to tantrum behavior in a student with autism. *Focus on Autism and Other Developmental Disabilities, 13,* 176–182.

Lancioni, G.E., O'Reilly, M.E., Speedhouse, P., Furniss, F., & Cunha, B. (2000). Promoting independent task performance by persons with severe developmental disabilities through a new computer-aided system. *Behavior Modification, 24,* 700–718.

Layton, T.L. (1988). Language training with autistic children using four different modes of presentation. *Journal of Communication Disorders, 21,* 333–350.

Lincoln, A.J., Dickstein, P., Courchesne, E., Elmasian, R., & Tallal, P. (1992). Auditory processing abilities in non-retarded adolescents and young adults with developmental receptive language disorder and autism. *Brain and Language, 43,* 613–622.

MacDuff, G.S., Krantz, P.J., & McClannahan, L.E. (1993). Teaching children with autism to use photographic activity schedules: Maintenance and generalization of complex response chains. *Journal of Applied Behavior Analysis, 26,* 89–97.

Marshall, J.K., & Mirenda, P. (2002). Parent–professional collaboration for positive behavior support in the home. *Focus on Autism and Other Developmental Disabilities, 17,* 216–228.

Martin, J.E., Elias-Burger, S., & Mithaug, D.E. (1987). Acquisition and maintenance of time-based task change sequence. *Education and Training in Mental Retardation, 22,* 250–255.

Martin, J.E., Mithaug, D.E., & Frazier, E.S. (1992). Effects of picture referencing on PVC chair, love seat, and settee assemblies by students with mental retardation. *Research in Developmental Disabilities, 13,* 267–286.

Mayer-Johnson, R. (1992). *The Picture Communication Symbol.* Solana Beach, CA: Mayer-Johnson.

McClannahan, L.E., & Krantz, P.J. (1999). *Topics in autism: Activity schedules for children with autism: Teaching independent behavior.* Bethesda, MD: Woodbine House.

Mechling, L.C., & Gast, D.L. (1997). Combination audio/visual self-prompting system for teaching chained tasks to students with intellectual disabilities. *Education and Training in Mental Retardation and Developmental Disabilities, 32,* 138–153.

Miller, J.F., Chapman, R.S., Branston, M.B., & Reichle, J. (1980). Language comprehension in sensorimotor stages V and VI. *Journal of Speech and Hearing Research, 23,* 284–311.

Mirenda, P. (2003). Toward functional augmentative and alternative communication for students with autism: Manual signs, graphic symbols, and voice output communication aids. *Language, Speech, and Hearing Services in Schools, 34,* 203–216.

Mirenda, P., & Brown, K.E. (2009). A picture is worth a thousand words: Using visual supports for augmented input with individuals with autism spectrum disorders. In J. Light & D.R. Beukelman (Series Eds.) & P. Mirenda & T. Iacono (Vol. Eds.), *AAC series: Autism spectrum disorders and AAC* (pp. 303–332). Baltimore: Paul H. Brookes Publishing Co.

Mirenda, P., MacGregor, T., & Kelly-Keough, S. (2002). Teaching communication skills for behavioral support in the context of family life. In J.M. Lucyshyn, G. Dunlap, & R.W. Albin (Eds.), *Families and positive behavior support: Addressing problem behavior in family contexts* (pp. 185–207). Baltimore: Paul H. Brookes Publishing Co.

Morrison, R.S., Sainato, D.M., Benchaaban, D., & Endo, S. (2002). Increasing play skills of children with autism using activity schedules and correspondence training. *Journal of Early Intervention, 25,* 58–72.

Morse, T.E., & Schuster, J.W. (2000). Teaching elementary students with moderate intellectual disabilities how to shop for groceries. *Exceptional Children, 66,* 273–288.

Myles, B.S., Ferguson, H., & Hagiwara, T. (2007). Using a personal digital assistant to improve the recording of homework assignments by an adolescent with Asperger syndrome. *Focus on Autism and Other Developmental Disabilities, 22,* 96–99.

Newman, B., Buffington, D.M., O'Grady, M.A., McDonald, M.E., Poulson, C., & Hemmes, N.S. (1995). Self-management of schedule following in three teenagers with autism. *Behavioral Disorders, 20,* 190–196.

Parsons, M.B., Reid, D.H., Reynolds, J., & Bumgarner, M. (1990). Effects of chosen versus assigned jobs on the work performance of persons with severe handicaps. *Journal of Applied Behavior Analysis, 23,* 253–258.

Peterson, S.L., Bondy, A.S., Vincent, Y., & Finnegan, C.S. (1995). Effects of altering communicative input for students with autism and no speech: Two case studies. *Augmentative and Alternative Communication, 11,* 93–100.

Pierce, K.L., & Schreibman, L. (1994). Teaching daily living skills to children with autism in unsupervised settings through pictorial self-management. *Journal of Applied Behavior Analysis, 27,* 471–481.

Quill, K. (1995). Visually cued instruction for children with autism and pervasive developmental disorders. *Focus on Autistic Behavior, 10,* 10–20.

Rehfeldt, R.A., Kinney, E.M., Root, S., & Stromer, R. (2004). Creating activity schedules using Microsoft PowerPoint. *Journal of Applied Behavior Analysis, 37,* 115–128.

Remington, B., & Clarke, S. (1983). Acquisition of expressive signing by autistic children: An evaluation of the relative effects of simultaneous communication and sign-alone training. *Journal of Applied Behavior Analysis, 16,* 315–328.

Remington, B., & Clarke, S. (1993). Simultaneous communication and speech comprehension: Part I: Comparison of two methods of teaching expressive signing and speech comprehension skills. *Augmentative and Alternative Communication, 9,* 36–48.

Reynhout, G., & Carter, M. (2007). Social Story efficacy with a child with autism spectrum disorder and moderate intellectual disability. *Focus on Autism and Other Developmental Disabilities, 22,* 173–182.

Robinson-Wilson, M.A. (1977). Picture recipe cards as an approach to teach severely and profoundly retarded adults to cook. *Education and Training of the Mentally Retarded, 12,* 69–73.

Romski, M.A., & Sevcik, R.A. (1991). Patterns of language learning by instruction: Evidence from nonspeaking persons with mental retardation. In N.A. Krasnegor, D.M. Rumbaugh, R.L. Schiefelbusch, & M. Studdert-Kennedy (Eds.), *Biological and behavioral determinants of language development* (pp. 429–445). Mahwah, NJ: Lawrence Erlbaum Associates.

Romski, M.A., & Sevcik, R.A. (1993a). Language comprehension: Considerations for augmentative and alterative communication. *Augmentative and Alternative Communication, 9,* 281–285.

Romski, M.A., & Sevcik, R.A. (1993b). Language learning through augmented means: The process and its products. In J. Reichle & M.E. Fey (Series Eds.) & A.P. Kaiser, & D.B. Gray (Vol. Eds.), *Communication and language intervention series: Vol. 2. Enhancing children's communication: Research foundations for intervention* (pp. 85–104). Baltimore: Paul H. Brookes Publishing Co.

Romski, M.A., & Sevcik, R.A. (1996). *Breaking the speech barrier: Language development through augmented means.* Baltimore: Paul H. Brookes Publishing Co.

Romski, M.A., Sevcik, R.A., Robinson, B., & Bakeman, R. (1994). Adult-directed communications of youth with mental retardation using the system for augmenting language. *Journal of Speech and Hearing Research, 37,* 617–628.

Romski, M.A., Sevcik, R.A., Robinson, B., Mervis, C.B., & Bertrand, J. (1995). Mapping the meanings of novel visual symbols by youth with moderate or severe mental retardation. *American Journal on Mental Retardation, 100,* 391–402.

Romski, M.A., Sevcik, R.A., & Wilkinson, K.M. (1994). Peer-directed communicative interactions of augmented language learners with mental retardation. *American Journal on Mental Retardation, 98,* 527–538.

Sansosti, F.J., & Powell-Smith, K.A. (2006). Using social stories to improve the social behavior of children with Asperger syndrome. *Journal of Positive Behavior Interventions, 8,* 43–57.

Sansosti, F.J., & Powell-Smith, K.A. (2008). Using computer-presented social stories and video models to increase the social communication skills of children with high-functioning autism spectrum disorders. *Journal of Positive Behavior Interventions, 10,* 162–178.

Sansosti, F.J., Powell-Smith, K.A., & Kincaid, D. (2004). A research synthesis of social story interventions for children with autism spectrum disorders. *Focus on Autism and Other Developmental Disabilities, 19,* 194–204.

Sarber, R.E., Halasz, M.M., Messmer, M.C., Bickett, A.D., & Lutzker, J.R. (1983). Teaching menu planning and shopping skills to a mentally retarded mother. *Mental Retardation, 21,* 101–106.

Schlosser, R.W., Belfiore, P.J., Nigam, R., Blischak, D., & Hetzroni, O. (1995). The effects of speech output technology in the learning of graphic symbols. *Journal of Applied Behavior Analysis, 28,* 537–549.

Schopler, E., Mesibov, G.B., & Hearsey, K. (1995). Structured teaching in the TEACCH system. In E. Schopler & G.B. Mesibov (Eds.), *Learning and cognition in autism* (pp. 243–268). New York: Plenum Press.

Sevcik, R.A., & Romski, M.A. (2002). Patterns of language development through augmented means in youth with mental retardation. In D.L. Molfese & V.J. Molfese (Eds.), *Developmental variations in learning: Applications to social, executive function, language, and reading skills* (pp. 257–274). Mahwah, NJ: Lawrence Erlbaum Associates.

Sevcik, R.A., & Romski, M.A. (2005). Early visual-graphic symbol acquisition by children with developmental disabilities. In L.L. Namy (Ed.), *Symbol use and symbolic representation: Developmental and comparative perspectives* (pp. 155–170). Mahwah, NJ: Lawrence Erlbaum Associates.

Sevcik, R.A., Romski, M.A., & Adamson, L.B. (2004). Research directions in augmentative and alternative communication for preschool children. *Disability and Rehabilitation, 26,* 1323–1329.

Sevcik, R.A., Romski, M.A., Watkins, R.V., & Deffebach, K.P. (1995). Adult partner-augmented communication input to youth with mental retardation using the system for augmenting language (SAL). *Journal of Speech and Hearing Research, 38,* 909–912.

Sigafoos, J., Didden, R., & O'Reilly, M. (2003). Effects of speech output on maintenance of requesting and frequency of vocalizations in three children with developmental disabilities. *Augmentative and Alternative Communication, 19,* 37–47.

Stromer, R., Kimball, J.W., Kinney, E.M., & Taylor, B.A. (2006). Activity schedules, computer technology, and teaching children with autism spectrum disorders. *Focus on Autism and Other Developmental Disabilities, 21,* 14–24.

Taylor, R.G. (1987). Teaching a severely handicapped deaf-blind young woman to prepare breakfast foods. *Journal of Visual Impairment and Blindness, 81,* 67–69.

Toplis, R., & Hadwin, J.A. (2006). Using social stories to change problematic lunchtime behaviour in school. *Educational Psychology in Practice, 22,* 53–67.

Vaughn, B., & Horner, R.H. (1995). Effects of concrete versus verbal choice systems on problem behavior. *Augmentative and Alternative Communication, 11,* 89–92.

von Mizener, B.H., & Williams, R.L. (2009). The effects of student choices on academic performance. *Journal of Positive Behavior Interventions, 11,* 110–128.

Watanabe, M., & Sturmey, P. (2003). The effect of choice-making opportunities during activity schedules on task engagement of adults with autism. *Journal of Autism and Developmental Disorders, 33,* 535–538.

Wilkinson, K.M., Romski, M.A., & Sevcik, R.A. (1994). Emergence of visual-graphic symbol combinations by youth with moderate or severe mental retardation. *Journal of Speech and Hearing Research, 37,* 883–895

Wood, L.A., Lasker, J., Siegel-Causey, E., Beukelman, D.R., & Ball, L. (1998). Input framework for augmentative and alternative communication. *Augmentative and Alternative Communication, 14,* 261–267.

The Use of Augmentative Strategies to Enhance Communication of Verbal Mode Users

Kathleen M. Feeley and Emily A. Jones

▷ CHAPTER OVERVIEW

Many learners with severe disabilities use speech as their primary mode of communication. Their speech may not always be intelligible, however; that is, the spoken utterance is not clear enough for the listener to know what it is the learner is communicating. Learners with disabilities that influence expressive communication production are particularly at risk for problems with intelligibility (Hustad, Auker, Natale, & Carlson, 2003; Kumin, 1994; Rosin, Swift, Bless, & Vetter, 1988). Augmentative and alternative communication (AAC) can facilitate productive communication by providing another mode with which to communicate a message (see Chapter 2).

▷ CHAPTER OBJECTIVES

After studying this chapter, readers will be able to

- Define *intelligibility* and *comprehensibility*
- Identify factors that affect intelligibility
- Assess intelligibility
- Use a multimodal approach to enhance intelligibility/comprehensibility

▷ KEY TERMS

- ▶ alphabet supplementation
- ▶ articulation
- ▶ communicative breakdown
- ▶ comprehensibility
- ▶ dysarthria
- ▶ intelligibility
- ▶ natural communicative gestures
- ▶ topic supplementation

INTELLIGIBILITY AND COMPREHENSIBILITY

Intelligibility and **comprehensibility** have been used to refer to the extent to which a communicative message is received by the listener, but they refer to different aspects of the communicative interaction. Dowden (1997) and Yorkston, Strand, and Kennedy (1996) describe intelligibility as a characteristic of the speech signal. Intelligibility is affected by intrinsic factors or signal dependent information, including **articulation,** rate of speech, length of utterance, and so forth. Intelligibility is often measured by having listeners transcribe spoken words or imitate a speech model. Sometimes, intelligibility is assessed by asking the listener to choose among a small group of potential target stimuli, one of which matches what the speaker communicated. Perceived intelligibility refers to a combination of the intrinsic factors associated with the speech signal as well as a host of contextual variables that may influence the listener's ability to discriminate the speech signal from others.

Comprehensibility refers to a listener's understanding of the speaker's utterance (Yorkston et al., 1996). Comprehensibility can be affected by both intrinsic factors as well as extrinsic factors such as environmental conditions and characteristics of the listener (e.g., knowledge of the topic, familiarity with the speaker) that, although they do not directly affect the speech of the speaker, affect the extent to which the listener is able to understand the message (Dowden, 1997). Comprehensibility is measured by the listener's ability to act on the speaker's communication (e.g., following directions, answering questions) (Drager, Reichle, & Pinkoski, 2010). Thus, comprehensibility is a measure of the extent to which the listener is able to gain meaning from the speaker's message, rather than just being able to transcribe or repeat the message. If the speaker says "What did you do last night?" and the listener responds by saying, "Last night, I went to the movies," then it is clear that the message was comprehended. The message was also intelligible, as otherwise the listener would not have been able to formulate a response.

Factors that Influence Perceived Intelligibility and Comprehensibility

Numerous variables influence intelligibility (actual and perceived) and comprehensibility, each of which can be the focus of strategies to improve intelligibility.

Competence of the Speaker

Many skills that a speaker may have, or can be taught, will enhance his or her ability to communicate messages to listeners. For example, using gestures or graphic symbols can assist in providing context for spoken utterances. Specifically, the topic of the conversation can be identified.

What Does the Research Say?
Gestures, Intelligibility, and Comprehensibility

Research generally shows positive effects of pairing gestures with speech on intelligibility. Garcia and Cannito (1996b) examined the intelligibility of an adult speaker with severe **dysarthria** who produced the same set of sentences with and without scripted gestures. Comprehensibility increased approximately 25% when gestures were used.

In a study examining natural use of gestures, Garcia, Crowe, Redler, and Hustad (2004) recorded a 12-year-old male with severe dysarthria producing several monologues of his own choosing with the spontaneous and natural gestures he added. The young man was part of an intervention program that included focusing on increasing his use of gestures to augment speech. Adding gestures significantly improved intelligibility scores (listener transcription of words) as well as comprehensibility (listener responses to questions about the monologue).

Hustad and Garcia (2005) examined the influence of gesture use and **alphabet supplementation** on the intelligibility of three adults with severe dysarthria secondary to cerebral palsy. In alphabet supplementation, the speaker specifically identifies the first letter of each word he or she is speaking by indicating the letter on an alphabet display. (Alphabet supplementation is described later in this chapter.) Speakers produced sentences using scripted hand gestures, alphabet supplementation, or neither cue. Both gesture use and alphabet supplementation resulted in significantly higher intelligibility scores than no cues. Two speakers showed no difference between alphabet supplementation and gesture use, consistent with other findings (Hustad & Garcia, 2002). Intelligibility was better with alphabet supplementation than gestures for one participant. Providing supplemental information, gestures, and alphabet supplementation may also result in slower speech and, as a result, improve intelligibility.

There is a wide range of material that can be used to supplement conversation.

What Does the Research Say?

Topic Supplementation

A number of studies examine **topic supplementation** in combination with and/or in comparison with alphabet supplementation. Using alphabet supplementation resulted in greater improvements in intelligibility than topic supplementation in a number of these studies. Their combined use often improves intelligibility even further (Hustad, Jones, & Dailey, 2003); however, there are some studies in which there is no advantage of the combined cues over alphabet supplementation alone (e.g., Hustad, Auker, et al., 2003).

Some supplementation provides information that may be related to the topic in general (e.g., providing "clothing" as a word class when speaking about "pants"). Beliveau, Hodge, and Hagler (1995) and Hustad and Beukelman (2001) found that adding topic information improved intelligibility for adults with dysarthria. Beliveau et al. showed that although alphabet supplementation also improved intelligibility, the combination of alphabet and topic supplementation (word class information) resulted in greater increases in intelligibility. Hustad and Beukelman reported that the combination of alphabet and topic supplementation cues resulted in the highest level of intelligibility for the four speakers with severe dysarthria secondary to cerebral palsy.

Gestures can be particularly helpful when a speaker can also take advantage of stimuli in the environment to provide even more information to the listener. For example, when speaking about something in the room, the speaker may draw the listener's attention to it (e.g., by moving toward it, pointing to it) as a means of informing the listener about what he or she is speaking. Adjusting the speech volume and rate can also influence intelligibility. Finally, using repair strategies that involve repeating or modifying communication acts following a breakdown in communication (i.e., when the listener has not understood what the speaker said) can improve intelligibility across speaking turns.

Repairing communication breakdowns is discussed in Chapter 11.

Characteristics of the Spoken Message

Linguistic redundancy increases the intelligibility and, in some instances, comprehensibility of an utterance. For example, sequences of topically related sentences forming a narrative tend to be better understood than single words spoken by individuals with mild dysarthria (Beukelman & Yorkston, 1979). Alternatively, linguistic redundancy can refer to the extent to which there are multiple words in an utterance that complement each other's meaning; for example, "I'm hungry. Let's eat." Intelligibility improves with longer utterances, even for synthesized speech (Drager, Clarke-Serpentine, Johnson, & Roeser, 2006; Mirenda & Beukelman, 1987, 1990).

Unfortunately, too often, many individuals with significant developmental disabilities have a relatively small vocabulary of different words that can be applied to the same topic and also have modest linguistic redundancy because of their limitations in producing multiple-word spoken utterances.

What Does the Research Say?

Characteristics of the Spoken Message and Intelligibility

Garcia and Cannito (1996a) and Garcia and Dagenais (1998) reported that contextually related utterances were more intelligible than unrelated utterances. Linguistic redundancy has also been shown to improve intelligibility in noise (Duffy & Giolas, 1974; Salasoo & Pisoni, 1985). Hustad and Garcia (2002) also found that highly predictive sentences were more intelligible than less predictive sentences. Hammen, Yorkston, and Dowden (1991) demonstrated that intelligibility increased with semantic context for 21 individuals with moderate, severe, and profound dysarthria. Hustad (2007a) reported that listeners of adults with mild to severe dysarthria who transcribed sentences with superimposed information about the first letter of the words the individual was speaking had improved intelligibility compared with a condition with no alphabet information.

Semantic class (e.g., modifiers, content words) is another factor that can directly affect intelligibility. Hustad (2006) found that modifiers (adjectives and adverbs) and

(continued)

content words (nouns, pronouns, and verbs) were less intelligible than function words (articles, prepositions, and conjunctions) when listening to speakers with moderate, severe, and profound dysarthria. Function words may be easier for the speaker to produce as they are often single syllables and consist of consonant-vowels or vowel-consonants. Function words are also highly predictable within sentences. In contrast, content words and modifiers tend to be more complex and less predictable (also see Hustad, Dardis, & McCourt, 2007).

Hustad (2007b) compared intelligibility for single words, unrelated sentences, and topically related sentences creating a narrative for speakers with dysarthria. Intelligibility scores were higher for narratives than single words or unrelated sentences. Sentences were more intelligible than single words, and unrelated sentences were more intelligible than single words when listening to learners with mild and severe dysarthria. Narratives were more intelligible than sentences or words for those listening to learners with moderate dysarthria, but no difference emerged between sentences and words. There were no significant differences in listening to words, sentences, or narratives for learners with profound dysarthria. Hustad's (2007a) findings highlight the need to consider unique learner characteristics in examining how characteristics of the spoken message affects intelligibility.

Characteristics of the Environment

The environment in which communicative interactions take place can greatly influence intelligibility.

- *Noise level*: The physical setting can enhance or detract from speech intelligibility as the message may be more difficult for listeners to hear. Background noise also negatively affects the intelligibility of synthesized speech (Koul & Allen, 1993).

- *Extent to which the learner is in view*: Simply seeing the speaker while he or she talks improves intelligibility (Hubbard & Kushner, 1980; Hustad et al., 2007; Monsen, 1983). In addition, situations in which the listener's view of the learner is interrupted (e.g., people walking by, while driving a car) can negatively affect receipt of the message (Yorkston, Bombardier, & Hammen, 1994).

Characteristics of the Listener

Listeners bring their own experiences/knowledge about communicative interactions that influence the extent to which communicative utterances are perceived as intelligible (Lindblom, 1990). Even the listener's age may influence intelligibility (Drager et al., 2010).

- *Familiarity with the topic of communication*: Listener familiarity with the topic enhances intelligibility.

- *Familiarity with the speaker's speech/communication system*: Repeated exposure to the speech of individuals with dysarthria (Tjaden & Liss, 1995) as well as to synthesized speech (McNaughton, Fallon, Tod, Weiner, & Neisworth, 1994) can result in increased intelligibility.

- *Motivation to communicate with the speaker*: Partner motivation and patience (Dowden, 1997) with the speaker can influence intelligibility. When a listener is motivated to understand the speaker, the listener may take actions such as positioning him- or herself closer to the speaker, focusing on the speaker while he or she is communicating, and ignoring distracting stimuli (e.g., not gazing past the speaker to view an interaction on the other side of the room) to increase the likelihood he or she will understand the message.

See Chapter 11 for information about teaching learners to introduce their AAC system to a communication partner.

What Does the Research Say?
Partner Familiarity with the Speaker's Communication System

Monsen (1983) compared experienced listeners who had day-to-day contact with talkers with hearing impairments to inexperienced listeners who may have heard someone with a hearing impairment speak, but not regularly. Lis-
(continued)

tener experience improved intelligibility, especially for the more unintelligible speakers and for more complex sentences. Tjaden and Liss (1995) found that a listener's familiarization with a speaker with dysarthria resulted in higher levels of intelligibility, which is consistent with others' findings (DePaul & Kent, 2000; Hustad & Cahill, 2003). Garcia and Cannito (1996a) familiarized listeners by exposing them to a sample of the speaker's speech prior to the test condition to evaluate intelligibility. They found differences in intelligibility across listener familiarity with the speaker.

ASSESSING INTELLIGIBILITY

Assessing speech intelligibility of an individual with severe disabilities will determine the extent to which the acoustic signal alone (i.e., the speech itself) is intelligible to listeners. Consider James, who works in the library at his local community college. His ability to effectively communicate with new co-workers/patrons (who will be less familiar with his speech) is important. A speech intelligibility assessment provides a baseline that will permit an evaluation of the effect that the addition of context or modifications to speech may improve intelligibility.

Using Evidence-Based Strategies to Assess Intelligibility

It is important to examine intelligibility using a systematic procedure. Below are steps that

Steps for assessing intelligibility

Step 1: Identify relevant questions or comments to which the speaker should respond.

Step 2: Identify relevant utterances the speaker can use to initiate an interaction

Step 3: Videotape the speaker communicating in the absence and presence of contextual cues.

Step 4: Have both familiar and unfamiliar partners listen to and write down what they perceive the speaker said.

Step 5: Determine the extent to which the speaker is intelligible from the listener's perspective.

will help ensure that the interventionist systematically examines intelligibility.

Step 1: Identify Relevant Questions or Comments to Which the Speaker Should Respond

The speaker's speech will be assessed responding to questions posed by the listener as well as when he or she produces spontaneous speech during interactions with the listener (see Step 2). Questions to assess a speaker's responses should be chosen that 1) are understood by the speaker (i.e., he or she will be able to respond appropriately) and 2) partners would typically pose to a speaker. The following sample questions are listed under the environment in which they might be relevant.

- *At home*: What did you do today? How was your field trip? What do you want for dinner?

- *At school*: What game do you want to play? What did you do this weekend? What did you do in physical education today?

- *In the community for younger children*: What's your name? What school do you go to? What's your teacher's name?

- *In the community for adults/adolescents*: How are you today? How can I help you? What are you looking for?

- *At work*: How was your weekend? What are you doing tonight? Where do you want to go to lunch?

It is also important to consider other specific environments the learner frequents (e.g., particular restaurants or stores, religious services) that may have predictable communicative phrases that occur during interactions that should be assessed.

Step 2: Identify Relevant Utterances the Speaker Can Use to Initiate an Interaction

Identify comments, directives, or questions that the learner is likely to use to initiate interactions with different communicative partners. The following are examples that might be important for learners to successfully communicate within specific environments.

- *At home*: Can I have ___? Where's Mom?
- *At school*: How was your weekend? Whose team am I on? May I have that?
- *In the community*: Hi, my name is ___. Where is the restroom? I'd like help please. My telephone number is ___.
- *At work*: How was your weekend? I'd like a break. I'd like help please.

☞ *Helpful Hint*

It may be necessary to prompt or otherwise set up the situation when assessing initiations so the learner produces target utterances.

- Prompt discretely to minimize the likelihood that the communicative partner gleans information (e.g., overhears a verbal prompt) that influences the results of the assessment.

- Interventionists may consider other assessment strategies. For example, "Pass the message" games involve the speaker passing a message as in the "telephone game." The speaker is given a message to pass to the next person who in turn reports the message to determine the speaker's intelligibility within that context. The exact message can be passed (e.g., "We live in New York State"), requiring the speaker to imitate the utterance. Because there is an increased likelihood of an imitated message being intelligible, however, the speaker could instead be asked to pass on the answer to a question (e.g., the first person says "Tell what state you live in"). In this case, the speaker is not imitating, but rather creating a uniquely generated utterance.

  Passing the message outside of a game format is another strategy that can be used. For example, the speaker can be asked to relay a message to a peer, co-worker, family member, or teacher. If the message is novel, then there is likely little contextual information on which the speaker or listener can rely. For example, the employee with a severe disability can approach his or her supervisor to request a piece of equipment he or she might need to complete his or her job. This provides an opportunity to determine the extent to which the speaker can communicate a novel message in an intelligible manner. If the communicative partner (the su-

pervisor in this case) does not understand the message and requests clarification, then the extent to which the speaker is able to respond to requests for clarification from communicative partners can also be determined.

Step 3: Videotape the Speaker Communicating in the Absence and Presence of Environmental Cues

Videotape the speaker engaging in each of the communicative responses and initiations identified in Steps 1 and 2 in two conditions.

1. Record the speaker in the absence of environmental cues that have the potential to enhance the communicative message to assess the extent to which speech alone is intelligible, in the absence of any additional information.

2. Videotape in the presence of environmental cues. Place related objects, drawings, or photographs within the speaker's view. Videotaping in the presence of these environmental cues will help determine the extent to which the speaker successfully uses environmental cues to enhance intelligibility.

Step 4: Have Both Familiar and Unfamiliar Partners Listen to and Write Down What They Perceive the Speaker Said

Involve both familiar and unfamiliar listeners in the assessment process to measure the extent to which the speaker is intelligible across a range of partners. Figure 13.1 shows a completed sample form (Form 13.1 is a blank version and is included on the accompanying CD-ROM).

Have both familiar and unfamiliar communicative partners listen to the audio (if videotaped, the audio recording only so that the listeners cannot see the speaker communicating) and write down what they perceive the speaker said on the audio-only section of Form 13.1. For example, if the question posed to the speaker is "Where do you live?" then the listener should document what he or she believes was said (e.g., "Smithtown").

Learner's name: __Liam__   Date: __10/15__

Listener (familiar or unfamiliar)	Utterance number	Speaker utterance Audio condition only in the absence of contextual cues
Mr. Jackson (unfamiliar)	1	Bike riding
	2	The bus
	3	Patriots
	4	?
	5	?
	6	I'd like cheeseburger and fries
	7	?
	8	?
	Total: 8	Total correctly recorded: 4

> Intelligibility in the absence of context
>
> Total number correctly recorded   [4]
> $\times$ 100 = [50] %
> Total number of utterances   [8]

Listener (familiar or unfamiliar)	Utterance number	Video/audio condition in the presence of contextual cues (note contextual cues)
Mr. Jackson (unfamiliar)	1	Bike riding (made motion with his arms and legs)
	2	The bus
	3	Patriots (pointing to logo on school jacket)
	4	Playing soccer (making kicking motion with his foot)
	5	?
	6	I'd like cheeseburger and fries (no contextual cues used)
	7	?
	8	Can you help me? (showing a difficult bag to open)
	Total: 8	Total correctly recorded: 6

> Intelligibility in the presence of context
>
> Total number correctly recorded   [6]
> $\times$ 100 = [75] %
> Total number of utterances   [8]

Figure 13.1. Completed Intelligibility Assessment Form for Liam. (*Note:* This is a filled-in version of Form 13.1, Intelligibility Assessment Form. A blank, printable version appears on the accompanying CD-ROM.)

Note a question mark if the utterance was completely unintelligible from the listener's perspective.

Have both familiar and unfamiliar communicative partners view the videotape and write down what they perceive the speaker said on the video/audio portion of Form 13.1. The listener should also note communicative acts (e.g., gestures, facial expressions, environment stimuli) that the speaker used to enhance his or her communicative message.

Step 5: Determine the Extent to Which the Speaker Is Intelligible from the Listeners' Perspective

Calculate percentage of intelligible utterances by dividing the number of communicative utterances the listener accurately recorded by the total number of utterances spoken and then multiply by 100. Calculate the following:

- An overall intelligibility score across the two conditions (absence and presence of environmental cues) in relation to both responses to questions and initiations of communicative interactions

- Separate intelligibility scores for the presence (audio and video viewing condition) and absence (audio-only condition) of environmental cues

- Separate intelligibility scores for familiar and unfamiliar listeners in each of the conditions

- Separate intelligibility scores for responses versus initiations

Figure 13.1 illustrates the intelligibility scores for Liam in the presence and absence of contextual clues.

CASE STUDY

Intelligibility Assessment

Liam was a 14-year-old student with Down syndrome who attended his local middle school. He was enrolled in academic courses as well as chorus, home economics, and computer and played soccer for his town league. Liam pri-

marily used speech; however, unfamiliar peers and many of his teachers had a difficult time understanding him. Liam's team identified four responses and four initiations that were likely to occur throughout his day at school (see Figure 13.1). An unfamiliar teacher understood only 50% of Liam's utterances when she listened only to the audio portion of the videotape. Then, she watched the video while listening to the audio and identified 75% of the utterances. A closer analysis of Liam's performance indicates that his intelligibility was better when he used environmental cues and that he used such cues more when responding to questions. Specifically, he successfully utilized environmental cues in response to three of the four questions but only once when initiating interactions. Liam was taught to supplement his speech using gestures and/or graphic symbols to enhance his initiations.

AAC APPLICATIONS TO ENHANCE INTELLIGIBILITY AND COMPREHENSIBILITY

The remainder of this chapter reviews select strategies particularly relevant to increasing intelligibility and comprehensibility. These intervention targets are based on the speaker's performance on the intelligibility assessment. Specifically,

- The parts of the messages or the specific answers to questions that were "unintelligible"

- Expanding use of specific strategies (e.g., gestures) that the speaker used spontaneously during assessment to enhance intelligibility

- Teaching the speaker to use specific strategies

Use of Natural Gestures

Some individuals with severe disabilities may fail to acquire **natural communicative gestures.** Pointing is one of the earliest developing gestures (Kita, 2003). Other natural gestures include shaking one's head as a means of negation, shrugging one's shoulders to indicate "I don't know," or giving the thumbs up as an indication of agreement. Teaching these widely recognized gestures can greatly enhance communicative interactions.

Helpful Hint

Beukelman and Mirenda (2005) suggested a gesture dictionary for speakers who use idiosyncratic gestures and others in their environment who must know the meanings of those gestures. The gesture dictionary could be displayed on a poster, in a portable alphabetized notebook, or provided in video format stored on a DVD or cell phone. The gesture dictionary should contain a description, photograph, or video of each of the speaker's gestures.

Who Might Benefit from Learning to Use Natural Gestures?

Any speaker with poor intelligibility might benefit from learning to use gestures. Speakers who use idiosyncratic gestures may particularly benefit from intervention by shaping those idiosyncratic gestures into ones that are more readily understood by multiple partners.

Using Evidence-Based Strategies to Teach the Use of Natural Gestures

As a strategy to supplement speech, gestures are natural, portable, and can be more quickly produced than supplementation strategies that involve the use of other communicative modes. Gestures that are used naturally by the learner's community of listeners represent viable intervention targets. The steps below outline a strategy to systematically implement gestural mode supplementation.

Steps for teaching the use of natural gestures

Step 1: Identify opportunities.
Step 2: Identify appropriate gestures.
Step 3: Develop intervention strategies.
Step 4: Implement intervention and monitor learner performance.

Step 1: Identify Opportunities Use the intelligibility assessment to identify communicative opportunities in which the speaker could use a natural gesture to enhance intelligibility/comprehensibility. Situations in which the speaker already used some gestures may be appropriate initial opportunities for intervention because the speaker is already spontaneously emitting the gestures, and intervention can focus on increasing the frequency of his or her use of those gestures.

Information regarding identifying and creating instructional opportunities is discussed in Chapter 5.

Step 2: Identify Appropriate Gestures Choose gestures related to the opportunities identified in Step 1. Consider the following:

- Are there any gestures already demonstrated by the speaker that could be expanded to support intelligible speech?

- Can pointing—a general and versatile gesture to help speakers indicate referents during interaction—be used? For example, teach the speaker to take advantage of things or people in his or her environment by pointing to them (Hustad, Morehouse, & Gutmann, 2002). Also, consider other general or versatile gestures, such as the speaker moving toward the referent of speech.

- Are there any gestures related to specific partner questions such as the following:

  Shaking one's head "yes" or "no" or using the thumbs up or thumbs down to illustrate "yes" and "no."

  Shrugging one's shoulders to indicate he or she does not know the answer to a question.

  Specific gestures that illustrate an object or action word(s) that is not intelligible. For example, teaching the speaker to use his or her hands to form the shape of a ball when saying the word *ball* or use actions when using words such as *eat* or *drink*.

- Are there any gestures that have the potential to compensate for environmental conditions (e.g., gesturing for the listener to come closer in a noisy environment)?

Step 3: Develop Intervention Strategies   Identify prompts and consequences for the speaker's use of gestures. See Chapter 5 for detailed information about developing prompting and reinforcement procedures.

Step 4: Implement Intervention and Monitor Learner Performance   Develop a performance monitoring procedure as described in Chapter 7.

Topic Supplementation with Graphic Symbols

Graphic mode topic supplementation has evidentiary support with both young learners with developmental disabilities and individuals with acquired disabilities (e.g., amyotrophic lateral schlerosis). Although potentially slower than gestural or alphabetic supplementation, graphic mode supplementation may place less cognitive load on the user. That is, gestures and alphabet require greater memory capabilities than the graphic mode, which does not have to require recall. Instead, graphic symbols require only recognition of the correct symbol.

Who Might Benefit from Using Topic Supplementation?

Using graphic symbols to supplement speech represents a good option to use with individuals who are not literate and have motor limitations making gestural mode supplementation impractical. Topic supplementation is particularly effective for speakers who have specific and predictable topics about which they are likely to communicate. For example, topic supplementation can be used to indicate a specific sport or hobby or a favorite television show or place to visit (e.g., zoo, amusement park).

Using Evidence-Based Strategies to Teach the Use of Topic Supplementation

The limited literature on topic supplementation provides some guidelines on its use.

> Steps for teaching the use of topic supplementation
>
> Step 1: Identify topics about which the speaker is likely to converse.
> Step 2: Determine the most appropriate symbol system and display.
> Step 3: Make the topic indicator available for easy access.
> Step 4: Plan for new vocabulary.
> Step 5: Identify intervention strategies.
> Step 6: Implement intervention, and monitor performance.

Step 1: Identify Topics About Which the Speaker Is Likely to Converse   Observe the speaker interacting within a variety of situations and note topics that naturally arise between him or her and a communicative partner. Also, consider people, activities, and objects that are preferred by the speaker. In addition, recent events (e.g., a holiday celebration, a field trip) may be important new topics benefitting from supplementation. It is also important to consider different audiences. For example, a speaker may speak often about his or her favorite action toys in the presence of peers, but never in the presence of strangers or his or her parents.

Step 2: Determine the Most Appropriate Symbol System and Display   Typical communicators make reference to things in their natural environments. For example, at breakfast while reading the newspaper, a man or woman may look at and point to something in the paper about which he or she then comments. Not all topics will have an environmental referent at all times. Portable systems can be developed for use across environments. For example, communication books containing graphic symbols can be used to extend the number of conversation turns between learners and their partners, as well as increase intelligibility (Hunt, Alwell, &

Goetz, 1988, 1991). Conversation books are described in more detail in Chapter 11.

Graphic mode supplementation can involve some portable and creative symbols carried by the speaker, such as charms on a bracelet or necklace, belt buckle, and digital displays (via a cell phone or camera). More traditional symbol systems with a range of display options include a wallet, notebook, photograph, agenda/date book, or key chain. Strategies to introduce a learner's mode of communication to unfamiliar partners are discussed in more detail in Chapter 11.

Step 3: Make the Topic Indicator Available for Easy Access   Identify where topic supplementation materials are necessary and ensure their availability.

Step 4: Plan for New Vocabulary   In addition to ongoing common topics (e.g., favorite sports, musician, television show), it is likely that new events will take place about which the speaker is likely to communicate. These may be the topics for which supplementation is most important because the words may be relatively novel to the speaker, and even familiar listeners may not have experience with the speaker using these words words, compromising intelligibility. To support new topics (Dowden, 1997)

- Clip pictures from the newspaper or magazines.

- Draw "instant" symbols using available materials (e.g., notepad, dry-erase boards).

- Use a souvenir (e.g., a movie ticket stub, a favorite store or restaurant logo).

- Print or store symbols (e.g., photographs) or even a video on a cell phone.

- Use a calendar across environments (e.g., family members, peers in school and community).

Step 5: Identify Intervention Strategies   See Chapter 5 to choose intervention strategies, including prompting, reinforcement, and error correction procedures.

Step 6: Implement Intervention and Monitor Performance   Develop performance monitoring procedures as described in Chapter 7.

CASE STUDY

Topic Supplementation

Liam's educational team decided he would benefit from learning to utilize topic supplementation to enhance the intelligibility of his initiations. Intervention procedures are described in detail in Figure 13.2 (Form 6.1 is a blank version and is included on the accompanying CD-ROM). For each class, Liam, his teaching assistant, teachers, and parents identified common topics of conversation that Liam was likely to initiate (e.g., good friends, favorite teams, restaurants) as well as course-related topics (e.g., appliances, utensils, food items). Symbols for the general topics were displayed on the outside of his daily agenda, and symbols for course-specific topics were displayed on the front cover of the corresponding course binders.

When Liam approached a peer or teacher, his teaching assistant pointed to his agenda or binder to prompt him to select a symbol to indicate the topic about which he was conversing. When Liam utilized topic supplementation by pointing to one of the symbols, his teaching assistant discretely showed him a thumbs up as he continued to converse with his peers and/or teachers. Figures 13.3 and 13.4 show Liam's performance learning to use topic supplementation in school.

Liam also used supplementation during soccer. Topic supplementation materials consisted of series of pins attached to Liam's sports bag that represented various topics about which he typically conversed with his teammates. Pins included a photograph of his close friend Adrian, his favorite sports (football, basketball, hockey, and baseball), and places that he enjoyed going. Liam's parents practiced using the pins in the same way Liam's teaching assistant had prompted Liam at school to use the symbols in his binder. Soon he used topic supplementation at soccer as well.

Learner's name: Liam   Start date: 11/1

Setting (circle one):   HOME   (SCHOOL)   COMMUNITY   WORK

Communication skill/function: Liam will point to line-drawn symbols stored in his class binders to indicate topic when conversing with peers and classroom teachers.

Opportunities

When: While initiating conversations with peers and classroom teachers

Where: In the classrooms and hallways

Minimum opportunities per day/session: 5 opportunities per day

Context for instruction: Naturally occurring opportunities within classes and during times of transition (e.g., while entering school, between classes)

Set up: Encountering a peer or teacher with whom Liam would like to converse

Materials: Line-drawn symbol display stored within class binders

Target Behavior

Mode: Graphic

Augmentative and alternative communication system features: N/A

Vocabulary: General vocabulary as well as course-specific vocabulary

Instructional Strategies

Skill sequence/steps: 1) Upon encountering a peer or teacher with whom Liam would like converse, Liam is prompted by his teaching assistant to use the symbols stored in his daily agenda and class binder to indicate the topic about which he wishes to communicate.

Prompts: The teaching assistant will use a gestural prompt (point to Liam's binder).

Consequences

Correct response: Immediately following Liam's use of his graphic display, his teaching assistant will discretely give him a thumbs up while smiling and nodding approvingly. After the communicative interaction, Liam's teaching assistant will deliver verbal praise and a high five, indicating how pleased she was that Liam used his pictures while he spoke to his friend/teacher.

Incorrect response (no response or error response): If Liam does not use topic supplementation and his communicative partner fails to understand him, then his teaching assistant will use another gestural prompt (i.e., tapping on the binder) to prompt Liam to select a symbol.

Prompt fading: Time delay will be used to fade the gestural prompt to select a symbol that corresponds to the topic of Liam's communicative initiation.

Generalization: Liam's parents will introduce a different topic supplementation aid at home for Liam to use at soccer.

Maintenance: Once mastery is achieved, Liam's teaching assistant will document Liam's performance once every two weeks to monitor maintenance.

Criterion for Mastery

Liam will independently use his topic supplementation strategy in the presence of unfamiliar peers and his teachers during 80% of his initiations (for which there is a corresponding symbol) across 2 days.

Performance Monitoring

Liam's teaching assistant will document Liam's performance.

Figure 13.2. Intervention Planning Form for teaching Liam to use topic supplementation strategies. (*Note:* This is a filled-in version of Form 6.1, Intervention Planning Form. A blank, printable version appears on the accompanying CD-ROM.)

Learner's name: __Liam__

Activity: __Classes and transitions__

Observer: __Maggie__   Prompt: __Teaching assistant points to binder__

Date	Environment/partner	Topic	Use of topic supplementation		Notes
11/1	Hallway/Jillian	Soccer	(Prompt)	Independent	0-second delay
11/1	Lockers/Marty	Soccer	(Prompt)	Independent	
11/1	Home economics/ Mr. Forest	Cooking	(Prompt)	Independent	
11/1	Chorus/Mr. Franklin	Concert	(Prompt)	Independent	
11/1	Social studies/Ed	Baseball	(Prompt)	Independent	
11/2	Science/Sam	Soccer	(Prompt)	Independent	
11/2	Hallway/Mrs. Scott	Web site	(Prompt)	Independent	
11/2	Computer/Mrs. Scott	Web site	(Prompt)	Independent	
11/2	English/Tom	Baseball	(Prompt)	Independent	
11/2	English/Mr. Knight	Computer	(Prompt)	Independent	
11/3	Hallway/Marty	Soccer	(Prompt)	Independent	5-second delay
11/3	Home economics/ Mr. Forest	Oven use	Prompt	(Independent)	
11/3	Lockers/Sam	Assembly today	(Prompt)	Independent	
11/3	Chorus/Angelo	Concert	Prompt	(Independent)	
11/3	Social studies/ Mr. Cringle	Writing help	Prompt	(Independent)	
11/4	Hallway/Mr. Sneef	Baseball	Prompt	(Independent)	
11/4	Science/Sam	Baseball	Prompt	(Independent)	
11/4	Computer/Mrs. Scott	Web site	(Prompt)	Independent	
11/4	English/Mr. Knight	Computer	Prompt	(Independent)	
11/4	English/Mr. Knight	Writing help	Prompt	(Independent)	
11/5	Hallway/Jillian	Lunch	Prompt	(Independent)	
11/5	Home economics/Bob	Favorite foods	Prompt	(Independent)	
11/5	Chorus/Mr. Franklin	Solo	Prompt	(Independent)	
11/5	Chorus/Angelo	Solo	Prompt	(Independent)	
11/5	Social studies/ Mr. Cringle	Project	Prompt	(Independent)	

Figure 13.3. Liam's performance with his peers and teachers during intervention.

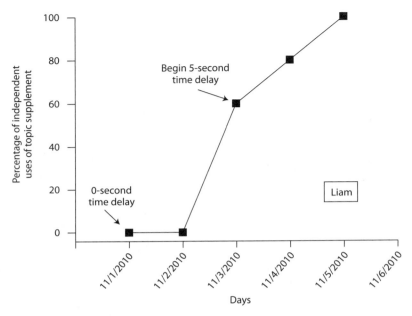

Figure 13.4. Percentage of opportunities for which Liam independently used topic supplementation to successfully initiate a conversation.

🏴 *Helpful Hint*

Alphabet Supplementation

A speaker uses alphabet supplementation by indicating the first letter of each word he or she is speaking on an alphabet display. The listener then often states the word to confirm the speaker's communication. If intelligibility remains poor when the speaker just indicates the first letter of the word spoken, then the speaker can spell out the entire word. Alphabet supplementation may help the listener narrow down potential words the speaker says and also separate the different words in a string (Hanson, Yorkston, & Beukelman, 2004).

Alphabet supplementation can result in intelligibility improvements (Beukelman & Yorkston, 1977; Hanson et al., 2004; Hunter, Pring, & Martin, 1991). In some studies, alphabet supplementation resulted in greater improvements than other strategies, such as topic supplementation. The combined use of different supports, however, often proves even more effective than individual types of supplementation alone in increasing intelligibility. Alphabet supplementation may be a consideration for

- Speakers who speak very quickly, as it not only provides the listener with additional informa-

tion, but it also often slows down the speaker's rate of speech, improving intelligibility (Beukelman & Yorkston, 1977; Hustad & Garcia, 2005)

- Speakers with mild impairments in intelligibility (Hustad, 2005)

- Speakers who can spell

Spelling ability may prohibit alphabet supplementation as an initial strategy for some learners. An alphabet board must be transported and available to the speaker. The listener must also attend as letters are identified and provide feedback (e.g., by saying the word the speaker is speaking) to ensure comprehension.

🏴 *Helpful Hint*

The examples provided in this chapter are based on situations in which the communicative partner clearly indicates a communicative breakdown occurred (i.e., he or she did not understand what the speaker said). In other situations, the communicative partner may not explicitly indicate the message is not understood or how it was not understood. For example, he or she might respond by leaning closer to the speaker, giving a questioning look, or saying, "What?" Chapter 11 contains strategies that can be used to teach speakers to recognize communicative breakdowns and respond to this variety of cues.

☞ Helpful Hint

How Can Partners Help Increase Perceived Intelligibility and Comprehensibility?

- Many speakers with severe disabilities take advantage of cues in the environment (e.g., look at the corresponding referent) and utilize gestures (i.e., facial, hand, body) while speaking. Because the use of these gestures enhances intelligibility, communicative partners must look at the speaker when he or she is formulating a message (Hunter et al., 1991).

- Partners may need instruction in the best way to convey to the speaker how to enhance his or her communicative message. For example, on a weekday, just before leaving for school, 9-year-old Michael remembered it was "pajama day" (a day in which teachers and students wear pajamas). He immediately asked for his pajamas. His mother did not understand him, however, as this request was not only out of the ordinary but also out of context (he was already dressed for school). After asking him to repeat it, followed by asking him to act it out, his mother finally asked him to go "get it," saying, "Michael, I don't understand. Go get what you are talking about." Michael retrieved his pajamas. His mother then realized what day it was at school. It also occurred to her to send the list of cues to school in the event students and staff experienced similar difficulties.

- Partners can also enhance intelligibility by altering the environment. For example, in the pajama example, while asking Michael to repeat what he had said, his mother also turned the television off and sent her other child out of the room to decrease background noise and increase the likelihood she would understand what Michael was saying.

SUMMARY

AAC strategies can enhance intelligibility and comprehensibility for learners with severe disabilities who rely on speech as their primary mode of communication so that a wide range of communicative partners can understand them. A careful assessment across both familiar and unfamiliar partners with and without additional information allows for the identification of specific communicative interactions that could be enhanced by AAC applications. Individually designed interventions can be used to teach supplemental strategies with the potential to improve intelligibility of learners with severe disabilities, thus enhancing their comprehensibility and increasing successful communicative interactions.

REFERENCES

Beliveau, C., Hodge, M.M., & Hagler, P.H. (1995). Effects of supplemental linguistic cues on the intelligibility of severely dysarthric speakers. *Augmentative and Alternative Communication, 11,* 176–186.

Beukelman, D.R., & Yorkston, K. (1977). A communication system for the severely dysarthric speaker with an intact language system. *Journal of Speech and Hearing Disorders, 42,* 265–270.

Beukelman, D.R., & Yorkston, K. (1979). The relationship between information transfer and speech intelligibility of dysarthric speakers. *Journal of Communication Disorders, 12,* 189–196.

DePaul, R., & Kent, R.D. (2000). A longitudinal case study of ALS: Effects of listener familiarity and proficiency on intelligibility judgments. *American Journal of Speech-Language Pathology, 9,* 230–240.

Dowden, P.A. (1997). Augmentative and alternative communication decision making for children with severely unintelligible speech. *Augmentative and Alternative Communication, 13,* 48–58.

Drager, K.D.R., Clark-Serpentine, E.A., Johnson, K.E., & Roeser, J.L. (2006). Accuracy of repetition of digitized and synthesized speech for young children in background noise. *American Journal of Speech-Language Pathology, 15,* 155–164.

Drager, K.D.R., Reichle, J., & Pinkoski, C. (2010). Synthesized speech output and children: A scoping review. *American Journal of Speech and Language Pathology., 19,* 259–273.

Duffy, J.R., & Giolas, T.G. (1974). Sentence intelligibility as a function of key word selection.

Journal of Speech and Hearing Research, 17, 631–637.

Garcia, J.M., & Cannito, M.P. (1996a). Influence of verbal and nonverbal contexts on the sentence intelligibility of a speaker with dysarthria. *Journal of Speech and Hearing Research, 39,* 750–760.

Garcia, J.M., & Cannito, M.P. (1996b). Top-down influences on the intelligibility of a dysarthric speaker: Addition of natural gestures and situational context. In D.A. Robin, K.M. Yorkston, & D.R. Beukelman (Eds.), *Disorders of motor speech: Assessment, treatment, and clinical characterization* (pp. 89–103). Baltimore: Paul H. Brookes Publishing Co.

Garcia, J.M., Crowe, L.K., Redler, D., & Hustad, K. (2004). Effects of spontaneous gestures on comprehension and intelligibility of dysarthric speech: A case report. *Journal of Medical Speech-Language Pathology, 12,* 145–148.

Garcia, J.M., & Dagenais, P.A. (1998). Dysarthric sentence intelligibility: Contribution of iconic gestures and message predictiveness. *Journal of Speech, Language, and Hearing Research, 41,* 1282–1293.

Hammen, V.L., Yorkston, K.M., & Dowden, P. (1991). Index of contextual intelligibility I: Impact of semantic context in dysarthria. In C. Moore, K.M. Yorkston, & D.R. Beukelman (Eds.), *Dysarthria and apraxia of speech: Perspectives on intervention* (pp. 43–54). Baltimore: Paul H. Brookes Publishing Co.

Hanson, E.K., Yorkston, K.M., & Beukelman, D.R. (2004). Speech supplementation techniques for dysarthria: A systematic review. *Journal of Medical Speech-Language Pathology, 12,* ix–xxix.

Hubbard, D.J., & Kushner, D. (1980). A comparison of speech intelligibility between esophageal and normal speakers via three modes of presentation. *Journal of Speech and Hearing Research, 23,* 909–916.

Hunt, P., Alwell, M., & Goetz, L. (1988). Acquisition of conversation skills and the reduction of inappropriate social interaction behaviors. *Journal of The Association for Persons with Severe Handicaps, 13,* 20–27.

Hunt, P., Alwell, M., & Goetz, L. (1991). Interacting with peers through conversation turn-taking with a communication book adaptation. *Augmentative and Alternative Communication, 7,* 117–126.

Hunter, L., Pring, T., & Martin, S. (1991). The use of strategies to increase speech intelligibility in cerebral palsy: An experimental evaluation. *British Journal of Disorders of Communication, 26,* 163–174.

Hustad, K.C. (2005). Effects of speech supplementation strategies on intelligibility and listener attitudes for a speaker with mild dysarthria.

Augmentative and Alternative Communication, 21, 256–263.

Hustad, K.C. (2006). A closer look at transcription intelligibility for speakers with dysarthria: Evaluation of scoring paradigms and linguistic errors made by listeners. *American Journal of Speech-Language Pathology, 15,* 268–277.

Hustad, K.C. (2007a). Contribution of two sources of listener knowledge to intelligibility of speakers with cerebral palsy. *Journal of Speech, Language, and Hearing Research, 50,* 1228–1240.

Hustad, K.C. (2007b). Effects of speech stimuli and dysarthria severity on intelligibility scores and listener confidence ratings for speakers with cerebral palsy. *Folia Phoniatrica et Logopaedica, 59,* 306–317.

Hustad, K.C., Auker, J., Natale, N., & Carlson, R. (2003). Improving intelligibility of speakers with profound dysarthria and cerebral palsy. *Augmentative and Alternative Communication, 19,* 187–198.

Hustad, K.C., & Beukelman, D.R. (2001). Effects of linguistic cues and stimulus cohesion on intelligibility of severely dysarthric speech. *Journal of Speech, Language, and Hearing Research, 44,* 497–510.

Hustad, K.C., & Cahill, M.A. (2003). Effects of presentation mode and repeated familiarization on intelligibility of dysarthric speech. *American Journal of Speech-Language Pathology, 12,* 198–208.

Hustad, K.C., Dardis, C.M., & McCourt, K.A. (2007). Effects of visual information on intelligibility of open and closed class words in predictable sentences produced by speakers with dysarthria. *Clinical Linguistics and Phonetics, 21,* 353–367.

Hustad, K.C., & Garcia, J.M. (2002). The influence of alphabet supplementation, iconic gestures, and predictive messages on intelligibly of a speaker with cerebral palsy. *Journal of Medical Speech-Language Pathology, 10,* 279–285.

Hustad, K.C., & Garcia, J.M. (2005). Aided and unaided speech supplementation strategies: Effects of alphabet cues and iconic hand gestures on dysarthric speech. *Journal of Speech, Language, and Hearing Research, 48,* 996–1012.

Hustad, K.C., Jones, T., & Dailey, S. (2003). Implementing speech supplementation strategies: Effects on intelligibility and speech rate of individuals with chronic severe dysarthria. *Journal of Speech, Language, and Hearing Research, 46,* 462–474.

Hustad, K.C., Morehouse, T.B., & Gutmann, M. (2002). AAC strategies for enhancing the usefulness of natural speech in children with severe intelligibility challenges. In D. Beukelman & J. Reichle (Series Eds.) & J. Reichle, D.R. Beukelman, & J.C. Light (Vol. Eds.), *AAC Series: Exemplary practices for beginning communicators:*

Implications for AAC (pp. 433–452). Baltimore: Paul H. Brookes Publishing Co.

Kita, S. (Ed.). (2003). *Pointing: Where language, culture, and cognition meet.* Mahwah, NJ: Lawrence Erlbaum Associates.

Koul, R.K., & Allen, G.D. (1993). Segmental intelligibility and speech interference thresholds of high-quality synthetic speech in presence of noise. *Journal of Speech and Hearing Research, 36,* 790–798.

Kumin, L. (1994). Intelligibility of speech in children with Down syndrome in natural settings: Parents' perspective. *Perceptual and Motor Skills, 78,* 307–313.

Lindblom, B. (1990). On the communication process: Speaker-listener interaction and the development of speech. *Augmentative and Alternative Communication, 6,* 220–230.

McNaughton, D., Fallon, K., Tod, J., Weiner, F., & Neisworth, J. (1994). Effect of repeated listening experiences on the intelligibility of synthesized speech. *Augmentative and Alternative Communication, 10,* 161–168.

Mirenda, P., & Beukelman, D.R. (1987). A comparison of speech synthesis intelligibility with listeners from three age groups. *Augmentative and Alternative Communication, 3,* 120–128.

Mirenda, P., & Beukelman, D.R. (1990). A comparison of intelligibility among natural speech and seven speech synthesizers with listeners from three age groups. *Augmentative and Alternative Communication, 6,* 61–68.

Monsen, R.B. (1983). The oral speech intelligibility of hearing-impaired talkers. *Journal of Speech and Hearing Disorders, 48,* 286–296.

Rosin, M., Swift, E., Bless, D., & Vetter, D. (1988). Communication profiles of adolescents with Down syndrome. *Journal of Childhood Communication Disorders, 12,* 49–64.

Salasoo, A., & Pisoni, D.B. (1985). Interaction of knowledge sources in spoken word identification. *Journal of Memory and Language, 24,* 210–231.

Tjaden, K.K., & Liss, J.M. (1995). The role of listener familiarity in the perception of dysarthric speech. *Clinical Linguistics and Phonetics, 9,* 139–154.

Yorkston, K.M., Bombardier, C., & Hammen, V.L. (1994). Dysarthria from the viewpoint of individuals with dysarthria. In J.A. Till, K.M. Yorkston, & D.R. Beukelman (Eds.), *Motor speech disorders: Advances in assessment and treatment* (pp. 19–35). Baltimore: Paul H. Brookes Publishing Co.

Yorkston, K.M., Strand, E.A., & Kennedy, M.R.T. (1996). Comprehensibility of dysarthric speech: Implications for assessment and treatment planning. *American Journal of Speech-Language Pathology, 5,* 55–66.

Conclusion

Joe Reichle and Susan Johnston

It is a far better time to be a recipient of communication intervention today than it was in the early 1990s, when Joe Reichle first gathered a group of graduate students together to write about augmentative and alternative communication (AAC) applications for individuals with severe developmental disabilities. In the years that have followed, Reichle and the coauthors of this book have had the opportunity to work with many excellent doctoral students. The current volume reflects the culmination of the incredibly strong work ethic of some of those individuals. There are also a number of extremely talented former doctoral students whose work is cited in this book. Dr. Jeff Sigafoos has made major contributions to the area of AAC among individuals with moderate and severe developmental disabilities. Dr. Kathy Drager has had a tremendous impact on the understanding of variables involved in successfully implementing speech-generating devices across a wide array of learners that include, but are not limited to, children and youth with developmental disabilities. Former University of Minnesota postdoctoral fellow Dr. Rachel Freeman has had a major influence on training/mentoring strategies in positive behavior support, whereas postdoctoral fellow Dr. Peggy Locke now influences public school service delivery in the area of autism spectrum disorders. Unfortunately, Dr. Scott Doss died far too young but will be remembered as one of the finest colleagues for which one could wish. In concluding this book, several topics that are currently receiving attention are mentioned briefly. Each one is important in furthering the effort to improve the quality of services to learners with severe developmental disabilities.

TECHNICAL ASSISTANCE AND TREATMENT FIDELITY

Although much "heavy lifting" has been accomplished in creating a plethora of innovative instructional strategies, less effort has been directed at developing systems to ensure that these strategies can be implemented efficiently in a range of home, school, and community environments. Researchers are often quick to point the finger at educators who fail to attend to and utilize evidence-based instructional procedures. Perhaps it would be better to question why more evidence-based procedures are not used by practitioners. In many instances, this may be because the procedures on which the evidence base was generated lacked a good "contextual fit" with the demands placed on interventionists or the conditions under which the instructional programs must be implemented. It is difficult to replicate some empirically validated intervention strategies due to a variety of reasons, including 1) the characteristics of the students, 2) the staffing pattern available for intervention implementation, 3) the equipment and materials required for implementation, and 4) the training and technical assistance to address challenges arising that were not discussed in validating literature. The latter point represents a huge gap in the ability to successfully implement validated instructional strategies and is likely attributable, in part, to weaknesses in preservice training. Postgraduate mentoring and technical assistance are the solutions to this challenge.

Providing technical assistance often is accomplished using an "expert model" in which the expert selects the intervention procedure that will be implemented. Dr. Leanne Johnson (personal communication, March 9, 2010) and her colleagues compared two different strategies for offering technical assistance. In the first, several choices of different intervention procedures were offered as examples of evidence-based instructional strategies from which the interventionist could choose. Technical assistance was then provided on the chosen procedure. In the second model, the technical assistance provider selected the procedure to be implemented and the same level of technical assistance was provided. Procedural fidelity was measured to examine differences between the choice and no-choice conditions. The hypothesis and some evidence to date suggests that initial fidelity is somewhat equal regardless of the strategy implemented. As the technical assistance is faded, however, fidelity appears to remain higher in the choice condition but, after a period of time, decays more rapidly in the no-choice condition.

These findings suggest that skill may be less implicated than contextual fit in sustaining the implementation of evidence-based practices in at least some instances. In this example, treatment fidelity represents an important method to determine the degree to which evidence-based instruction is being delivered. Unfortunately, treatment fidelity and treatment adherence are areas that are often overlooked and/or receive limited attention in applying intervention procedures.

Treatment (procedural) fidelity often is not carefully monitored in school and community environments, which, in turn, can have a significant effect on intervention outcomes. The fidelity with which staff implemented components of positive behavior support strategies was examined in the context of implementing positive behavior support procedures. Procedural fidelity was found to be less than 40% (Johnson, Reichle, & Monn, 2009). It is impossible to troubleshoot a program without procedural fidelity because one does not know what portions of

an intervention strategy were actually implemented. Failure to monitor procedural fidelity can result in an interventionist concluding that a strategy did not work when, in fact, it had never really been implemented. Learner performance data are difficult to troubleshoot when procedures are not implemented with fidelity because it is not clear whether the need is for a program troubleshoot or for the interventionist(s) simply to implement with greater fidelity. If fidelity is good, then monitoring learner performance becomes important.

OBJECTIVELY MONITORING LEARNER PERFORMANCE

In a survey completed with preschool teachers and speech-language pathologists (Reichle, 2004), 83% reported that they valued objective data and believed that it should be the basis for decision making in education. However, only 17% responded affirmatively when asked whether they regularly obtained objective data for learner performance on instructional objectives. This outcome is puzzling and causes one to wonder how objective data get reported in a relatively high proportion of individualized education programs even though such a low proportion of staff report obtaining data. One of the reasons why interventionists struggle in troubleshooting instructional programs is that they do not objectively monitor learner performance in order to determine what is working and what requires change. Furthermore, many educators have never experienced the reinforcement of seeing trends in learner performance change in accordance with changes in objective data. With the substantial effort that good interventionists expend in implementing an intervention strategy, it seems important to consider how best to maximize gains from the implementation. Acquiring desirable behavior and decelerating undesirable collateral behavior as a result of intervention implementation is one area that is receiving increasing attention.

COLLATERAL EFFECTS ASSOCIATED WITH INTERVENTION

Several chapters in this book discussed collateral effects of intervention strategies. A collateral acquisition occurs when behavior that was not the intended focus of intervention is acquired and related to the intervention implemented. The potential for acquiring related collateral behavior in other communicative modes is of particular interest to communication interventionists. As discussed in earlier chapters, collateral communicative behavior is a particularly important topic given the common fear among parents that implementing AAC may impede spoken communicative development. As pointed out previously, although the data are limited (Millar, 2009), there is good reason to believe that this is not the case. Both speech production and comprehension of speech have been cited as collateral behavior associated with the initiation of AAC systems (e.g., Bondy & Frost, 2001; Yoder & Layton, 1988).

Examining the mechanisms that account for collateral acquisitions is a particularly important area for future scrutiny. Doing so may help interventionists predict who will acquire collateral behavior as well as offer clues regarding pivotal skills that, if taught, could enhance the probability of collateral acquisitions. For example, imitation has been strongly implicated as a factor in acquiring spoken vocabulary as a collateral acquisition associated with AAC (see Yoder and Layton, 1988). Although yet to be demonstrated, implementing a high-tech AAC system may provide more consistently modeled speech output for a learner than what occurs when humans model spoken words. Thus, with respect to spoken language models, there may be a technological advantage (although the speech produced may be less intelligible than human speech) (see Drager, Reichle, & Pinkoski, 2010, for a systematic review). When issues such as these are more fully investigated, it may improve the ability to better ensure collateral acquisitions. With respect to collateral comprehension of spoken vocabulary, Harris and Reichle (2004) demonstrated that speech comprehension improved by systematically pairing speech while teaching graphic symbol use. This suggests that production can precede comprehension of spoken language in graphic mode communication systems. This may have implications for strictly adhering to normal development as a model when designing intervention strategies.

Finally, collateral acquisitions as a result of implementing AAC are not limited solely to forms and modes of communicative behavior. Investigators (Derby et al., 1997) found the emergence of collateral behavior, including toy play and social interaction, is contingent on acquisition of communicative behaviors. Thus, establishing an initial repertoire of communicative functions may foster social interaction skills for some learners who find social contact with others to be reinforcing.

Decelerating undesirable behavior has been the focus of numerous investigations in the area of positive behavior support (see Bambara & Kern, 2005; Reichle & Wacker, 1993). When one considers collateral communicative acquisitions related to challenging behavior, one must consider the conditional use of the communicative behavior and its effect on collateral gains such as increased task engagement that might result from the deceleration of problem behavior. For example, if a learner is taught to request a break rather than have a tantrum during a less preferred task, then it is likely that the learner's use of break requests will skyrocket. This increase in requesting decreases opportunities for independent engagement. When the learner's request is denied, however, the challenging behavior will reemerge. Thus, the learner needs to be taught when to use and when not to use newly taught behavior. Thus teaching the conditional use of new behaviors taught becomes very important. Unfortunately, it is often overlooked during intervention implementation.

CONDITIONAL USE OF NEWLY ESTABLISHED BEHAVIOR

As discussed in several chapters, there are often two or more concurrently available response options when producing communication. For example, when the ketchup is far away and a person wants it, he or she may request that someone pass it. When it is nearby, however, the person picks it up and uses it. Being able to choose between these options as a function of environmental and reinforcement conditions is what separates a competent communicator from a person who communicates, as some would say, "rotely." Individuals learn to communicate conditionally because there are two different reinforcement schedules associated with each response. Reichle and McComas (2004) examined this issue with a 10-year-old boy who experienced emotional disturbances. As pointed out in an earlier chapter, the learner's requests for assistance continued to be emitted even though he had learned to independently complete math problems that originally necessitated teaching him to request assistance. As a troubleshoot, interventionists delivered a more powerful reinforcer for independent work and a less powerful reinforcer when the learner requested assistance. Subsequently, the child learned to request assistance with tasks that he was not competent in independently completing, but he was able to independently complete those tasks in which he was competent. Although it appears to be effective, the strategy just described seems to have been used sparingly by interventionists in applied settings (see Johnston, Reichle, & Evans, 2004; Reichle & Johnston, 1999; Reichle & McComas, 2004). When an intervention strategy has supporting evidence but has not been widely embraced in educational practice, one must consider the degree of contextual fit (mentioned earlier) with the range of interventionists who could use it. Contextual fit, in turn, is likely to be influenced by the efficiency of the intervention from the interventionist's perspective.

RESPONSE EFFICIENCY/CONTEXTUAL FIT

In all likelihood, there are a variety of parameters that represent efficiency that factor into the degree of contextual fit between an intervention strategy and an educators' "intervention strategy comfort zone" (Johnston et al., 2004). Some considerations that directly relate more to effort expended for outcome achieved may include

- How quickly is the intervention apt to result in change?

- How similar is the procedure to instructional techniques that are already used fluently?

- What is the likelihood that other classroom educators (paraprofessionals) can be easily mentored in the implementation of the procedure?

- Are all of the components of the procedure necessary to achieve a desired outcome?

Despite the increasing demands placed on validating instructional technology in natural environments, the area of contextual fit in applied settings by practitioners has received limited attention. Although response efficiency has been addressed experimentally from a learner's perspective (e.g., Horner & Day, 1991), less effort has been expended examinining it from an interventionist's perspective.

One important aspect of response efficiency is implicated in interventionists' efforts to extend intervention into home and community environments. When generalization of learned behaviors does not occur in these environments, there seems to be a propensity for interventionists to attempt to completely replicate the intervention that resulted in original acquisition. That may not be necessary, however, as a lower dose intervention may be sufficient.

LOW-DOSE INTERVENTION

Performance in new environments may be achieved in low-dose intervention by implementing only a portion of an original intervention that was required to establish a new behavior. For example, Drasgow, Halle, and Ostrosky (1998) found that the newly established communicative behavior did not sufficiently generalize to home settings when teaching learners with significant developmental disabilities to use more socially acceptable requests for toys. Instead of reimplementing the teaching procedure in its entirety, however, home interventionists were coached to refrain from reinforcing the old (more socially unacceptable) communicative forms. This had a propensity to result in the newly taught (more socially acceptable) forms to be used. In working with families, this may speak to having skilled interventionists initially establish a new behavior in one environment. Then, secondary interventionists can be taught to implement a lower dose intervention when intervention begins in an environment where the same level of intervention effort that was applied in the original environment cannot be expended. This strategy requires far more attention than it is currently receiving in the intervention literature. Low-dose intervention is part of a larger area of inquiry that is beginning to gain traction among communication interventionists. Specifically, there is a need for a careful evaluation of the role that treatment intensity plays in the acquisition, maintenance, and generalization of new skills.

TREATMENT INTENSITY AND ITS INTERACTION WITH RESPONSE EFFICIENCY

Warren, Fey, and Yoder (2007) delineated a set of treatment intensity parameters, including dose, dose form, dose frequency, total intervention duration, and cumulative intervention intensity. They suggested that these parameters are important in evaluating the efficacy of intervention strategies. The literature often compares two different instructional strategies that were implemented with varying levels of treatment intensity yet concludes that one has a superior outcome.

It is challenging to compare the efficacy of the actual components of an intervention strategy, however, unless aspects of treatment intensity are either carefully controlled or are the focus of applied investigations. The parameters described by Warren et al. warrant more careful consideration in designing programs. Although there is insufficient space here to adequately deal with each of the parameters listed, they represent an area that will be critically important in identifying intervention protocols that are better individualized to specific learner needs.

SUMMARY

As stated previously, it is a far better time to be a recipient of communication intervention today than it was in the early 1990s. In spite of best efforts, however, communication intervention does not yet allow finely tuned algorithms to completely customize procedures to a particular learner based on an evidence base. Numerous applied researchers are feverishly working with practitioners to find a well-defined continuum of evidence-based approaches from which skilled interventionists can craft a strategy that has a high probability of being successful in establishing or enhancing a learner's communication ability. To be truly successful, however, professionals must be able to use the evidence to guide the delivery of intervention and to influence the needed troubleshoots to keep selected interventions on track. There is much heavy lifting yet required. The good news is that it can be done.

REFERENCES

Bambara, L.M., & Kern, L. (2005). *Individualized supports for students with problem behaviors.* New York: Guilford Press.

Bondy, A., & Frost, L. (2001). The Picture Exchange Communication System. *Behavior Modification, 25,* 725–744.

Derby, K., Wacker, D.P., Berg, W., DeRaad, A., Ulrich, S., Asmus, J., et al. (1997). The long-term effects of functional communication training in home settings. *Journal of Applied Behavior Analysis, 30,* 507–531.

Drager, K.D., Reichle, J., & Pinkoski, C. (2010). Synthesized speech output and children: A scoping review. *American Journal of Speech-Language Pathology, 19*(3), 259–273.

Drasgow, E., Halle, J., & Ostrosky, M. (1998). Effects of differential reinforcement on the generalization of a replacement mand in three children with severe language delays. *Journal of Applied Behavior Analysis, 31,* 357–374.

Harris, M., & Reichle, J. (2004). The impact of aided language stimulation on symbol comprehension and production in nonverbal children with moderate cognitive disabilities. *American Journal of Speech-Language Pathology, 13,* 155–167.

Horner, R., & Day, H.M. (1991). The effects of response efficiency on functionally equivalent competing behaviors. *Journal of Applied Behavior Analysis, 24,* 719–732.

Johnson, L., Reichle, J., & Monn, E. (2009). Longitudinal mentoring with school-based positive behavioral support teams: Influences on staff and learner behavior. *Evidence Based Communication Assessment and Intervention, 3*(2), 113–130.

Johnston, S., Reichle, J., & Evans, J. (2004). Supporting augmentative and alternative communication use by beginning communicators with severe disabilities. *American Journal of Speech-Language Pathology, 13*(1), 20–30.

Millar, D.C. (2009). Effects of AAC on the natural speech development of individuals with autism spectrum disorders. In J. Light & D.R. Beukelman (Series Eds.) & P. Mirenda & T. Iacono (Vol. Eds.), *AAC series: Autism spectrum disorders and AAC* (pp. 171–194). Baltimore: Paul H. Brookes Publishing Co.

Reichle, J. (2004). *Survey of preschool educators.* Unpublished manuscript. University of Minnesota, MN.

Reichle, J., & Johnston, S. (1999). Teaching the conditional use of communicative requests to two school-age children with severe developmental disabilities. *Language, Speech, and Hearing Services in Schools, 30*(4), 324–334.

Reichle, J., & McComas, J. (2004). Conditional use of a request for assistance. *Disability and Rehabilitation, 26,* 1255–1262.

Reichle, J., & Wacker, D. (Vol. Eds.). (1993). *Communication and language intervention series: Vol. 3. Communicative alternatives to challenging behavior: Integrating functional assessment and intervention strategies.* Baltimore: Paul H. Brookes Publishing Co.

Warren, S.F., Fey, M.E., & Yoder, P.J. (2007). Differential treatment intensity research: A missing link to creating optimally effective communication interventions. *Mental Retardation and Developmental Disabilities Research Reviews, 13*(1), 70–77.

Yoder, P., & Layton, T. (1988). Speech following sign language training in autistic children with minimal verbal language. *Journal of Autism and Developmental Disability, 18,* 217–229.

Index

Page numbers followed by *f* indicate figures; those followed by *t* indicate tables.